What People are Saying *Conquering Arthritis*:

"Conquering Arthritis is a book in a category of its own—easy to understand and detailed step-by-step instructions. A great strategy for managing such a complex and "Conquering Arthritis is a book in a category of its own - puzzling disease as arthritis. A must read for anyone not satisfied with their current treatment."
—**Monica Tegeler**, medical student with rheumatoid arthritis, St. Louis, Missouri

"Of enormous importance, is that this book teaches a lesson to all of us who ever have been, or ever will be, told by our health care provider that we are afflicted with a disease for which there is no certain cure."
—**William C. Mootz, M.D.,** Saint Louis University School of Medicine

"You need this book; or someone you know needs this book. Not only has Barbara Allan found, compiled, and correlated vital information that was not widely disseminated before her work. She also has put it in easily understood terms, in logical and appropriate order, and has added inspiring encouragement based on her own miraculous cure and those of others. She helps you commit to your own cure and stay the course. I feel privileged to know Barbara and to support her in her effort to share this miracle."
—**Wayne Mosher**, business consultant, St. Louis, MO

"This is awesome stuff! I find it impactful for me and have already decided to look into some of the things you write about."
—**Les Harwell**, ankylosing spondylitis, Morristown, Arizona

"It's beautifully written. It's very clear and easy to follow. WOW. This is a very important book - putting together all these kinds of information in one place. What a gift to the world."
—**Jan Adamson**, extensive food allergies, Ottawa, Canada

"This is EXCELLENT!!!"
—**Gail Furman**, former arthritis sufferer, Saint Louis, Missouri

Exercise Chapter
"I loved this chapter and think everyone who has had surgery or any major physical set back should read it."
—**Mary Hamilton**, CPA, Glendale, California

Fasting and Testing for Problem Foods Chapters

"Having guided many individuals through therapeutic fasts as well as nutritional programs, I am pleased to see such thorough and scientifically based instructions on therapeutic fasting and positive nutritional strategies. Ms. Allan has truly grasped the essence of the benefits of fasting and proper nutrition in order to heal what is often considered "non-curable". Often medicine can only provide symptom management for chronic systemic inflammatory conditions. She has shown that CURE is not only possible but very "doable" for anyone who applies themselves to their self healing. As a practitioner of 22 years, I have yet to see such a well-written book supporting anyone who wishes to do so, to take responsibility for their own health and healing in order to reclaim their life. This book will be a well used resource in my office!

—**Naide Bruno**, Chiropractor and Naturopath, Cave Creek, Arizona

Hidden Allergen Chapters

"The hidden allergen lists alone are worth the price of the book."
—**Helen Eisen**, poet, St. Louis, Missouri

Healing Food Chapter

"This chapter is very reader friendly, practical and thoroughly documented."
—**Kelly Standing**, Chrone's disease, Sunset Hills, Missouri

Meditation Chapter

"I loved it!"
—**Mary Hamilton**, Glendale, California, meditation facilitator with Vipassana Support Institute

"The scope of information and personal experience is quite impressive."
—**Carol Wilson**, Meditation Teacher at Insight Meditation Society in Barre, Massachusetts

Myofascial Release Chapter

"Several years ago, I had a message therapist who was learning myofascial massage, and used it on me. It really was amazing. Thanks for the reminder."
—**Mary Hamilton**, CPA, Glendale, California

Conquering
Arthritis
first edition

Conquering Arthritis:

What Doctors Don't Tell You Because They Don't Know

(9 Secrets I Learned the Hard Way)

By Barbara D. Allan

Shining Prairie Flower Productions
Saint Louis, Missouri

Conquering Arthritis:
What Doctors Don't Tell You Because They Don't Know
by Barbara D. Allan

Published by:
Shining Prairie Flower Productions
Post Office Box 63353
St. Louis, MO 63163
314-776-4827
orders@ConqueringArthritis.com
http://www.ConqueringArthritis.com

This book contains information gathered from many sources. It is published for general reference and not as a substitute for independent verification by users when circumstances warrant. It is sold with the understanding that neither the author nor the publisher is engages in rendering any psychological or medical advice. The publisher and author disclaim any personal liability, either directly or indirectly, for advice or information presented within. Although the author and publisher have used care and diligence in the preparation, and made every effort to ensure the accuracy and completeness of information contained in this book, we assume no responsibility for errors, inaccuracies, omissions, or any inconsistency herein. First Printing 2002

Allan, Barbara Diane
Conquering arthritis: what doctors don't tell you because they don't know / Barbara D. Allan.
p.cm.
Includes bibliographical references and index.
ISBN 0-9718897-0-8
1. Health & Fitness.   2. Self-Help.   3. Body, Mind and Spirit   4.   Biography   &
Autobiography

ATTENTION: HMOs, EDUCATIONAL ORGANIZATIONS, ARTHRITIS ADVOCACY GROUPS AND OTHERS: Quantity discounts are available on bulk purchases of this book for reselling, educational purposes, subscription incentives, gifts, or fund raising. Special books or book excerpts can also be created to fit specific needs. For information, please contact our Special Sales Department at P.O. Box 63353, St. Louis, MO 63163, 314-776-4827

Dedication

I dedicate this book to everyone suffering from arthritis.

It is the book I wish had been available when I developed arthritis. It would have saved me years of pain and incapacitation. May it help others find their own way back to health.

Table of Contents

Chapter 3: Food Sensitivities—How to Test for Them 45

Chapter 4: Calming your Inflammation and Activating your Healing Potential—How to Therapeutically Fast 61

Chapter 5: Food Sensitivities—How to Avoid Offending Foods and Food Additives in a World of Vague, Incomplete and Confusing Food Labels..79

Chapter 6: Super-Important Information–Names on Food Labels that Can Indicate Hidden Allergens.................................95

Chapter 7: Food Sensitivities—Products that Can Contain Hidden Allergens...106

Chapter 8: Additives to Avoid...119

Chapter 9: Strategies for Restocking Your Kitchen with Safe Food 126

Acknowledgements

This book is the result of input from many people.

I relied heavily on the books, research articles and teachings of many people for my inspiration. These works are cited frequently in this book.

I relied heavily on my family and friends during the years I was sick. They helped me in so many ways, including financially, physically, emotionally, mentally and through prayer. I especially want to acknowledge my mother and father, who have always been there for me, and my St. Louis friends, who made it possible to continue living on my own during those hard years.

I also relied heavily on family and friends during the discovery and writing process. This help came in the form of providing information, granting interviews, helping clarify ideas through discussions, giving advice, and providing feedback. It included reading and commenting on chapter drafts. It included moral support. The following is a partial list of the many people who have provided substantial help: Inge Allan, Barry Allan, Karen Williams, Kathy Wysack, Helen Eisen, Carol Hwang, Shirley Crenshaw, Angela Crenshaw, Gail Furman, Marion Rood, Linda Small, Kris Dolgas, Shinzen Young, Carol Wilson, Mary Hamilton, Jan Adamson, Les Harwell, Ginger Gall, members of the St. Louis writing group organized by Judy Miller, members of Midtown Clayton Toastmasters Club No. 283, especially Wayne Mosher and Carol Weisman, and members of the St. Louis chapter of the National Speakers Association, especially Terry Jo Gile, Kelly Standing and Kristi Franke. Thanks also to photographer Susie Gorman for the great cover photo.

Thank you all for your help. May this project make it easier for all those with arthritis to find their way quickly back to better health.

Prologue by Shinzen Young

"All over the world in traditional cultures, men and women voluntarily subject themselves to pain as a vehicle for radical spiritual transformation. The Sundances and sweat lodges of native North America are examples of this. As cultures become more complex, the shamanic ordeals of the tribe evolve into systems of ascetical and contemplative practice.

But what about involuntary pain? In theory, this too could be turned into a purifying ceremony or a sacred meditation. In practice it is exceedingly difficult to do this unless you are fortunate enough to encounter a competent guide in this area.

In this area, the qualifications for a competent guide are severe. The guide must be a person who has successfully used non-consensual pain to transcend their limited identify and unite with the source. Furthermore, to be a competent guide, one must have the creative communication skills to clearly convey to others how they could also do this.

Such people are very rare. Barbara Allan is one of them. And this, her book, will be a godsend to those in pain who are ready for radical growth."

—Shinzen Young, director of Vipassana Support Institute, Burlington, Ontario, Canada

Foreword by William C. Mootz, M.D.

A good book teaches us more than one lesson. Sometimes an author presents a lesson in an overt manner. At other times, a lesson is presented more covertly. Covert lessons are those that may require us to 'read between the lines', or perhaps, to recognize a common theme, never explicitly stated, but which, nonetheless, runs like an undercurrent, throughout a book.

Overtly, Barb Allan's book contains lessons for those of us who have been diagnosed with arthritis. In particular, it teaches us nine secrets that Barb 'learned the hard way'. Less obvious, but of enormous importance, is that Barb's book teaches a lesson to all of us who ever have been, or ever will be, told by our health care provider that we are afflicted with a disease for which there is no certain cure. This covert lesson is the way in which Barb reacted to her own health situation. In a nutshell, she adopted a *proactive attitude*. Unwilling to remain passive, when her expectations for restoration of her health were not forthcoming, she took action. She read widely about arthritis, and in so doing, she learned about other treatment options previously unknown to her, as well as to her doctors. She applied her intellect to allow her to discern which of the treatments she learned about were worthy of serious consideration, and which were not. She applied the lessons she had learned, and then she listened to her body, and allowed it to offer guidance. She altered her dietary habits, she incorporated meditation into her treatment regimen, and she exercised. She refused to let her arthritis have its way, unchallenged. In so doing, she altered her life for the better.

As a graduate of an 'allopathic' medical school, I could well be described as one of the 'Doctors who don't tell you, because they don't know'. In fact, I can recall no medical schools classes on food sensitivity, and cannot claim expertise in this area. However, 25 years of practicing 'allopathic' medicine has taught me that how a patient approaches her/his illness, and the attitude that she/he takes towards restoring her/his health is usually the single most important factor influencing the prognosis. Barb Allan took charge of her own well-being and refused to surrender to her arthritis. Her overt lessons are there to help those with arthritis. Her covert lesson stands as an example to us all. Congratulations Barb.

William C. Mootz, M.D.
Saint Louis University School of Medicine

Foreword by my Parents

To our daughter Barbara,

Your book is completed at last! We want to congratulate you and tell you how proud we are of you for taking time out of your now so-busy schedule to persevere and see it through. If it helps even one person to recover, as you did, it will be worth all the time and effort that you have put into it.

It still seems like such a miracle that you are finally well. You were barely functioning outside of your bed for a few hours each day and using an electric cart whenever you managed to go out. We remember how we planned our outings with you so carefully to get you close to doors and helped you assemble your cart quickly. Now you are full of energy! Whenever you came to visit us, I spent a whole day removing all the foods you could not have and scrubbing the whole kitchen so that no stray crumbs or dusting of flour could contaminate your food. Still, we had accidents. I felt so bad when I forgot to read a label and used frozen vegetables, unaware that they contained salt with dextrose and made you sick. Now you can eat anything!

We learned so much from you, not only about your food allergies but also about good nutrition and exercise. We feel healthier because of your patient teaching. When people say to us, "you don't look your age," we just smile. Now we can say, "Read Barbara's book and you may look and feel younger too!"

We used to feel so sad after talking to you on the phone. So many nights your Dad would talk you through your pain and try to keep your courage up. Now when you call it is usually to tell us of the exciting things you have just done, like long bicycle rides, great hikes and kayaking trips. We used to pray that some day you might again be able to just walk into a grocery store unaided!

Barbara, when none of the doctors' medicines helped, you didn't give up and feel sorry for yourself. You read, you studied, and you used the brain that had always kept you at the head of your class in school, and when you found something that made sense to you, you had the courage to try it. It was a bumpy road of trial and error and some luck, like the article you happened to be translating for your business which caused you to realize that you were allergic to the filler in your medication. But you persevered and now you are really well!

For a long time we were so afraid it would not last, and I was really frightened when you tested yourself on a pizza, of all things. But here you are two years later, healthy and strong, and you have just recorded all the information it took you years to gather into a well-organized book. As usual you have done a very thorough job! May it be of great help to the many people who are still suffering from food allergies and arthritis.

With all our love,
Your Mama and Daddy

Preface—My Story

At age 25 I became one of the more than 9.1 million people in the United States with an autoimmune-type arthritis. My arthritis was triggered by a bout of bacterial dysentery caused by eating food tainted with a bacterium called *Shigella*. I was vacationing in Michigan at the time.

The onset of my arthritis, about 6 weeks after the dysentery, was sudden and left me in chronic, overwhelming pain that often made it difficult to walk even a few steps without passing out. Sometimes it was so bad that I was incapable of rational thought, or any thought at all. Sometimes my hands were so bad I couldn't hold silverware well enough to feed myself. For years I lived with the loss of many things that I had valued highly: my health, my mobility and to some extent, the use of my mind. I lost friendships, status, the ability to continue as a graduate student, and the ability to hold a regular job.

Usually this type of arthritis, called reactive arthritis, goes away within a month; my case went on for years. My doctors didn't know what to do with me. Nothing they tried did much good.

My illness led me to devote 11 years of my life to systematically researching and personally testing promising alternative therapies until I perfected the strategies that cured my own difficult disease.

After I got sick, I started reading everything I could get my hands on related to the latest scientific research on the causes of arthritis and possible new treatments. Because I was in a doctoral program in molecular biology at Washington University in St. Louis, one of the major medical research universities in the country, this type of information was readily available to me. When I was in too much pain to leave my apartment, friends brought copies of journal articles to me. Unfortunately, the most promising research was years away from possible clinical trials, and the current cutting-edge treatments were not very effective.

After four and a half years of conventional treatments that did little or nothing to improve my condition, I decided that if I continued to follow the conventions dictated by the current medical model, I was unlikely to get well. Even those in the medical field are aware that few patients treated by rheumatologists can expect lasting or substantial improvements. I needed a new plan.

In my next phase of the search, I started evaluating everything I came across in the lay press that promised to help arthritis, pain, or rebuild health.

Not surprisingly, much was silly or potentially dangerous. In this category are claims that arthritis can be cured by burial in horse manure, taking cocaine, topical application of motor oil, brake fluid, gasoline, kerosene and lighter fluid, and sitting in inactive uranium mines.

However, as I avidly read material targeted to the lay public, I did find many modalities that made sense and that were supported by studies published in reputable research journals. I applied these promising alternative therapies to my own condition. Some helped and some didn't.

Eventually I was able to completely overcome my arthritic condition using the *nine secrets* discussed in detail in this book. Each method provided a lasting and dramatic improvement in my condition. After years of having difficulty just walking from one room to another, I now walk many miles a week without difficulty and go on 30 to 50 mile bike rides for fun. I have regained full use of my hands and my hips. The pain and fatigue are gone. In addition, my health has improved each of the last 8 years since I discovered these methods. I credit this to the fact that I have continued to use and refine the health-promoting measures described in *Conquering Arthritis*, allowing my body to heal at deeper and deeper levels.

Disclaimer

The information contained in this publication is solely intended to communicate information about possible treatment options for arthritis and food sensitivities. It is hoped that this information will be helpful and educational to the reader, but it is in no way intended to replace medical diagnosis or treatment. Please consult your physician—preferably a naturopath, holistic physician or osteopath, chiropractor, or other natural health care specialist—for medical advice before undertaking any treatment, making any change in your medication or making any change in your diet.

The author and publisher declare that to the best of their knowledge all information in this publication is accurate; however, although unknown to the author and publisher, some of the treatment options discussed may be harmful to some people. The information provided here is intended to help you make informed decisions about your health, not act as substitute for or override medical advice and care provided by medical professionals.

There are no warranties which extend beyond the educational nature of this publication. Therefore, we shall have neither liability nor responsibility to any person with respect to any loss or damage alleged to be caused, directly or indirectly, by the information contained in this publication.

The 9 Secrets: One or More Will Help You

1. How food sensitivities can cause arthritis
2. How to test for food sensitivities
3. How to therapeutically fast and why this is such a powerful aid to healing
4. How to manage food sensitivities
5. How to rid yourself of food sensitivities
6. How to use superior nutrition to facilitate healing from arthritis
7. How to use meditation as a powerful aid in healing
8. How to gain maximum benefits from exercise even if you are still very sick
9. How to use myofascial trigger point release to clear up residual pain and stiffness

Who Should Read this Book?

This book is primarily for two groups of people:

1. People with an **autoimmune type of arthritis**, such as that caused by rheumatoid arthritis, juvenile rheumatoid arthritis, reactive arthritis, Reiter's syndrome, inflammatory bowel disease arthritis, systemic lupus erythematosus, ankylosing spondalytis, psoriatic arthritis, chronic fatigue syndrome and fibromyalgia. Doctors are just starting to recognize that a sizeable number of these cases are caused by food-related problems. This brings us to our second group of readers.

2. People with **food allergies, food sensitivities or food intolerances.** More than 70 medical conditions have been linked to food-related problems. These conditions include arthritis, myalgia, fatigue, edema, hypoglycemia, diabetes, being overweight or underweight, premenstrual syndrome, sleep disorders, candiditis, depression, and respiratory conditions such as hay fever, asthma, bronchitis, recurring ear infections, sinus conditions, rhinitis, laryngitis, allergic sore throat and hoarseness. Other conditions include digestive problems such as gastroenteritis, irritable bowel syndrome, celiac disease, inflammatory bowel disease, diarrhea, constipation, colic and malabsorption; cerebral conditions such as headaches, dizziness, learning disorders and irritability; and skin-related conditions such as dermatitis, eczema, hives and rashes. By identifying and treating or eliminating food allergies, food sensitivities and food intolerances, many seemingly hopeless chronic health problems can be improved or eliminated.

This book is also for the following groups:

1. **Friends and family who provide major physical and emotional support to someone with arthritis, food allergies, food sensitivities, or food intolerances**. Since these conditions can make a person too sick and tired to do a good job of finding out about options for healing, such caregivers often make all the difference in whether someone gets well or remains sick. Armed with the knowledge in this book, caregivers can help loved ones learn about how to get well, and help them implement these proven strategies.

2. **Healing professionals who work with people with autoimmune arthritis and food-related problems**. Much unnecessary suffering still goes on because the knowledge in this book has not yet fully reached all levels and branches of the healing professions. This book can serve as "continuing education" on the latest and most effective complementary therapies that are now available. Because it is written in lay language, it may also serve as a valuable resource for their clients. References to the scientific literature are also included.

3. **HMO administrators interested in lower treatment costs**. Autoimmune arthritis and food-related problems can lead to a lifetime of frequent doctor's visits, medical tests and interventions, and expensive medications. These patients don't go away, they just get sicker, angrier, more desperate, and more aggressive in demanding medical care. Many of the interventions described in this book are inexpensive. Many are steps that patients can take at home, without running up medical bills. Providing this book as a resource for patients with autoimmune arthritis, and food allergies, food sensitivities, and food intolerances could greatly increase cure rates and significantly lower treatment costs.

Introduction: Why This Book Was Written And How To Best Use It

This is the book I wished had been available when I got sick.

Through luck and perseverance I was eventually able to find simple ways to restore my health, some of which my doctors said would never work. Some of these methods specifically remedied the underlying causes of my arthritis, and some are applicable to anyone who wishes to feel better, no matter their current state of health.

My personal miracle is that I found ways to get well. This book will show you, step by step, how you can get better, too.

Benefits Offered by this Book

Conquering Arthritis:
- Provides hard-earned, practical, detailed information that is critical for successful healing of arthritis, but that is not found in any other book. Without this information many people with arthritis will not get well.
- Presents this information in a clear, simple fashion.
- Organizes this information into a well-researched, easy to follow plan for getting well again.
- Explains how to carry out simple adjustments to restore health, some of which the author's doctors said would never work. I spent hundreds of hours in medical school libraries finding well-done studies that clearly demonstrate the effectiveness of these methods, even though my doctors scoffed at them. I have included more than 130 references, so you don't have to take my word for it.

Conquering Arthritis:
- Can shave years off your attempts to find a way to get well again.
- Is based on the experience of people with dramatic and lasting recoveries from arthritis.
- Is not based on overselling a single magic bullet as a cure.
- Focuses not just on coping with arthritis, but on curing it.
- Screens out silly or potentially dangerous "cures".
- May just be the answer to your prayers.

The methods in this book are of two types:

- Some specifically remedy the underlying causes of arthritis.
- Others, which are equally powerful for healing arthritis, are more general health builders applicable to anyone who wishes to feel better.

Conquering Arthritis includes:
- Clear descriptions of why the strategies work.
- Clear descriptions of the scientific studies that prove their effectiveness.
- A glossary, so that even if you don't have a science background, you can still understand what it all means.

Conquering Arthritis provides:
- A way to bypass the current allopathic medical model, where patients with autoimmune disorders are unlikely to get well. Even those in the medical field are aware that, short of joint replacement, very few patients treated by rheumatologists can expect any lasting or substantial improvements.
- A new plan, one that cures by correcting the underlying problems, not just covers up symptoms or relies on drugs that perpetuate the problem.

Questions this Book Answers
- Of the many alternative treatments touted for healing arthritis, which treatments actually have a good track record? Which have been tested scientifically?
- How can all the various proven treatments be combined into a comprehensive, easy to understand, step by step plan?
- Is there such a thing as an arthritis diet?
- Why is it necessary to identify food sensitivities to recover from arthritis?
- How can I use fasting to test for food sensitivities? Why would I want to?
- What are the benefits of a fast and how can I retain them once it is over?
- Is fasting really necessary?
- What are hidden allergens and why is it important that I avoid them? Where are they found?
- Once I know what my food sensitivities are, how can I find safe food?
- How can I get safe food at restaurants? When traveling?
- How can I get rid of food sensitivities?

- What foods help heal arthritis? How?
- What vitamins and supplements help heal arthritis? How?
- Why is exercise important? How can I possibly exercise when I am this sick?
- What does meditation have to offer in terms of pain management and relief? Is there a simple way to get started?
- What are trigger points and why is knowing about them important for making a complete recovery from arthritis?

How to Best Use this Book

All of the nine secrets in this book work together synergistically.

Because of the synergy, you can benefit from implementing many of the strategies in any order. However, experience and common sense dictate that implementing the strategies in the order of the chapters is most likely to bring about the quickest results.

By following this order you **first** eliminate food sensitivities, one of the major causes of arthritis. **Next** you give your body the nutritional support it needs to heal. **Finally** you give yourself: 1) a meditation practice that allows you to retrain your response to pain; 2) a gentle exercise program that allows your body to regain strength and flexibility and to avoid further damage; 3) massage work that allows your muscles to release the restrictive pain patterns that they have been holding, often below the level of conscious awareness. If you want to do still more, carry out some of the additional suggestions in the conclusion.

Chapter 1: False Friends—How Some Of Your Favorite Foods May Be Perpetuating Your Pain

Certain foods can trigger arthritis. Not only that, but the exact list of foods that trigger arthritis tends to vary from one person to the next.

My doctors were hostile to these ideas. They insisted there was absolutely no connection between arthritis and diet. This despite the fact that there was already a solid body of evidence in the medical literature supporting these ideas.

However, if you really understand what is going on, you realize that elimination diets can sometimes work miracles. The specific foods to be eliminated must be individually identified. Favorite foods are often the culprit, because they are eaten frequently enough to trigger ongoing attacks in your joints. These attacks cause arthritis. Eliminate the attacks and the body spontaneously heals.

The following case histories illustrate how people in two families eliminated arthritis by eliminating problem foods.

Notice:
- How each of these people found support from a book describing an elimination diet that just happened to correspond to the foods she personally needed to eliminate.
- How the foods needing to be eliminated among family members are often exactly the same or very close.
- How autoimmune diseases such as rheumatoid arthritis and insulin-dependent diabetes tend to run in families. The autoimmune disease(s) developed need not be the same as autoimmune disease(s) of other family members. This tendency toward autoimmune disease seems to be related to problems triggered by food sensitivities.
- How the foods that trigger arthritis in adulthood can be some of the same foods that triggered childhood allergies.
- How eliminating problem foods can mean the difference between being in the grips of a crippling case of arthritis and living an active, productive life.

Just by looking at your family tree, you can often detect whether you are likely to be dealing with an autoimmune type of arthritis. Just by looking at your childhood allergies, you can predict foods that may be a problem now. And if you are lucky enough to have someone in your family who has already cured themselves of arthritis by eliminating problem foods, there is a high probability that your list of problem foods will be nearly the same.

Case Histories

Gail Furman

Gail Furman is the friendly, high-energy, 43-year-old director of the Clinical Skills Lab at St. Louis University School of Medicine. To look at her you would never suspect a history of arthritis. Indeed, you would be more likely to wonder how even very healthy people manage to keep up with her.

The truth is that the key to Gail's high-energy lifestyle is a careful avoidance of certain foods. Her body reacts poorly to tomatoes, potatoes, eggplant, chocolate, and dairy products such as milk, yogurt and cheese. Within 8 to10 hours of eating any of these she becomes achy all over, particularly in her knees, ankles and elbows. After about seven days back on her anti-arthritis diet, her symptoms disappear again.

At age 33 her symptoms prompted her to start visiting physicians, who treated her painful symptoms as sports injuries. She was given various anti-inflammatory pills, all of which upset her stomach, so she never took these pills for long. Once she was treated with physical therapy to "correct" the way she was walking, but this treatment also did nothing to improve her knee pain.

At 35 she received her first diagnosis of arthritis and also first made the connection between food intolerance and her joint pain. Another friend who had brought her rheumatoid arthritis under control through selective elimination of problem foods gave Gail some written information on food allergies. Gail says that for the first time she made the connection between her childhood food allergies and her adult joint pain. Many of the same foods were triggering both.

As a child Gail broke out in a rash on the inside of her elbows whenever she had foods high in citric acid such as oranges, grapefruit juice or tomatoes. She was also allergic to chocolate, and, although not lactose intolerant, she absolutely refused to drink milk. In third grade she had her first asthma attack. At that time citrus, tomatoes, chocolate, mildew, dust, pollen and horses were found to be allergic triggers for her asthma. Gail has not had a full-blown asthma attack since childhood but on rare occasions has shortness of breath and chest tightness during aerobics. In her gym bag she keeps an inhaler that quickly and effectively relieves this exercise-induced asthma.

Gail is the person who first told me about Dr. Peter J. D'Adamo's work with blood-type-specific diets. (See Chapter 2 for more information on Dr. D'Adamo's work.) It turns out that Gail has type A blood and her list of food intolerances closely follows Dr. D'Adamo's list of foods that are problematic for people with type A blood. Her response to his book was, "Finally someone has been able to explain theoretically what I already knew experimentally from my own body."

Like many people with arthritis, the illness runs in Gail's family. Gail's mother has rheumatoid arthritis, as did her mother before her.

Although Gail's mother, Gert Furman, 75, has rheumatoid arthritis, it started relatively late in life and is rather mild. Because of Gail's experience, Gert has tried cutting out nightshade vegetables (potatoes, tomatoes, eggplant, peppers) from her diet, but has not noticed that it makes a difference in her arthritis. The reason the change in diet has not helped may be because she has never tested to see if more foods need to be eliminated.

Shirley and Angela Crenshaw

Shirley Crenshaw, 50, is a social worker and psychotherapist. Although she was once quite sick, she now looks so youthful and energetic she is still occasionally "carded" at restaurants and bars. As a single mother who completed a master's degree in social work while working full time and taking on additional part-time jobs, Shirley is another very busy person who takes little time to rest. That Shirley has managed to do all this is all the more amazing given that rheumatoid arthritis runs in her family.

Shirley's mother developed rheumatoid arthritis at 25. Shirley remembers her mom groaning with each step as she slowly walked down the hall with the aid of crutches. Later her mom was so severely affected that she was restricted to a wheelchair.

For Shirley, symptoms started at about 37. She was diagnosed with a classic case of traveling rheumatoid arthritis about four years after her symptoms first appeared in her jaw. About a year later it moved to her neck, a year later to her shoulders, a year later to her wrists, and finally a year later to her hips. Once the arthritis moved into her wrists, Shirley says, her arms swelled up like those of the cartoon character, Popeye the Sailorman. She had nearly continuous pain, tingling and numbness in her hands and had great difficulty with tasks such as writing, driving and brushing her teeth. In addition, Shirley also suffered from profound fatigue and a sense of defeat.

When Shirley's arthritis started, her daughter Angela was 13. Angela's father had just died and Angela was afraid that her mother would be in constant pain and unable to care for herself or for Angela. Angela says that it seemed like the end of Shirley's life, even though she was not literally dying. Shirley herself says the arthritis was like her worst nightmare come true, since in her pain she was now groaning uncontrollably in front of her own daughter, just like her own mother had done.

Shirley read as much as she could about possible cures. Her medical doctor gave her the anti-inflammatory drug Anaprox, but that did little to help and caused stomach problems. She tried all sorts of vitamins and nutritional supplements but they also had little effect. Finally her brother Hu, who had developed rheumatoid arthritis in his early 20s, called her with an elimination diet that was helping him. He had read about this diet in the book *Prescription for Nutritional Healing* by James F. Balch, Jr. and Phyllis A. Balch[1].

Shirley eliminated potatoes, tomatoes, eggplant, green peppers, paprika, red meat, milk products, sugar, salt and citrus fruit from her diet, just like her brother had done. The results were a miracle. She started feeling better within a month and actually felt good after two months, when she noticed that she was also very sensitive to wheat and cut this out of her diet. Within two weeks of not eating wheat she was able to take off her arm braces and stop taking Anaprox.

Angela began to develop rheumatoid arthritis around age 15. Shirley is extremely grateful that Angela witnessed her miraculous recovery; otherwise, she doubts that she could have gotten a teenager such as Angela to stick with such a restrictive diet that eliminates most fast food. It turns out that Angela and Shirley (and Shirley's brother) have exactly the same food sensitivities. The consequences of a single ingestion of a problem food is so immediately apparent (considerable pain, stiffness and fatigue within about eight hours that last about one week) that it has been relatively easy for them to stay on their anti-arthritis diet.

Angela is now 23 and is a daughter of whom it is easy to be proud. She is friendly, beautiful (she has worked professionally as a model) and made

---

[1] James F. Balch, Jr. and Phyllis A. Balch, *Prescription for Nutritional Healing* (Garden City Park, NY: Avery Pub. Group, 1990).

excellent grades at Harvard while also working part time. She now lives and works in San Francisco. When she has symptoms they are mostly in her knees, shoulders, jaw and hands. Without her anti-arthritis diet it would probably not have been possible for her to attend college at all, much less thrive there. When she stuck to her diet and got enough rest, she had no symptoms. Unfortunately, not having her own kitchen when in college made it difficult to always stay on her anti-arthritis diet, and being very busy made it difficult to always get enough sleep. When I last talked with her, she told me how happy she is to have her own kitchen and more control of her time.

Angela's arthritis probably began so early because she likely inherited the tendency toward autoimmune disease not only from her mother's side of the family but also her father's side. Her father also had rheumatoid arthritis and her paternal grandmother and uncle had insulin-dependent diabetes that began in their early 20s.

Angela's maternal grandmother, Shirley's mother, was never willing to try changing her diet. Despite conventional medical treatment, her condition never improved. She slowly deteriorated until her death at age 77.

The Lessons

The lessons to be learned from these case histories are:

- If food sensitivities are causing your arthritis, you will need to eliminate your problem foods. Your list may or may not look like anyone else's, although problem foods tend to run in families.
- If you are lucky enough to have someone in your family who has already cured themselves of arthritis by eliminating problem foods, there is a high probability that your list of problem food will be nearly the same.
- By looking at your family tree, you can often detect whether you are likely to be dealing with an autoimmune type of arthritis. If so, definitely check to see if food sensitivities are causing your symptoms. (See Chapter 3 for how to test yourself for food sensitivities.)
- Childhood allergies can often predict foods that may be a problem now.
- Eliminating problem foods can eliminate even crippling cases of arthritis.

Chapter 2: Food Sensitivities—
What They Are, How They Develop
and What to Do About Them

Highlights:

The differences between classical food allergies and food sensitivities.
- Four factors known to cause both food sensitivities and arthritis.
- How to test for each of these four factors.
- How to correct the underlying causes or at least minimize the damage caused by each of these factors.

Effort Involved:

- Read this chapter. Understand the information.
- Educate your doctor, if necessary.
- Take steps to correct any underlying causes of food sensitivities you might have.

Payoff:

- Improved understanding of the underlying problems that cause arthritis and how to correct them.
- Knowledge you need to take an active and effective role in ensuring that you get the best and most appropriate care.

It's Not All in Your Mind—Get the Treatments You Need to Correct Underlying Physical Problems

My doctors were not able to help me get well because the tests they used were just not capable of detecting the problems going on in my body. The therapies they prescribed were only capable of suppressing my symptoms, not treating my underlying problems. They falsely concluded that since they could find nothing wrong and their therapies didn't work, I must be a slacker, clinically depressed, or suffering from a mental illness. Furthermore, they concluded that there was simply nothing further that could be done to get me well again. In reality, none of this was true.

Their training had simply not included the methods presented in this chapter and in Appendix A for finding and treating what was actually wrong. They only had standard allopathic medical strategies available to them. In my case, these strategies were helpful only in ruling out problems, not in detecting the actual problem and not in restoring health.

After a bone scan, standard blood tests, treatment with various nonsteroidal anti-inflammatory drugs (NSAIDs), treatment with an anti-ulcer drug to combat the side effects of the NSAIDs, and treatment with prednisone, I was still quite ill. Because of the suspicion that I was clinically depressed, I was put on Prozac. My choice was to take Prozac or have my doctor refuse any further treatment. The fact was I did not need to be on Prozac or any other anti-depressant. Despite my low dose, I suffered unpleasant overdose effects that my doctor was very slow to recognize or acknowledge. This was despite the fact that I was very concerned about these side effects and brought them to my doctor's attention many times. Finally, my doctors ran out of treatments and went into denial that anything was physically wrong. I continued to get worse.

This chapter will help dispel the kind of ignorance that prevents arthritis sufferers with underlying food sensitivity problems from getting the treatment they need to get well.

I urge you to read this chapter. I know the information in this chapter is complex, but it is the key to your recovery.

A glossary is included in the back of this book. Even if you don't have a scientific or medical background, the glossary is there to help you follow what is presented here.

If your doctor is not familiar with these treatments, you may want to show him or her this chapter, Chapter 13 and Appendix A. This will provide a good introduction to the body of research that has already been done in this area.

If you, your family or your friends are not up to the effort that it might take to familiarize your doctor with this information, you may want to look for a naturopathic doctor, recognized by the initials N.D. Naturopathic doctors should already be familiar with these treatments. Unfortunately, naturopaths are still relatively uncommon in the United States. To find naturopaths and other holistically oriented doctors in your area, you can visit the Holistic Healing Web page: www.HolisticMed.com.

Learning the Lingo–Terms Used in the Discussion of Food Sensitivities

Many terms are commonly used to designate adverse reactions to food. These terms include food sensitivity, food hypersensitivity, food intolerance, food toxicity and food allergy. Unfortunately, no consensus has developed on their exact meaning. In this book I use the term **food sensitivity** to refer to an adverse reaction to food that usually become apparent not minutes but hours or days after ingesting a problem food. I use the term **food intolerance** to mean any an adverse reaction to food.

Austrian physician Clems Von Pirquet coined the term allergy in 1906 from two Greek roots meaning "altered reactivity."[2] Alternative medical practitioners and the general public tend to use the term allergy with its broad original meaning. Many physicians use the term allergy ONLY when the immune system is known to be involved. Though I refer to the part of a food that triggers an intolerance reaction as an "allergen," I avoid the term food allergy since what I write about is not universally recognized as involving the immune system. However, there is solid evidence that the immune system does play a role in food sensitivity and food intolerance.

The definitions of these and other terms used to discuss food sensitivities are given in the glossary at the back of this book. Flip to the glossary whenever you encounter a term with which you are unfamiliar.

Important Information Your Doctor May Not Know–Differences Between Classical Food Allergies and Food Sensitivities

The phenomenon I write about in this book is not a "classical" or "true food allergy". In these cases a small amount of food, such as peanuts or shrimp, causes a near-immediate response, such as intense local inflammation or anaphylactic shock, that is sometimes fatal. The allergic response usually dissipates within a few hours. In classical allergy, laboratory tests also show high levels of the **IgE antibody** class. These antibodies are a special part of the immune system that guards the body by latching onto foreign matter and flagging it for destruction. (IgE is pronounced by saying the name of each letter: I-G-E.)

---

[2] Marilyn Gioannini, *The Complete Food Allergy Cookbook* (Rocklin, CA: Prima Publishing, 1996.)

In classical allergy, these IgE levels are high both for IgE antibodies that bind specifically to allergy-triggering foods <u>and</u> also for the total amount of IgE antibodies in the bloodstream.

There are THREE CRUCIAL DISTINCTIONS between classical food allergies and the type of food sensitivities described in this book. First, food sensitivity reactions usually become noticeable not minutes but hours to days after ingesting an offending food, and may take several days to resolve. Second, patients with food sensitivities do not have high IgE levels in their bloodstream. Third, commonly available allergy skin testing, which is how many people are tested for allergies, reliably detects classical allergies but is unreliable in cases of food sensitivities.[3]

Differences Between Classical Food Allergies and Food Sensitivities

	Onset of Symptoms	IgE Antibody Against Specific Allergen	Total IgE Antibody in Blood	Skin Prick Allergy Testing
Classical Food Allergy	Within minutes	High	High	Reliable
Food Sensitivity	Within hours or days	Sometimes slightly elevated	Low	Unreliable

4 Factors that Cause Food Sensitivities

Although the case histories in Chapter 1 show how there can be great similarities in food sensitivities within families, these sensitivities are actually complicated phenomena whose symptoms and triggers are seldom exactly the same from one person to the next. Because digestion can be disrupted in many ways, many factors contribute to food sensitivities. Not all of these are well understood.

---

[3] Linda Gamlin, "Another Man's Poison," *New Scientist* 123 (1989)48-53.

Enough medical research has been done to identify the following four factors that cause or exacerbate food sensitivities:

1. Leaky gut syndrome
2. Breakdown of oral tolerance
3. Low levels of certain detoxification enzymes
4. Dietary lectins

Each of these factors, except low levels of certain detoxification enzymes, directly involves the immune system in some way.

This chapter gives a brief overview of these four factors. If you are interested in more detail, see Appendix A.

1. Leaky Gut Syndrome

In leaky gut syndrome, a large number of food particles pass either totally undigested or partially undigested into the bloodstream. This passage of undigested food occurs in the small intestine, where virtually all absorption of fully digested food also occurs. All people, even very healthy people, have some undigested food that leaks into their bloodstream. However, most food-sensitive individuals have much higher levels.[4]

Things that can trigger leaky gut syndrome are use of nonsteroidal anti-inflammatory drugs (NSAIDs), alcohol, anti-ulcer drugs such as Zantac and Tagamet, antacid tablets and/or antibiotics (including antibiotics taken years ago), diets high in simple carbohydrates, gulping food without chewing thoroughly, presence of parasites in the digestive tract, and a personal or family history of allergies or food sensitivities.

Symptoms can include any of the following: poor digestion, gas and bloating, food sensitivities, yeast infections, fatigue, joint pain, cloudy thinking, and difficulty maintaining weight.

A doctor can easily determine if leaky gut syndrome is present using the test described later in this chapter.

---

[4] Charlotte Cunningham-Rundles, M.D., Ph.D., "Dietary Antigens and Immunologic Disease in Humans," *Rheum Dis Clin North Amer* 17(2) (1991):287-307.

The most effective way to treat leaky gut syndrome is to avoid any foods to which you have an adverse reaction. In addition, you correct underlying problems that contribute to developing food sensitivities. If you don't correct these problems, you run the risk of continuing to develop sensitivities to more foods. Measures for correcting these underlying conditions are described throughout this chapter and in Chapter 13.

Four Ways to Avoid Leaky Gut Syndrome

1. Avoid NSAIDs

All nonsteroidal anti-inflammatory drugs (NSAIDs), except aspirin and nabumetone[5] and the new class of NSAIDs known as COX-2 inhibitors, are known to increase the permeability (leakiness) of the intestinal wall and may be capable of causing food sensitivities or increasing their severity. In fact, conventional NSAIDs almost always cause acute lesions in the mucosal lining of the stomach and upper part of the small intestine (called the duodenum), although only 50 percent of patients with these lesions have upper abdominal discomfort[6]. This means you can have these stomach and intestinal lesions without even knowing it.

If you have been using conventional NSAIDs for a long time, the biochemical damage, which results in increased intestinal permeability, may take months to heal even after you stop taking the drugs.[7] In a study at Karolinska Hospital in Stockholm, Sweden, intestinal permeability increased in every single rheumatoid arthritis patient treated with

---

[5] I. Bjarnason and T. J. Peters, "Influence of Anti-Rheumatic Drugs on Gut Permeability and on the Gut Associated Lymphoid Tissue," *Baillieres Clin Rheumatol.* 10(1) (1996):165-76.

[6] P. Bertschinger, G. F. Zala and M. Fried, "Effect of Nonsteroidal Antirheumatic Agents on the Gastrointestinal Tract: Clinical Aspects and Pathophysiology
Schweiz Med Wochenschr. 126(37) (1996):1566-8.

[7] I. Bjarnason and T. J. Peters, "Influence of Anti-Rheumatic Drugs on Gut Permeability and on the Gut Associated Lymphoid Tissue," *Baillieres Clin. Rheumatol.* 10(1) (1996):165-76.

conventional NSAIDs.[8] It is therefore best to avoid using conventional NSAIDs whenever possible.

A new class of NSAIDs, called COX-2 inhibitors, may be an exception to the avoid NSAIDs rule. Preliminary work shows two drugs of this class, celecoxib and refecoxib, seem to lower inflammation without causing as much gastrointestinal bleeding as conventional NSAIDs.[9] These drugs are still new enough that the jury is still out on their safety, but they do, at least, seem easier on the stomach than conventional NSAIDs.

2. Avoid Alcohol

Consuming alcohol increases the permeability of the intestinal wall. If you have food sensitivities, avoid beer, wine and all other forms of alcohol until your condition has improved.

3. Try to Avoid Pathogenic Bacteria

Any one of a number of gastrointestinal pathogens, particularly the bacteria *Shigella, Salmonella, Campylobacter, Yersinia* and *Clostridium*, can cause a form of arthritis known as reactive arthritis. My reactive arthritis was triggered by a bout of bacterial dysentery caused by eating food contaminated with the *Shigella* bacteria.

The arthritis caused by these types of bacteria seems to be dependent on the ability of these pathogens to give off toxins that increase intestinal permeability. These bacteria generally cause diarrhea. In my case, the diarrhea was over within a week, but I felt under the weather for several weeks. About six weeks after the initial diarrhea, I developed the sudden onset of arthritis. One day I could walk for miles. The next I had difficulty walking across my living room without passing out from the pain. Even though the bacteria was presumably gone from my system after the first week, the arthritis it caused persisted for years until I applied the healing strategies detailed in this book, including those for correcting leaky gut syndrome.

---

[8] Hans Oman et al., "Increased Intestinal Permeability to Polysucrose in NSAID-Treated Patients," *Eur J of Gastroenterol Hepatol* 4(3) (1992):235-240.

[9] B. Everts, P. Wahrborg and T. Hedner, "COX-2-Specific Inhibitors—the Emergence of a New Class of Analgesic and Anti-Inflammatory Drugs," *Clin Rheumatol* 19(5)(2000):331-43.

As an interesting sideline, although diarrhea can certainly be caused by many things besides pathogenic bacteria, the fact that these bacteria cause both diarrhea and arthritis has resulted in a long history of the two being linked in the medical literature. This includes a report about Christopher Columbus getting arthritis after a bout of diarrhea in 1496 during his second voyage to the New World.[10]

To try to protect yourself from exposure to these arthritis-causing bacteria:

☐ Drink only disinfected water and eat only food that has been stored and prepared under proper sanitary conditions.
☐ Avoid restaurants that do not have good health department ratings.
☐ Avoid food at gatherings that has been sitting out too long at room temperature.
☐ Be cautious what you eat and drink when traveling in Third World countries or anytime you are in primitive conditions.
☐ Don't eat food from cans that look swollen.
☐ Don't eat food that may be spoiled. When in doubt, throw it out!

4. Correct the Factors Which Lead to Bacterial Overgrowths

People with healthy digestion have more than 400 kinds of bacteria living in their intestines, most of them "friendly" types.[11] This healthy balance of bacteria is critical for good health. It prevents the growth of an unhealthy array of intestinal flora, the kind that can cause food sensitivities. The way this works is similar to the way a lush, thick lawn is resistant to weeds because there is simply no place for the weeds to put down roots.

However, it is not only the unhealthy types of intestinal flora discussed above cause leaky gut syndrome; but sometimes normally healthy types of bacteria can as well. This happens when certain normally healthy strains grow so vigorously that they upset the normal balance or spill over into areas of the digestive tract where they do not belong. People with food sensitivities often have an overgrowth of usually harmless organisms,

---

[10] D. J. Allison, "First Case of Reiter's Disease in the Old World," *Lancet* 2 (1980):1309.

[11] Gary L. Simon and Sherwood L. Gorbach, "Intestinal Flora in Health and Disease," *Gastroenterol* 86 (1984):174-93.

especially protozoan parasites, yeast or bacteria, living in their intestines.[12,13]

These overgrowths can be the result of parasitic infestations, a diet high in flesh protein, a diet high in sugar, a diet low in plant fiber, poor digestion, low gastric acid secretion, or repeated or long-term use of antibiotics. Each of these factors affects the complex balance of what is growing and where.

A study by Dr. A.E.K. Henriksson from the Department of Rheumatology at Karolinska Hospital has demonstrated that many patients with rheumatoid arthritis exhibit bacterial overgrowth in the small intestine and that the degree of overgrowth is associated with the severity of symptoms and disease activity.[14]

The upper part of the human small intestine is designed to be relatively free of bacteria. When bacteria overgrowths are present, bacteria compete with their host (the human body) for nutrition. They ferment carbohydrates and produce excessive gas, bloating and abdominal distention. They prevent fat and fat-soluble vitamins from being absorbed properly. They putrefy proteins and form certain kinds of amines (vasoactive amines) that, in excess, can cause leaky gut syndrome. Frequently, anemia results due to vitamin B-12 deficiency.

When intestinal flora is returned to a healthy balance, digestion improves and food sensitivities often spontaneously disappear.

If you suspect that bacterial overgrowths might be a problem, see Chapter 13 for a list of easy steps to return intestinal flora to a healthy balance. This list is found on page 205.

---

[12] Nicolette M. Dumke, *5 Years Without Food: The Food Allergy Survival Guide* (Louisville, CO: Adapt Books, 1997, 18).

[13] J. O. Hunter, "Food Allergy–or Enterometabolic Disorder?" *Lancet*, 338 (1991):495-496.

[14] A. E. K. Henriksson et al., "Small Intestinal Bacterial Overgrowth in Patients with Rheumatoid Arthritis" *Annals Rheumatic Dis* 52 (1993):503-10.

How To Test for Unhealthy Intestinal Flora and Poor Digestion

A laboratory method called comprehensive digestive stool analysis (CDSA) consists of a battery of integrated diagnostic laboratory tests that evaluate digestion, intestinal function, intestinal environment and absorption by carefully examining the stool.[15] It is useful for pinpointing the exact nature of digestive disturbances. In addition to giving a great deal of information on the digestive process itself, CDSA also provides information on the presence of various friendly and/or pathogenic microorganisms in the intestines and on the presence of bacterial overgrowth in the small intestine.

The test involves following a special diet for at least two days before submitting a stool sample.

Laboratories that provide CDSA are:

❑ Great Smokies Diagnostic Laboratory (800-522-4762)
❑ Diagnos-Techs (800-87-TESTS)

To have a CDSA run for you, contact a naturopathic doctor or have your health practitioner arrange to have this test run for you in cooperation with one of the laboratories listed above. Many M.D.s are unfamiliar with this test; if you wish to arrange this test through an M.D., you may have to introduce him or her to the concept. You may even have to shop around until you find one who is willing to work with you on this.

How to Test for Leaky Gut Syndrome

The test for diagnosing leaky gut syndrome involves administering two sugars – mannitol and lactulose.[16] Mannitol is a small molecule that is quickly taken up by intestinal cells. Lactulose is a larger molecule that should not be taken up by intestinal cells. However, if leaky gut syndrome is present, lactulose is taken up. Since neither sugar is metabolized, they can be measured by urine analysis of a sample collected six hours later. Normal absorption rates are 5 to 25 percent for mannitol and 0.1 to 0.8 percent for lactulose. If the levels of both sugars are increased, it indicates

---

[15] S. Barrie, "Comprehensive Digestive Stool Analysis" in: *A Textbook of Natural Medicine,* edited by J.E. Pizzorno and M.T. Murray (Seattle, WA: Bastyr University Publications, 1986).

[16] Michael T. Murray, N.D., *Chronic Candidiasis: The Yeast Syndrome,* (Rocklin, CA: Prima Publishing, 1997).

generally increased intestinal permeability. If levels of both sugars are decreased, it indicates malabsorption. In a sense, malabsorption is the opposite of leaky gut syndrome. It means that normal absorption of nutrients is somehow being blocked. If the level of lactulose is increased and the level of mannitol is decreased, it may indicate damage to the absorptive surfaces of the small intestine.

Because the measures for correcting leaky gut are all health-promoting measures that are relatively easy to carry out, you may want to skip the time and expense involved in taking this test and move immediately to the remedy.

2. The Breakdown of Oral Tolerance

Oral tolerance refers to training the immune system **not** to react to molecules of food that leak through the gut into the bloodstream of everyone, even healthy people. In healthy people the training is successful, so food molecules are not attacked. However, for some reason the process of oral tolerance does not work as well in food-sensitive individuals.

See appendix A if you are interested in more details on how oral tolerance is established and maintained.

How to Reestablish Oral Tolerance

❑ Follow the steps given in Chapter 13 for correcting leaky gut syndrome.

3. Low Levels of Certain Detoxification Enzymes

A series of enzymes is important in detoxifying certain types of food molecules. These enzymes convert a toxic type of chemical group (sulfide group) into a nontoxic type of chemical group (sulfoxide group). The name of the reaction occurs is sulfoxidation.

A related detoxification pathway is called sulfation. Sulfation detoxifies another type of toxic group called a phenolic. It needs sulfate produced by sulfoxidation to work properly. Not surprisingly, impaired sulfation has been found in many of the same conditions associated with poor sulfoxidation.

Acetaminophen is often used to treat rheumatoid arthritis and other arthritic conditions. Acetaminophen is the generic name for a drug sold under 97 brand names, including Tylenol®. It is also sold combined with other drugs in more than 100 brands, including Sinutab®.[17]

For individuals with impaired sulfation, this drug is a bad idea. In high doses acetaminophen saturates the sulfation pathway, making it impossible for the pathway to handle all the other dietary substances it should be detoxifying. Saturating the pathway also depletes the amount of sulfate available. Sulfate is required for maintaining the structure of the glycosaminoglycans within joints, and a lack of sulfate may impair joint repair.

Medical writer Linda Gamlin notes that among people with both food intolerance and intolerance to common synthetic chemicals, such as chlorine, natural gas, exhaust fumes and solvents, about 90 percent have a reduced ability to carry out sulfoxidation reactions.[18] The correlation of difficulty carrying out sulfoxidation reactions with food and chemical sensitivities is interesting because it suggests a possible reason why people with food intolerance are often also chemically sensitive.

Detoxification of synthetic compounds probably relies on both sulfoxidation and sulfation enzymes, whose original function was to break down bacterial products and certain substances in food. Those of us with slightly suboptimal detoxification enzymes do fine as long as our toxic load does not exceed the ability of our enzymes to detoxify it. However, with increased exposure to toxic chemicals in our environment, our enzyme systems become overwhelmed and can no longer detoxify all the chemicals, problematic bacteria and problematic food substances to which we are exposed.

Many people find that if they can avoid the chemicals to which they are sensitive, they can better cope with foods that were previously a problem.

For a more extensive discussion of detoxification pathways, see Appendix A.

---

[17] *1998 Mosby's GenRx: The Complete Reference for Generic and Brand Drugs, 8th Edition* (St. Louis, MO: Mosby, 1998.)

[18] Linda Gamlin, "Another Man's Poison," *New Scientist* 123 (1989):48-53.

See Chapter 13 for steps you can take to reduce toxic loads and increase your body's ability to handle toxic substances.

4. Dietary Lectins and Blood Type Reactions

Dr. Peter J. D'Adamo, author of *Eat Right for Your Type*[19], believes that blood type is an important factor in your body's response to food. According to Dr. D'Adamo, this is because foods contain proteins called lectins that tend to make cells stick together or agglutinate.

Improper agglutination caused by lectins can harm the body in several ways, depending on which of the body's cells are improperly clumping together. First, if you eat a food containing a type of lectin that is incompatible with your blood-type antigen, blood cells begin to agglutinate improperly in the organ or body system (kidneys, liver, brain, stomach, etc.) targeted by that particular lectin. Second, other lectins can settle at various locations in the body and cause nonblood cells there to clump together and be targeted for destruction as if they were foreign invaders. Third, still other lectins can interact with the surface receptors of lymphocytes (blood cells such as T-cells and B-cells), causing them to multiply at an inappropriately rapid rate.

There is evidence that lectin-induced agglutination and proliferation can cause many problems, including arthritis. Dr. D'Adamo states that injections of lentil lectin into the knee joint cavities of nonsensitized rabbits resulted in the development of arthritis that was indistinguishable from rheumatoid arthritis. Other work suggests that RA symptoms can be reduced by avoiding dietary sources of problem lectins.[20]

Many people with arthritis feel that avoiding nightshade vegetables such as tomatoes, eggplant and white potatoes seems to help their arthritis. That is not surprising, since most nightshades are very high in lectins that affect

---

[19] Peter J. D'Adamo with Catherine Whitney, *Eat Right for Your Type: The Individualized Diet Solution to Staying Healthy, Living Longer & Achieving Your Ideal Weight,* (New York: G. P. Putnam's Sons, 1996).

[20] L. Cordain, L. Toohey, M. J. Smith and M. S. Hickey, "Modulation of Immune Function by Dietary Lectins in Rheumatoid Arthritis," *Br J Nutr* 83(3)(2000)207-17.

people with type A blood adversely, and people with type A blood seem to be more susceptible to autoimmune types of arthritis than people with other blood types (O, B and AB). For extensive lists of foods that are thought to be good and bad for people with each blood type, see Dr. D'Adamo's book.

As mentioned above in the discussion of leaky gut syndrome, normally only a small percentage of food particles from the diet make their way undigested into the bloodstream. For people suffering from leaky gut syndrome, this percentage can be much higher. Since lectins in the diet only wreak havoc when they get into the bloodstream undigested, they are much more likely to do damage in people with leaky guts. If you know or suspect that you have food intolerances, it is probably worth your while to try Dr. D'Adamo's diet plan for your blood type to see if it helps. It is also important to do everything in your power to help heal your digestive tract. This includes:

❑ Avoiding alcohol.
❑ Avoiding conventional nonsteroidal anti-inflammatory drugs (NSAIDs).
❑ Avoiding protease inhibitors which further impair digestion (protease inhibitors are found in the raw and undercooked forms of the following foods: soybeans, peanuts, lentils, rice, corn and potatoes).
❑ Avoiding any other foods to which you react poorly.
❑ Maximizing the digestive process by chewing each bite of food until it is liquefied.

Dr. David L.F. Freed[21], an allergy specialist at Beaumont Hospital in England, has pointed out that the current fashion for sprouting beans is good because it reduces lectins in the diet. In most cases sprouting causes a sharp drop in lectin content within a few days. He also says that beans soaked overnight before cooking lose all lectin activity after 10 minutes of boiling, but without this presoaking some lectin activity remains even after 45 minutes of boiling. Although many lectins are destroyed by normal cooking (this is why cooked grains and beans are edible by humans), many are not. In fact, a few lectins, such as banana agglutinin are actually enhanced by heating, so it is better to enjoy bananas raw.

There are also nonfood sources of lectins. The bacteria *Bordetella pertussis* causes blood cells to clump and causes damaging IgE responses. Influenza virus has a similar effect. Many patients with food intolerance associate the

---

[21] David L. F. Freed, "Dietary Lectins and Disease," in *Food Allergy and Intolerance,* edited by Jonathan Brostoff and Stephen J. Challacombe (London: Bailliere Tindall, 1987).

onset of their illness with an attack of influenza. Presumably this is due to an inappropriate IgE antibody response in the intestines caused by the influenza and a resulting breakdown of oral tolerance.

How to Avoid Damage from Lectins

- ☐ Use the lists from Dr. D'Adamo's book, *Eat Right for Your Type,* to avoid foods that contain lectins that are thought to be bad for people with your blood type (A, B, AB or O).
- ☐ Soak beans and grains overnight before cooking.
- ☐ Cook all beans and grains thoroughly.
- ☐ Follow the steps listed in the section titled "Correcting Leaky Gut Syndrome" in Chapter 13.

Questions and Answers About Food Sensitivities

1.
Q: My doctor says I couldn't possibly have food allergies because I don't have an immediate reaction to the foods I eat. However, I feel lousy the day after I eat certain foods. What is going on?

A: Although you don't have a classical food allergy, you very likely have food sensitivities. Unlike classical food allergies, the symptoms of food sensitivity often take hours or days to appear.

2.
Q: For one person profiled in Chapter 1, tomatoes, potatoes, eggplant, chocolate and dairy products cause symptoms. For two others, wheat, potatoes, tomatoes, eggplant, green peppers, paprika, red meat, milk products, sugar, salt and citrus fruit cause symptoms. I have heard of other people with yet other lists of what causes their arthritis. Why are there so many different claims as to what foods cause arthritis?

A: Each person's body is unique. Immune systems, how well the digestive system is working, enzyme levels, blood type, and many other factors determine whether a person develops food sensitivities. Since these factors vary from person to person and over time for the same person, it is not surprising that the list of foods to which a person is sensitive tends to vary from one individual to another.

3.
Q: Intestinal permeability seems really important. If the small intestine lets incompletely digested food into the bloodstream all sorts of bad things

happen. Oral tolerance can break down leading to an overactive immune system, too many circulating immune complexes (CICs) can lead to painful deposits in the joints and other places, undigested lectins can wreak havoc by causing cells to clump together and be targeted for destruction. What can I do to make my small intestine less permeable?

A:

- First, chew your food well. Don't swallow until your food has completely turned into liquid. Ideally, the carbohydrates in your food should reach the small intestine in a completely digested state. This will only happen if food is chewed completely and the digestive enzymes that are added to food while chewing have a chance to mix with the food while still in the mouth. Digestion of carbohydrates depends on contact time with these enzymes while still in the mouth. When you consume soy drinks or any other kind of soup or drink, swirl each mouthful around in your mouth before you swallow to make sure these digestive enzymes have a chance to mix with your food. Although digestion of protein and fat occurs in the stomach, complete digestion of these substances still depends on food being broken into very small pieces, so chew well.
- Second, avoid anti-inflammatory drugs and antibiotics whenever possible, because they can cause increased intestinal permeability. After a round of antibiotics reseed your intestines with friendly bacteria by eating a live culture yogurt or other source of friendly bacteria (nondairy cultures are also available in health food stores).
- Third, eat a healthy diet low in refined carbohydrates and animal protein and high in plant-derived foods like fruits, vegetables, whole-grain products and beans.
- Fourth, don't eat anything to which you know you are intolerant, as this will tend to irritate your intestines and perpetuate over-permeability.
- Fifth, don't eat the following foods raw or undercooked: soybeans, peanuts, lentils, rice, corn and potatoes. In their raw form they contain protease inhibitors that interfere with digestion.
- Sixth, don't consume alcoholic beverages (or at least very rarely and only in small quantities); alcohol makes intestines more permeable.
- Seventh, don't drink coffee or consume any other form of caffeine if you find that caffeine causes you abdominal pain or discomfort.
- Eighth, be checked by a doctor for any possible intestinal infestations or remaining digestive difficulties. If these conditions exist, have them treated.

4.

Q: Why can avoiding exposure to toxic chemicals improve my food sensitivities?

A: Some of the same enzymes that are used to process food are used to detoxify toxic chemicals. If your enzymes are capable, for instance, of processing a total of 100 units a day and no more, as long as your total exposure is less than 100 units, you have no symptoms. Say you eat 90 units of food that need to be processed by these enzymes. If you have no exposure to any toxic chemicals, your enzymes get the job done and you feel just fine. If you have up to 10 units of exposure to toxic chemicals requiring these enzymes for detoxification, your enzymes are working at maximum capacity but still get the job done. You still feel just fine. However, if you have 11 or more units of chemical exposure, your enzymes can no longer handle the load and you start to have food sensitivity and/or chemical-exposure symptoms.

5.
Q: Some of your advice sounds like advice my mother gave me as a kid: chew your food, get to bed on time, eat your vegetables, don't smoke or drink. I expect that next you will be telling me to sit up straight. Haven't I outgrown such restrictions?

A: Mothers help their children establish healthy habits. Those same habits are useful in maintaining and restoring health to adults as well. If you are sick, returning to such basic, healthy habits will aid you in getting well again. And by the way, the importance of good posture in alleviating pain is addressed in Chapter 17 on myofascial trigger points.

Long-Term Benefits

Understanding the factors that contribute to food sensitivities puts you in an excellent position to get the best and most appropriate care for your condition. You can talk much more knowledgeably with physicians and you can make better treatment choices.

By combining the understanding you gain from this chapter with the strategies in Chapter 13 for ridding yourself of food sensitivities, you will very likely be able to minimize or even eliminate any food sensitivities and the arthritis that they are causing.

Chapter 3: Food Sensitivities— How to Test for Them

Highlights:
- How to test for food sensitivities.

Effort Involved:
- **Elimination of all problem foods from your diet for up to a week,** either by fasting or by eating only a small group of foods that is generally safe.
- **Elimination of consumption of and/or exposure to vitamins and mineral supplements, most medicines, sugar, caffeine, smoking, alcohol, pollen, dust, animal hair and toxic chemicals while testing.** Testing can last from a few weeks to several months, depending on the number of foods to which you react adversely. (Warning: never quit taking prescription medicine without consulting a doctor first.)
- **Careful reintroduction** of not more than one new food a day, sometimes not more than one new food once every three days, during the reintroduction phase of testing.
- **Keeping a food journal** that includes information on your energy level and any adverse reactions you might be having.

Payoff:
- **Exact identification of problem foods.** Eliminating problem foods often leads to a seemingly miraculous recovery.

An Overview—How to Test
Testing for food sensitivities is done in two steps—an elimination step and a reintroduction step. In the elimination step all potentially offending foods are eliminated from the diet. After all possible problem foods are eliminated, a person with food sensitivities generally feels much better. In fact, major improvement after one week indicates that food sensitivities are indeed the cause. In the next step, foods are reintroduced, one by one, to precisely identify which foods are ACTUAL problems for you.

Step 1 of Testing—Elimination of Problem Foods

One of two strategies is used to eliminate offending foods. The first strategy is fasting (either a complete water fast or a juice fast). The second strategy, referred to as selective elimination, is eating only a small number of foods that are unlikely to trigger food intolerance reactions. You will need to choose one strategy. I recommend juice fasting, but the choice is yours.

Advantages of Fasting

Fasting has four major advantages. The first is that complete fasting (water only) is the most reliable method of testing, since all foods are eliminated. The second is that both complete fasting and juice fasting induce healing changes that do not occur when one is eating. The third is that adverse reactions during the reintroduction phase of testing come and go more quickly and are easier to identify. (See Chapter 4 on fasting for details.) The fourth is that you get to the testing phase much more quickly than with an elimination diet. It takes only 3-5 days to clear out problem food from your system while fasting, but up to a week while still eating.

Juice fasting, which is much easier for most people than complete fasting, is in many ways therapeutically superior to complete fasting. Since it relies on only one or a few foods (for instance, carrot juice and/or cabbage juice and/or celery juice) that seldom trigger food sensitivities, it is almost as reliable as carrying out elimination with complete fasting.

Juice fasting is the method I used to discover my food sensitivities. Because one of my food sensitivities is to rice, a food that is often allowed on selective elimination diets, I may never have discovered my food sensitivities if I had not used fasting. Some people with extreme sensitivities react poorly to more than 20 foods. Fasting is often the only reliable way to uncover multiple sensitivities.

Disadvantages of Fasting

The disadvantages of fasting are mostly at the level of emotional reaction. Preconceived ideas about fasting sometimes trigger negative emotions. Some people think it will be too hard. Others are frightened of going without solid food for a few days. Still others simply do not like the idea of enemas.

I know from personal experience that juice fasting is unexpectedly easy and pleasant. My one minor hang-up is that I do not like the idea of enemas. This is a quirk of human nature, because I also know from repeated experience that the actual procedure is no big deal. It is only the thought of an enema that bothers me. The actual enema doesn't bother me at all.

Enemas are necessary because the body throws off waste at an accelerated rate during fasting. Enemas replace the cleaning function of the bulk that normally moves though the bowels. This cleaning keeps the waste from being reabsorbed through the intestines.

If you have negative ideas about what fasting will be like, consider doing it anyway. Fasting is actually likely to be much more pleasant than you think.

Advantages of Selective Elimination
Selective elimination of food has four major advantages. The first is that the individual being tested can still eat, something many people prefer. A second advantage is that if withdrawal symptoms from offending foods occur, for example, headaches, they tend to be milder than when fasting. A third advantage is that you avoid the unpleasant body odors that occasionally accompany fasting. These body odors come from material sometimes being cleared from your body so quickly that your normal means of elimination are overwhelmed, leading to temporary, unusually high concentrations of odors on the breath. A fourth advantage of selective elimination is that if it works, you have a built-in list of foods you already know to be safe.

Disadvantage of Selective Elimination
Unless you eliminate every single one of your problem foods, especially the foods to which you are most intolerant, you may not notice an improvement. You may falsely assume that food sensitivities are not a problem, even though they most definitely might be.

Requirements for the Elimination Phase of Testing
Both the fasting and the selective elimination strategies require that you:
- Eliminate all vitamin and mineral supplements and most prescription drugs. (They often contain binders or tableting ingredients such as corn or wheat. In addition, commercially produced vitamins such as vitamin C and folate[22] trigger sensitivity reactions in some people.)
- Eliminate sugar. (Many people react adversely to sugar without knowing it. Sugar can also cause an overgrowth of certain microorganisms in the intestine that cause food intolerance.)

---

[22] "Folate Supplements Needed but Allergenic," *Science News*, 149 (1996):198.

- Eliminate all caffeine, smoking and alcohol. (Caffeine, smoke and alcohol all contain substances that commonly trigger intolerance reactions. They also cause changes in the gastrointestinal tract that can contribute to food intolerance.)
- Limit your exposure to other nonfood substances that you find allergenic, such as pollen, dust and animal hair.
- Avoid toxic chemicals. Toxic chemicals are found in new paint and carpet, exhaust fumes, some newspaper inks and many cleaning products. Debra Lynn Dadd's book *Home Safe Home: Protecting Yourself and Your Family from Everyday Toxics and Harmful Household Products* gives practical advice that you can use to minimize toxic exposure. You do not want adverse reactions to toxic chemicals masking any improvement you might experience in the elimination phase of food sensitivity testing. The section on detoxification enzymes in Chapter 2 and Appendix A details how exposure to toxic chemicals affects food sensitivities.

Preparing for the Elimination Phase of Testing

- High doses of vitamins should be gradually ceased. Suddenly stopping high doses of vitamin C can create a temporary condition known as rebound scurvy.
- Depending on your condition, you might not be able to stop your prescription medicines during the food-sensitivity testing. If you are on prescription medicine, talk with your doctor about whether short-term elimination of your medicine is an option. You might also explain your need to eliminate tablet binders and ask if the active ingredient for your prescription is available in another form.
- Gradually decrease caffeine intake. For some people suddenly stopping caffeine can lead to headaches, vomiting and other flu-like symptoms.
- Gradually decrease sugar intake. Sugar has druglike effects on the body and alters brain chemistry.[23] Large, sudden drops in sugar intake can lead to difficulty regulating mood and energy level. During the withdrawal period, food may also taste less appealing.
- If need be, seek help in eliminating tobacco and alcohol use. Use support groups if necessary.

---

[23] S. N. Young, R.O. Pihl and F.R. Ervin, "The Effect of Altered Tryptophan Levels on Mood and Behavior in Normal Human Males," *Clin Neuropharmacol* 11 Suppl 1 (1988):S207-215.

Directions for Elimination Method No. 1: Fasting

Follow the directions in Chapter 4 for juice fasting. If you feel markedly better after three to five days, you can slowly break the fast (as described in Chapter 4). Then move directly into the second step of food sensitivity testing—the reintroduction phase.

If you do not notice any improvement after five days of juice fasting, you may want to switch to complete fasting (water only) for a few days to make certain you are not sensitive to the juice you are using. If there is still no improvement, either food sensitivities are not causing your arthritis, or adverse reactions to nonfood substances, such as pollen, dust, animal hair or toxic chemicals, are so strong they are masking any improvement.

Directions for Elimination Method No. 2: Selective Elimination

Selective elimination of foods is accomplished by following a special diet that eliminates most common problem foods. The most restrictive is the "lamb and pears" type, where two foods you seldom eat are eaten exclusively for the duration of the elimination phase. Plans become more complicated as more foods are allowed. There are many such diet plans and many good books describing how to carry out both the first phase of elimination and second phase of reintroduction. One such book is *The Allergy Discovery Diet: a Rotation Diet for Discovering your Allergies to Food* by John E. Postley with Janet M. Barton. Another is *The Complete Guide to Food Allergy and Intolerance* by Jonathan Brostoff and Linda Gamlin.

If you use a selective elimination diet, remember it is crucial to totally eliminate suspected foods, including those from unexpected sources such as toothpaste. Even trace amounts can cause reactions to continue and can invalidate the test. To eliminate trace amounts of foods, carefully read the sections in Chapters 5-8 on food labeling and hidden allergens.

The Healing Crisis—It's Actually Good News

If you have food intolerances, you may feel worse for a few days on a fast or elimination diet until your body clears all traces of the offending substances from in your system. If this withdrawal reaction happens, feel glad. It is a strong indication that food sensitivities are present and therefore that your illness has a cure. If your symptoms improve dramatically by the end of the first week, that is proof that food sensitivities are indeed causing your problems.

Step 2 of Testing—Reintroduction of Suspect Foods

The second step of testing is to challenge your body by reintroducing the foods you have been avoiding, one at a time, to see which foods cause your symptoms to reappear.

How to Reintroduce

During the reintroduction phase it is important to test with only a small amount of a reintroduced food. That's because the body deprived of the substances to which it is intolerant may be hypersensitive to these substances. During my reintroduction phase I sometimes shifted from feeling great to being in a state of major pain and fatigue within an hour of testing a single bite of reintroduced food.

Do not reintroduce foods too quickly. Because of the nature of food sensitivity reactions, at most only one food can be tested per day. Some grains, such as wheat, must be tested for as long as three days, because intolerance reactions may take that long to appear. To be on the safe side, test all grains in the grass family (Gramineae) to which wheat belongs with three days between the introduction of the grain and the introduction of the next food to be tested. The grains in the grass family are wheat, kamut, spelt, corn, rye, oats, barley, millet, rice, wild rice and teff.

Reintroduce plain, simple foods, not commercially processed foods with several ingredients. For instance, do not test wheat by reintroducing a piece of bread. Instead, reintroduce plain, cooked grains of wheat from a health food store. Bread may have many different ingredients and you have no way of knowing if an adverse reaction is to wheat or some other ingredient. If you test with grains of wheat cooked in nothing other than pure water and you react adversely, you know for sure the problem is wheat. If you do not react adversely, you know wheat is OK. If you later test a piece of bread and react adversely, you know you are reacting to something in the bread besides the wheat.

When a reaction does occur, no new testing can take place until you are well again. Getting well often takes three or four days, but sometimes up to a week.

If you use a selective elimination diet to clear out your system before testing, you will already have a core group of safe foods to which you can revert after suffering an adverse testing reaction. This is a very good thing. You have a relatively quick way to get well again. Just stick to the elimination diet. If you need to, you can also take a break from testing by sticking just to your safe foods.

If you use a fast to clear out your system before testing, it is important to quickly establish a core group of safe foods so you can stay well or get well again without fasting. First, test foods that are unlikely to be causing a problem. Don't risk wheat, corn, milk, eggs, or other likely troublemakers at this stage. See the list titled "Foods that Most Commonly Trigger Food Intolerance Reactions" later in this chapter for a more extensive list of these troublemakers. Instead, test foods like meats, fish, fruits and vegetables that you seldom or never eat and that to your knowledge have never caused a problem. This way you can (hopefully) quickly build a satisfactory list of safe food before your first adverse food reaction. If you are sensitive to many different foods and react adversely to a food before you have identified safe foods, you may have to fast again to be symptom-free before you resume testing.

Identifying all of your specific problem foods can be a difficult process. It takes patience. Because of the time necessary for the elimination phase, the slow rate of reintroduction during testing, and time out from testing to get well again after an adverse reaction, it can easily take six weeks or more to test all the foods commonly in your diet.

How to Avoid Hidden Allergens

Since I had many different food intolerances and didn't know about the many sources of hidden allergens in my diet, I had a hard time getting well enough to test additional foods once I had an adverse testing reaction. It usually took another fast for me to get well enough to test again and I generally didn't fast more than once every month. It therefore took more than six months to identify the foods I couldn't tolerate.

If you avoid commercially processed food during the reintroduction testing phase, your testing should go much more quickly and smoothly than mine. The reason I relied so heavily on fasting is that the only time I was not inadvertently getting trace amounts of problem foods was during fasting and immediately after fasting. During this time I prepared everything myself, using only fresh fruits and vegetables and unprocessed or minimally processed foods from a health food store. It was largely additives (especially corn derivatives) in commercially processed foods that were keeping me sick. I didn't know that additives as simple as salt (table salt contains dextrose which is derived from corn) were keeping me so sick.

Eliminating hidden sources of allergens in your diet is a critical step in your recovery. Even after I identified the foods to which I am intolerant, it took more than three years and much research and further testing to finally eliminate all the minor sources of hidden allergens in my life. It wasn't until I eliminated all traces of corn products that I left the gray borderland between sickness and wellness and moved deep into wellness territory. The final hidden source was my toothpaste — it contained at least one corn product. Once I switched to baking soda, I needed an hour less sleep at night. My energy levels skyrocketed. I was finally well.

My lists of hidden allergens (see Chapters 5-8) should allow you to quickly eliminate those minor sources of hidden allergens that aren't enough to keep you fully sick, but also don't let you get fully well, either. These lists may also help you eliminate major sources of allergens you didn't previously recognize.

Eliminating major sources of allergens is like calling a cease-fire. However, with only partial elimination, violence can still erupt at any moment. Eliminating the minor sources of allergens is like eliminating the sniper fire, car bombs, and other acts of terrorism that still take place during the so-called cease-fire. Only when the violence has ended can a nation or a body heal on a deep level.

Remember that even seemingly insignificant sources of allergens are enough to keep your body in an ongoing state of hypersensitivity. Not only the food you eat, but also food odors and touching food can trigger food sensitivities. The same is true of allergens in products such as toothpaste, antiperspirants and soap.

How to Keep a Food Diary

Keep a food diary with notations about your energy level, symptoms and activities. This will allow you to identify problem foods with more certainty. If you notice that you are stiffer, achier, or crankier the morning after testing a new food, but you also spent the day doing more gardening than usual, you might want to retest the suspect food again in a week or two. If you notice that on the third day after reintroducing a certain grain that you are having more symptoms, you are likely having a delayed reaction to that grain. Write down even minor symptoms. They can be significant, especially if they are part of a recurring pattern.

Foods that Most Commonly Trigger Food Intolerance Reactions[24, 25]

- **Corn** (Corn derivatives are in many products that you might not suspect, including soft drinks, table salt, fruit juice, aspirin and other medicines in tablet form, antacids, baking powder, breath sprays, toothpaste and many "low fat" versions of foods.)
- **Eggs**
- **Milk** (Milk derivatives commonly found in processed foods include whey and casein.)
- **Nuts** (Nuts from trees as well as peanuts.)
- **Soy** (Soy and soy derivatives such as lecithin are found in many products, including most processed food.)
- **Sugar** (Sugar is commonly made from cane or beets. You may be able to tolerate sugar from one source but not the other.)
- **Wheat** (Wheat can be found in unexpected places, such as in dust from sanding drywall and on hard candies.)

---

[24] Ranjit Kumar Chandra, "Food Hypersensitivity and Allergic Disease: a Selective Review, " *Am J Clin Nutr*, 66 (1997):526S-529S.

[25] Peter J. D'Adamo with Catherine Whitney, *Eat Right for Your Type: The Individualized Diet Solution to Staying Healthy, Living Longer & Achieving Your Ideal Weight* (New York: G. P. Putnam's Sons, 1996.)

- **Yeast** (Yeast is found in many baked goods and fermented products such as beer, wine, vinegar and soy sauce. It can grow on ripe and dried produce, especially fruits and berries. It can be present in vitamins and foods labeled as enriched with vitamins unless labeled as yeast-free. It can be found in antibiotics derived from yeast. Yeast overgrowth in the intestines can also contribute to food sensitivities, including yeast sensitivities.[26] If you suspect yeast overgrowth, avoid milk and other dairy products and any foods high in sugar, including fruits and fruit juices.)

Foods that Often Trigger Food Intolerance Reactions

- **alcohol**
- **apples**
- **bacon**
- **beans, dried**
- **beef**
- **berries**
- **buckwheat**
- **caffeine** (Some people react adversely to caffeine, no matter what its source. Others react not to caffeine but to other ingredients in caffeine-containing foods. Thus, it is possible to react poorly to one or a few caffeine-containing foods and be quite tolerant of other caffeine-containing foods.)
- **cheese**
- **chocolate**
- **coffee**
- **cola drinks**
- **cinnamon**
- **coconut**
- **some types of fish**
- **food additives** (including but not limited to food dyes, preservatives, MSG, etc.)
- **lettuce**
- **mustard**
- **nuts**

---

[26] There are many good books available on how to identify and treat yeast overgrowth in the intestines. One such book is *The Complete Candida Yeast Guidebook* by Jeanne Marie Martin with Zoltan Rona, M.D. (Rocklin, CA: Prima Publishing, 1996).

- onions
- oranges (citrus)
- peanuts
- peas
- pork
- tomatoes (and other nightshade vegetables such as potatoes, peppers and eggplant)
- raisins
- rye
- shrimp
- sugar
- tea

Foods that Sometimes Trigger Food Intolerance Reactions

- alfalfa
- amaranth
- bananas
- barley (malt)
- celery
- cherries
- chicken
- chilies
- cloves
- cottonseed
- garlic
- lobster
- melons
- mushrooms
- oats
- oysters
- pears
- pineapples
- plums/prunes
- quinoa
- rice
- sesame seeds
- spices
- spinach
- strawberries
- sunflower
- turkey
- vinegar

Foods that Seldom Trigger Food Intolerance Reactions[27]

- **any food you seldom or never eat** (unless this is because it once caused a severe food reaction or otherwise makes you feel unwell)
- **asparagus**
- **apricots**
- **beets**
- **cabbage**
- **carrots**
- **cassava**
- **cauliflower**
- **cranberries**
- **grapes**
- **honey**
- **Jerusalem artichoke**
- **lamb**
- **lotus roots**
- **malanga**
- **milo**
- **olive oil**
- **peaches**
- **plums**
- **rabbit**
- **safflower oil**
- **salmon**
- **sea salt**
- **squash**
- **star fruit**
- **sweet potatoes**
- **tapioca**
- **taro root**
- **true yams**
- **water chestnuts**

Caution: Any food is capable of triggering a food sensitivity reaction, regardless of how infrequently it triggers reactions in the general population. If you react to one or more of these foods, trust the signals from your body and eliminate the offenders from your diet.

---

[27] Items made from some of the more unusual foods listed here, such as malanga, cassava, true yams, lotus roots, Jerusalem artichoke, milo, water chestnut and star fruit, are available from a company named Special Foods, 9207 Shotgun Court, Springfield, VA 22153, 703-664-0991.

Cautionary Note—Cross-Reactions, Concomitant Reactions, Synergistic Reactions and Reactions to Whole Classes of Foods

At first glance the reactions mentioned in this section may seem depressing.. However, the fact is that you are unlikely to experience more than a few of these reactions, if any. Having this knowledge may mean the difference between being able to function well in the world (after taking reasonable and achievable precautions) and suffering frequent relapses due to factors you don't understand and have no idea how to control.

A cross-reaction is a reaction that initially developed in response to one substance but is then triggered in response to a different substance. Some food sensitivities are associated with cross-reactions. As the use of latex in the health care industry has grown, so have latex allergies and cross-reactions to bananas. People allergic to ragweed pollen cross-react with bananas, watermelon, zucchini, honeydew, cucumber and other members of the gourd family, even if they have never eaten these foods before. People allergic to birch pollen cross-react to potatoes, carrots, celery, hazelnuts and apples.

People sensitive to beans, peanuts or black-eyed peas tend to react not just to one but to all three. Sensitivity to a certain food, such as oranges, makes reaction much more likely to other closely related foods, like other citrus fruit, such as lemons, grapefruits, limes, tangelos, tangerines, clementines, kumquats and ugli fruit.

Concomitant reactions occur only when another allergen, such as pollen, dust or mold, is present. An example is milk sensitivity or mint sensitivity that occurs only when ragweed pollen is present. Concomitant reactions can occur up to six weeks after pollen season is over. Sometimes prescription drugs can provoke reactions to normally safe foods. A few of the many other concomitant reactions that can occur are to legumes and grains when any grass pollen is present; to milk, mint, onion, chocolate and nuts when a viral infection is present; and to lettuce when cottonwood pollen is present.

Synergistic reactions occur only when two foods are eaten in the same meal. An example is a reaction to corn and banana when they are eaten together but not when they are eaten separately. Proven synergistic foods include: corn and banana, beef and yeast, cane sugar and orange, milk and mint, egg and apple, and pork and black pepper. For more information on concomitant and synergistic food reactions I recommend the book *The Whole Way to Allergy Relief and Prevention* by Jacqueline Krohn, et al.

Some people react to a wide spectrum of foods such as all fermentation products. Fermentation products include buttermilk, vinegar, soy sauce, miso, tempeh, alcohol, yogurt and aged cheese. Others react to any trace of mold or yeast. Products that can contain mold or yeast are numerous and include the fermentation products mentioned above as well as sprouts, fruit, fruit juices, nuts, coffee, tea, citric acid, ketchup, vanilla extract, any foods enriched with vitamins including enriched flour (the vitamins are often derived from yeast), malted products and sour cream. Because molds and yeasts are also in the air, the best one can hope for is to keep exposure from ingestion and inhalation very low.

Remember that not everyone who has food sensitivities has these or any of the other reactions mentioned in this section. The way to test for these reactions is the same way you tests for any food sensitivity reaction: elimination and then reintroduction. When pollen or other airborne allergens are involved, you might have to remove all dust, dander and/or pollen from your home and wear a mask designed to filter out dust and other airborne allergens when outside.

Keep a long-term food diary with frequent notations on everything you eat, how you feel, your activities during the day and any other allergens or chemicals you might have been exposed to is as useful aid in identifying complex patterns of food sensitivity. Patterns sometimes emerge that were not obvious at the time the notations were being made. In addition, it is useful to keep track of factors such as the season, weather changes, menstrual cycle, infections, medications, exercise, alcohol, and amount and quality of sleep. These factors can also contribute to whether an adverse food reaction occurs and how severe it is.

Checklist: Testing for Food Sensitivities

Preliminary

❑	Get a notebook for recording all food eaten, energy level, activities during the day, pollen counts, etc.

❑	Eliminate smoking, alcohol, refined sugar, and sources of caffeine such as coffee, tea, soft drinks and chocolate. This can be done gradually if necessary. In fact, for caffeine gradually cutting back is recommended. Some heavy caffeine users experience severe headaches, flu-like symptoms and even vomiting if they stop caffeine too suddenly.

- ❏ If you are on prescription medicine ask your doctor if it is possible to eliminate your medicine during a testing period of one to several weeks.
- ❏ Reduce toxic exposure to cleaning products, exhaust fumes, tobacco smoke, etc.
- ❏ Familiarize yourself with the information in Chapters 5-8 on avoiding offending foods and other problematic substances.

Elimination Phase of Testing if Juice Fasting

- ❏ Get a juicer and suitable vegetables for juice fasting (see Chapter 4 for instructions),
- ❏ Carefully follow the guidelines for juice fasting (Chapter 4).

Elimination Phase of Testing if Using an Elimination Diet

- ❏ Select an elimination diet plan (from your doctor or one of the many books available on the topic) and get the specifically required types of fresh, unprocessed food (organic if possible) that will be needed.
- ❏ Carefully follow the guidelines for the elimination diet plan you choose.

Reintroduction Phase of Testing

- ❏ Buy pure, simple, preferably organically grown forms of foods to be tested; for instance, wheat berries, rye berries, plain popcorn or cornmeal, plain soybeans, etc. Prepare these foods with only water and perhaps sea salt. You may have to go to a health food store to find these items.
- ❏ Carefully follow the guidelines given in this chapter for the reintroduction phase of testing, including keeping a detailed record of everything you eat, your energy level and your activities.

Long-Term Benefits

Identifying your food sensitivities is a major empowerment. Knowing exactly which foods trigger your problems is an important first step in systematically eliminating any exposure to these troublemakers. This elimination, in turn, stops the damage they trigger in your body. It allows your body to heal from arthritis and from underlying food sensitivities.

Once you have identified your problem foods, use the information in Chapters 5-12 to eliminate any exposure while still eating well in the process.

Resources

Minimizing Exposure to Toxic Chemicals
Debra Lynn Dadd, *Home Safe Home: Protecting Yourself and Your Family from Everyday Toxics and Harmful Household Products* (New York: Jeremy P. Tarcher/Putnam Books, 1997).

Juice Fasting
Chapter 4

Elimination Diets
John E. Postley with Janet M. Barton, *The Allergy Discovery Diet: a Rotation Diet for Discovering your Allergies to Food* (New York: Doubleday, 1990).

Jonathan Brostoff and Linda Gamlin, *The Complete Guide to Food Allergy and Intolerance* (New York: Crown Publishers, 1991).

Sources of Hypoallergenic and Unusual Foods
The resource section at the end of Chapters 9 and 10

Eliminating Hidden Sources of Allergens
Chapters 5-8

Cross-Reactions, Concomitant Reactions, Synergistic Reactions
Jacqueline Krohn et al., *The Whole Way to Allergy Relief and Prevention* (Point Roberts, WA: Hartley & Marks, 1991).

Chapter 4: Calming your Inflammation and Activating your Healing Potential—How to Therapeutically Fast

Highlights:
- How to fast.
- How to test for food sensitivities after a fast.

Effort Involved:
- One to two days on a cleaning diet.
- Four to five days on a fast.
- Three days of carefully breaking the fast and testing for food sensitivities by selective reintroduction of food.
- Two weeks or so of eating normally but still testing for food sensitivities by selective reintroduction of food.

Payoff:
- Correction of sluggish elimination, a major underlying cause of arthritis.
- Healing of the digestive tract and of the joints.
- Strong anti-inflammatory effect that can be held indefinitely if problem foods are avoided.
- Exact identification of problem foods.

A Brief History of Fasting—How Therapeutic Fasting Is Different from Water or Religious Fasting

Fasting has been used by many cultures through the ages for many purposes. Religious seekers from the dawn of human history to the present day have used it to help gain access to spiritual realms. Political protesters have used it to draw attention to their causes. Men and women have also used it with great success to help heal many physical conditions, including arthritis.

Religious fasting and fasting as a means of political protest usually involve abstaining from all food and drink other than water.

Therapeutic fasting is sometimes done with just water, but more often includes small amounts of freshly made vegetable juice and/or vegetable broth. The vegetable juice and/or broth offer vitamins, minerals and alkalinity. The vitamins and minerals aid healing. The alkalinity also aids healing by helping the body avoid becoming overly acidic.

In addition, the juice and broth tend to minimize hunger. When drinking only water, fasters are often hungry the first three to five days until the body completely switches over to fasting mode. With juice and broth, fasters are generally only hungry the first day, if at all.

Long History of Success—Juice Fasting in European Clinics

There is a long history of using juice fasting in European natural-cure clinics to successfully treat many conditions, including arthritis. In a respected journal, Rheumatic Disease Clinics of North America, Norwegian doctors Jan Palmblad, Ingiäd Hafström and Bo Ringertz state:

"Total fasting may represent the most rapid and most available way of inducing relief of arthritis pain and swelling for patients who have rheumatoid arthritis. It can be administrated with a minimum of discomfort and is safe if not prolonged beyond 1 week (provided that the patient has no complicating disorders)."[28]

The book I used as a guide for my fasts is *There is a Cure for Arthritis* by Paavo O. Airola, N.D. This book details the fasting regimes used to cure arthritis at the Bircher-Benner Clinic in Zurich, Switzerland and in several famous Swedish clinics. It includes interviews with many former patients who completely recovered from arthritis through the fasting and other natural-cure treatments offered at these clinics. The treatments other than fasting vary somewhat from clinic to clinic but include a follow-up diet of healthy, minimally processed food (see Chapter 14), and, when the patient is able, exercise such as walking (see Chapter 16).

---

[28] Jan Palmblad, Ingiäd Hafström and Bo Ringertz, "Anti-Rheumatic Effects of Fasting," *Rheum Dis Clin North Amer*, 17(2), (1991):351-361.

Treatment at these health clinics is based on the philosophy that most diseases are of man's own making and are the result of health-destroying habits, wrong nutritional patterns and harmful environmental factors. Their success is based on replacing these destructive patterns with healthy patterns and allowing the body to naturally heal itself.

Miraculous Relief—How Fasting Stops Chronic Inflammation Better than Anti-Inflammatory Drugs

Fasting works so well for arthritis because it is more anti-inflammatory than any known drug. By turning off the body's autoimmune attacks upon itself, fasting stops the damage and gives the body a chance to heal.

The Miracle

My experience with fasting was MIRACULOUS. Three days into my first fast I was pain-free for the first time in 4½ years. The fatigue vanished. I could move around freely without bringing on pain and inflammation. I could think more clearly than I had in years. It reminded me of the verse in the Bible where the healed were commanded to pick up their beds and walk. Suddenly, after years of crippling illness, I could finally pick up and walk. Fasting had done what arthritis drugs had not. Fasting stopped the inflammation and gave me the boost I needed to get well.

Why Fasting is So Anti-inflammatory

Fasting turns off both biochemical pathways that lead to inflammation. Most drugs affect only one of these pathways. This means that they only turn down part of the inflammatory process. For instance, aspirin and other nonsteroidal anti-inflammatory drugs only interfere with the action of an enzyme called cyclooxygenase but not with the action of the enzyme called lipoxygenase. This means that they reduce inflammation caused by a substance called prostaglandin E_2 but not inflammation caused by leukotriene B_4. Fasting offers much better relief because it reduces levels of both prostaglandin E_2[29] and leukotriene B_4.[30]

---

[29] O. Adam, G. Wolfram and N. Zöllner, "Prostaglandin Formation and Platelet Aggregation During Fasting and Linoleic Acid Intake," *Res Exp Med (Berl)* 185 (1985): 169-172.

[30] Ingiäd Hafström, Bo Ringertz, Hans Gyllenhammar, Jan Palmblad and Mats Harms-Ringdahl, "Effects of Fasting on Disease Activity, Neutrophil Function, Fatty Acid Composition, and Leukotriene Biosynthesis in

Fasting's superior anti-inflammatory effect has been known by the medical community for a long time, but dismissed because doctors did not know how to retain these benefits at the end of a fast. The following statement by Dr. Lars Sköldstam and Dr. Karl-Eric Magnusson, is typical of those found scattered in the medical literature:

> "We and others showed that prolonged fasting for 7 to 10 days induced decreases in RA-associated inflammatory activity and a remarkable improvement in patient status. A modified fasting regimen supplemented with diluted fruit and vegetable juices seemed equally effective and had more appeal to the patient.
>
> The health benefits obtained from fasting disappeared shortly after eating was taken up again and, with regard to the chronic character of RA, were of little therapeutic significance."[31]

How to Hold the Anti-inflammatory Benefits of a Fast

I discovered, contrary to the prevailing medical opinion, that it was possible to hold the anti-inflammatory benefits of a fast long after ending the fast. As long as I did not eat something that triggered the inflammation, I remained INFLAMMATION-FREE. By identifying and then avoiding all of my problem foods, I was able to hold the benefits of a fast indefinitely. (Chapter 3 details how to test for problem foods. Chapters 5-11 detail how to avoid problem foods.)

I later found support for this in the literature. For instance, in a controlled study from Norway, patients with rheumatoid arthritis were initially put on a therapeutic fast very similar to the one I describe in this book. Dietary intake during the fast consisted of herbal teas, garlic, vegetable broth, a concoction of potatoes and parsley, and juice extracts from carrots, beets and celery. No fruit juices were allowed. Patients fasted for seven to 10 days and were then put on an individually adjusted gluten-free vegan diet for three to five months. The food was then gradually changed to a

---

Patients with Rheumatoid Arthritis," *Arthritis Rheum*, 31(5) (1988):585-592.

[31] Lars Sköldstam and Karl-Eric Magnusson, "Fasting, Intestinal Permeability, and Rheumatoid Arthritis," *Rheum Dis Clin North Am*, 17(2), (1991):363-371.

lactovegetarian diet. The benefits of the fast were still present after one year.[32]

To my mind, the key to the retention of the fasting benefits in the Norwegian study was the identification and elimination of problem foods. The fine print in this study notes that after the fast, patients:

> "reintroduced a 'new' food item into their diet every 2nd day. If they noticed an increase in pain, stiffness, or joint swelling within 2-48 hours, this item was omitted from the diet for at least 7 days. If symptoms were exacerbated on reintroduction of this food item, it was excluded from the diet for the rest of the study period. During the first 3-5 months the patients were asked not to eat food that contained gluten, meat, fish, eggs, dairy products, refined sugar, or citrus fruits. Salt, strong spices, and preservatives were avoided—likewise alcoholic beverages, tea, and coffee. After this period the patients were allowed to reintroduce milk, other dairy products, and gluten-containing foods in the way described above."

The benefits of fasting in the Norwegian study were still present after one year in part because of an individually adjusted post-fast diet. Because of this, patients avoided foods that re-triggered their arthritis. The authors of this study estimated that 37 percent of the patients in the fasting-diet group had food allergy/intolerance. They attributed the rest of the improvement to the vegetarian diet causing an extensive change in the profile of fatty acids in serum phospholipids. As explained in Chapter 14, this is a fancy way of saying that the types of fats and oils in a healthy diet, such as used in this study, can greatly reduce inflammation. Chapter 14 also details 12 other healing effects of this type of diet that the authors of the Norwegian study neglected to mention.

Because I did not have the information discussed in Chapters 3-4, and 6-11 on identifying and eliminating problem foods when I started, it took me years to identify all the hidden sources of problem foods in my diet. That first year I fasted for three to five days about once a month to keep my inflammation under control. I had to because I kept inadvertently re-triggering my inflammation. Once I learned to avoid all my problem foods, I no longer needed to fast to keep my inflammation in check.

---

[32] Jens Kjeldsen-Dragh, Margaretha Haugen, Christian F. Borchgrevink, Even Laerum, Morten Eek, Peter Mowinkel, Knut Hovi and Oystein Forre, "Controlled Trial of Fasting and One-Year Vegetarian Diet in Rheumatoid Arthritis," *Lancet* 338 (1991): 899-902.

As you will discover in Chapter 13, once you learn to avoid all your problem foods or at least eat them on a rotation diet schedule it is also possible to minimize or eliminate food sensitivities. In other words, many people are eventually able to eat without problem the very foods that formerly caused adverse reactions.

My hope is that the information in this book will allow you to quickly identify and eliminate whatever triggers your inflammation. What took me years to discover should only take you a week or at most several months. Even the price I paid (years of experimentation and research) is a small price to pay for recovery.

A Call to Health—4 Ways Fasting Activates your Body's Natural Ability to Heal

1. Stopping Autoimmune Attacks

As detailed earlier in this chapter, fasting is more anti-inflammatory than any known drug. It stops autoimmune attacks on the body and gives the body a chance to heal.

2. Freeing Energy Normally Used for Digestion for Healing

Digestion takes energy. After a big meal, people often become sleepy. This is because much of the body's resources are diverted to the digestive tract and away from the rest of the body. During fasting the energy that is normally devoted to digestion becomes available for healing.

3. Correcting Sluggish Elimination

Although most people don't realize this, arthritis is not localized to the joints but is a systemic problem. One of the predisposing conditions is sluggish elimination. Fasting allows the body to catch up on housecleaning. The body has a lot of wisdom. During fasting it will selectively eliminate toxins and superfluous cells and other material that it doesn't need. Healthy cells become healthier. Old, sick and diseased cells are eliminated.

4. Healing the Digestive Tract

For most people with food sensitivities, the autoimmune attack on their bodies begins right in the digestive tract. Withdrawal of all foods, especially problem foods, gives the digestive tract a chance to heal. Freshly made cabbage juice accelerates this process. As explained in greater detail in Chapter 14, cabbage juice contains compounds called mucins that form a protective coating in the stomach that promotes healing.

Healing the digestive tract also helps the body reverse any leaky gut syndrome that may be present. Healing a leaky gut means that fewer allergens get into the bloodstream where they can trigger autoimmune attacks throughout the body, including in the joints. Leaky gut syndrome is discussed in more detail in Chapter 2 and Appendix A. Additional steps to promote the healing of leaky gut syndrome are detailed in Chapter 13.

The Mechanics—6 Simple Skills for Successfully Undertaking a Therapeutic Fast

1. Making Fresh Vegetable Juice

Chapter 12 contains a recipe for freshly made **vegetable juice**. You will need an **electric juicer**. Juicers range in price from about $30 to $250. Cheaper juicers work just fine, but don't stand up to heavy, long-term use. Expensive juicers are slightly easier to use and clean and built well enough to stand up to years of frequent use. I recommend a cheaper juicer if you intend to use it only for the fasting described in this book. Get a more expensive juicer if you anticipate frequent and long-term use.

You also need **fresh carrots, cabbage and, optionally, celery**, all organically grown if possible.

2. Making Vegetable Broth

Chapter 12 also has a recipe for **vegetable broth**. You will need vegetables of your choice, based on personal taste and low probability of triggering an intolerance reaction. See the list in Chapter 3 titled "Foods that Seldom Trigger Food Intolerance Reactions."

3. Making Herbal Tea

Herbal tea is optional but easy to make. Add a tea bag or loose tea to a cup, pour in hot water and let it steep for 10-15 minutes. It is important to initially **use tea made out of a single, pure ingredient**. You may need to go to a health food store for this. Rosehips, alfalfa, mint and clover all support healing from arthritis and are some of the many types of herbal teas available. Once you know that you do not react adversely to several of these single-ingredient teas, you can combine them to suit your tastes. I find that adding a little mint to alfalfa makes for a better tasting tea.

Avoid herbal teas that are mixtures of several ingredients, especially with added flavorings, even "natural flavorings." You have no way of knowing what these additives might be. Every extra ingredient ups the likelihood that your food sensitivities will be triggered. This is something you want to avoid, especially during a fast.

4. Taking an Enema

Enemas are available at drugstores. Follow the instructions on the package. Enemas are important because during a fast the body is working overtime eliminating toxins and wastes. Enemas flush out these toxins and wastes and prevent them from being reabsorbed.

Most European fasting clinics provide two to three enemas a day during fasting. I used two enemas a day. I used a commercial enema for my first enema of a fast. I cleaned the top well and then reused the bottle to deliver four bottles full of plain warm water for all subsequent enemas. The European fasting clinics mentioned in Dr. Airola's book also provided one or two sessions of colonic irrigation during the first week of a fast for their patients with a history of chronic constipation. Colonic irrigation washes out the colon much more thoroughly than an enema. If you have a history of chronic constipation, you may want to arrange for colonic irrigation during your fast. Alternative healers sometimes offer this service.

Continue taking daily enemas until your bowel movements resume after the fast.

5. Maintaining a Positive Attitude

A positive attitude is a must during a therapeutic fast. A positive attitude helps unlock your body's healing potential. A negative attitude shuts down your ability to heal.

If you have a negative attitude, it is better not to undertake a fast at home, or perhaps at all. If you feel strongly that fasting is something that you want to do but are scared, find a medical professional with experience supervising fasts. See if talking with them helps calm your fears.

6. Finding Social Support through Activities other than Eating

Like it or not, human beings are social creatures. The support of family and friends is critical to our well-being. For most of us, deep in our subconscious we link eating together with social acceptance. Sharing food symbolizes a deep mutual acceptance. Refusing to share food symbolizes deep rejection.

If you do not find ways to give and receive social support that do not involve eating, you are likely to find fasting emotionally distressing. Subconsciously, your family and friends may also feel alienated.

Alternative activities can satisfy the same deep needs that are met by eating together. These alternatives include eye contact, smiling, talking, holding hands, hugging and sharing in joint activities such as walking or running errands together.

If you are creative, sometimes you can still share in the comforts of gathering for food or beverage, even while fasting. When I was giving up coffee, I found the hardest time of the day was in the morning when all my co-workers were still gathering for their coffee. What I discovered was that if I filled my coffee mug up with hot water instead of coffee, I still had all the comforts of sipping a hot beverage and being included in the group. More than anything, what I craved were the creature comforts of sipping from a hot mug while sitting in a group and hearing what was on everyone's mind.

Just telling your family and friends why you are fasting and that it is in no way a rejection of them can go a long way toward dispelling tensions on both sides. Sometimes a friend or family member might even volunteer to help you or even fast with you as a show of support. If this happens, count yourself lucky. That kind of support can go a long way toward making your fast more fun and successful.

How to Fast at Home—An Overview

Length of Fast

European fasting clinics vary in the length of fasts that they recommend. Some recommend a series of short fasts (approximately three to five day fasts repeated at once a month or so intervals). Depending on the patient, some recommend fasts of 20 or 30 days or longer. The sicker you are, and the more that conventional medicine has damaged your body's natural ability to heal itself, the longer you may need to fast to activate your healing powers. If you are very sick or just like the idea of having a trained, professional staff take you through the healing process, I recommend you undertake fasting with the support and supervision of a fasting clinic. I certainly would not undertake a fast of longer than a week without close medical supervision. Consult with your physician before any kind of fast, to make sure that it is safe for you to do so. Some of the many conditions that rule out fasting are pregnancy, emaciation, advanced heart disease, cancer, diabetes, tuberculosis, or being highly afraid of fasting.

Ideal Surroundings and Exercise

Fasting clinics are generally in quiet, beautiful surroundings. They encourage those who are able to go on long walks, slow bike rides and swims. Extremely fast or vigorous exercise is not appropriate, but slower sustained exercise is. Gentle exercise improves circulation and promotes the elimination of wastes. It strengthens and relaxes the body. It lifts the spirit. If you fast at home, try to create a pleasant, tranquil atmosphere and engage daily in gentle exercise, such as walking.

Naps

An afternoon nap is the norm at fasting clinics. Getting enough rest is important during therapeutic fasting. Although some moderate exercise is important, most of your body's resources should be dedicated to cleaning out and healing the body. Rest and quiet time facilitates this healing.

Before the Fast Begins

The information in this section has already been given in Chapter 3. However, it is so important that it is repeated here to make sure you don't miss it.

Before the fast begins and for the duration of the fast and food sensitivity testing:

- ❑ Eliminate all vitamin and mineral supplements and most prescription drugs. (They often contain tableting ingredients such as corn or wheat that are common triggers of food sensitivities. Vitamins that are synthesized in a lab are sometimes subtly different from their natural counterparts and trigger sensitivities. Even vitamins isolated from natural sources can contain traces of allergens left over from the source material.)
- ❑ Eliminate sugar. (Many people react adversely to sugar without knowing it. Sugar can also cause an overgrowth of certain microorganisms in the intestine that cause food intolerance).
- ❑ Eliminate all caffeine, smoking and alcohol. (Caffeine, smoke and alcohol all contain substances that commonly trigger intolerance reactions. They also cause changes in the gastrointestinal tract that can contribute to food intolerance.)
- ❑ Limit your exposure to other nonfood substances that you find allergenic, such as pollen, dust and animal hair.

□ Avoid toxic chemicals. Toxic chemicals are found in new paint and carpet, exhaust fumes, some newspaper inks and many cleaning products. You do not want adverse reactions to any substance masking any improvement you might experience in the elimination phase.

See Chapter 3 for pointers on the best way to accomplish this.

While on the Fast—What to Expect

Lack of Hunger

You probably won't feel very hungry while fasting. On a juice fast there is usually only slight hunger the first day or two. Usually by day three your body switches over to fasting mode and hunger disappears. Although you aren't physically hungry, you may still notice that you have a desire to eat out of habit. If this is the case, try to notice when you have the desire to eat despite not being hungry, because that is also likely to be the case even when you are not fasting. One of the rules you must follow after breaking a fast is to only eat when you are hungry. This helps hold the benefits of the fast.

Surprisingly, it is actually much easier to fast than to eat a low-calorie diet. On a fast the hunger goes away after the first few days. On a low-calorie diet, hunger is an issue for the entire length of the diet.

Energy and Alertness

You might imagine that fasting will leave you tired or weak. This is not the case. In fact, you may find that you have a more steady and reliable stream of energy. You may also notice that you become sharper mentally and/or experience a feeling of euphoria from an increase in endorphins.

Healing Crises

Sometimes during fasting there is a feeling of lightheadedness or a passing feeling of disorientation or feeling bad. Although it might not seem like it at the time, this is generally a good sign. It is referred to as a healing crisis. As fat is metabolized during a fast, the toxins that were formerly stored there pour into the bloodstream. When a pocket of these toxins releases very quickly, it can temporarily exceed the body's ability to remove them. The healing crisis will pass on its own, usually in a few hours or within a day, as the body flushes these toxins from your system.

Sometimes the body will go through a healing crisis that is actually a withdrawal reaction from problem foods, similar to a drug withdrawal reaction. This can feel very much like getting the flu. In extreme cases this type of healing crisis can go on for days. This is rare, but happened to a friend of mine who had extensive food allergies.

If you experience an extended healing crisis (longer than one day), you might want to strongly consider ending your fast early or continuing only with expert support and supervision. Instead of fasting, a more appropriate first measure would be to use one or more of the strategies given in Chapter 13 for minimizing or eliminating food sensitivities. In particular, start with the suggestions for healing leaky gut syndrome.

Hygiene

During the beginning of a fast, the tongue will often become coated. This is normal. It reflects the amount of waste that your body is eliminating. Simply brush your teeth and tongue with a soft toothbrush. Avoid using toothpastes or mouthwashes with artificial colors, flavors or sweeteners during the fast. Use a natural toothpaste or plain baking soda.

Bathe or shower at least once a day. This is important because the body also eliminates toxins through the skin. Stimulating the skin by rubbing a washcloth or brush all over your body will also aid this elimination process.

After about three days on a fast, you might notice a funny, slightly sweet smell on your breath. This is due to ketosis. It signals that your body has entered a metabolic state where it is using fat as its primary fuel. It has run out of the carbohydrates that are usually part of this process. As long as you are not diabetic, this is nothing to worry about. In fact, if you are interested in losing weight, you will like ketosis. Once you enter this state you are likely to lose a pound or more a day.

Body Temperature

When fasting, the body conserves energy by lowering body heat slightly. This means you are more likely to become chilled when fasting. Compensate by dressing a little bit warmer and using more covers when you are sleeping or resting.

Daily Schedule

Short Cleansing Diet For a Day or Two Before the Fast Starts

Prepare yourself for a fast with cleansing foods. For a day or two before eat nothing but raw vegetables and fruits, and perhaps a few cooked vegetable dishes. Vegetables and fruits (especially apples) contain fiber that helps sweep clean the intestines and colon.

Evening Before the Fast Starts

Skip the last meal of the day. Instead, take a double enema to further clean the colon and lower intestines. Shortly before going to bed for the night, take in about 1 pint of body-temperature water into the bowel and then release it again. Repeat this procedure with a full quart of water.

Sample Schedule for Fasting Days

Upon rising: single enema, 1 quart plain, body-temperature water
8 A.M.: bowl of vegetable broth
9 A.M.: 30 minutes or more walking or other suitable exercise
11 A.M.:   optional cup of herbal tea (no sweetener allowed)
1 P.M.:   1 glass fresh pressed vegetable juice
1:30 P.M.:   nap or rest in bed for about an hour
4 P.M.:   optional cup of herbal tea (no sweetener allowed)
7 P.M.:   1 glass fresh pressed vegetable juice
9 P.M.:   single enema, 1 quart plain, body-temperature water

During the day, whenever you are thirsty, drink freely of plain water, either warmed or at body temperature.

The Critical Step—How to Successfully Break a Fast

The most critical phase of fasting is breaking the fast. If you eat too much too soon, you can totally undo the benefits of the fast. You can even leave yourself worse off than before. However, if you break your fast correctly, you lock in the benefits of the fast and develop patterns of moderation that will serve you well long after the fast is over.

Eat Small Portions

The reason you need to reintroduce food slowly is because your body requires time to switch from fasting back to eating mode. The reason that most people find breaking a fast difficult is because it reactivates all the old patterns around wanting to eat (even if you are not particularly hungry) and all the preconceived notions about how much food it takes to satisfy you. Once we start eating again, most of us find it hard to eat only small, infrequent amounts even if we are not particularly hungry. However, for three days that is exactly what it takes to break a juice fast.

Chew Well

When you break a fast it is important to start with small amounts of food and to chew so thoroughly that your food is liquefied before you swallow. This is a very good habit anyway and one that promotes good digestion. Also, make sure you do not eat when you are rushed or anxious. Create a calm time and space that will allow you to focus on and savor the taste and texture of your food.

Only One New Food Every 24 to 36 Hours

Fasting provides an excellent opportunity to test for food sensitivities. If you have food sensitivities, by the end of the fast you will likely feel better than you have in ages. The contrast when you reintroduce a problem food is likely to be quite noticeable. Any adverse reaction, such as the return of arthritis pain, fatigue or poor mood, is an indication of a problem food. To maximize your ability to identify problem foods, follow the testing guidelines in Chapter 3. In brief, keep a daily log of exactly what you eat and how you feel. Keep reintroduced foods simple. For example, when testing milk use plain milk instead of a milk product like cottage cheese or ice cream that contains several ingredients, any of which might trigger a reaction. Reintroduce a new food only once every 24 to 36 hours.

Reintroducing a new food once every 24 hours (instead of 36 hours) is useful in terms of quickly developing a repertoire of safe foods. For quick responders this works fine. If you are a quick responder, any adverse reaction will happen within the first 24 hours. There will be a clear-cut association between reintroduced foods and any symptoms that were triggered.

Slow responders should reintroduce new foods once every 36 hours. If you have no idea if you are a slow responder, but have the patience, use 36 hour intervals. You will get a clear cut association between reintroduced food and symptoms

For slow responders at least 36 hours between new food reintroduction is mandatory. Otherwise, even with a journal, it will quickly become too difficult to pinpoint problem foods.

Some people respond quickly to one problem food and slowly to another. The foods most likely to trigger a delayed response are in the grass family (Gramineae) to which wheat belongs. To be on the safe side, even if you are usually a quick responder, test all grains in the grass family with 36 hours between the introduction of the grain and the introduction of the next food to be tested. The grains in the grass family are wheat, kamut, spelt, corn, rye, oats, barley, millet, rice, wild rice and teff.

Be Aware of the Possibility of Hypersensitivity

While breaking a fast, many people are hypersensitive to problem foods. I used to go from feeling very good to a ball of pain within 30 minutes to three hours of eating something to which I reacted adversely. Although this hypersensitivity is not pleasant, it is useful because it allows you to clearly identify problem foods. The quicker and the more severe, the easier it is to know exactly what caused the problem. When eating a normal diet, these reactions are often masked or delayed, making it much more difficult to pinpoint the problem.

Because of hypersensitivity, use only a small amount of a test substance, perhaps only a bite or two. If you do have a hypersensitivity reaction, it will pass more quickly if you have eaten only a little.

Menus for Breaking a Juice Fast

Day 1:

Follow the usual juice and broth menu that you used while fasting. To this add one whole apple or other sweet fruit and a small bowl of fresh vegetable salad (no dressing, only raw vegetables).

Apples are good because they are high in pectin and thus provide soft bulk to help sweep clean the intestines. However, fruits such as peaches, plums, and grapes trigger fewer food sensitivities than apples. The trade-off is that they do not provide the same benefits of bulk. If you have no reason to suspect a sensitivity to apples, feel free to take advantage of the benefits of breaking the fast with an apple. Otherwise, pick another sweet fruit.

Most people do not have food sensitivities to most vegetables, and especially not to lettuce. The exception is that many people with arthritis do have food sensitivities to tomatoes and peppers. Unless you already know from previous fasting and selective reintroduction that you are not sensitive to tomatoes or peppers, avoid these vegetables for at least a few days until you build up a fall-back list of safe foods that you know you won't react to. Chapter 3 has lists of foods that most commonly trigger food sensitivities and those that rarely do. Until you have a list of safe foods, avoid those on the "Foods that Most Commonly Trigger Food Intolerance Reactions" list in Chapter 3.

If you still feel good on the second day, proceed to eat from the menu for the second day. In the extremely rare event that the fruit or salad triggered an adverse reaction, go back on the fasting regime for a day or two until you feel OK again. Then try again with a different fruit and/or vegetable. Once you still feel good the day after, proceed to the menu for the second day.

On rare occasions, the body has difficulty holding down solid food until after it has absorbed enough carbohydrates to reverse ketosis. Your first line of defense against this is chewing extremely well. Don't swallow until your food has become liquefied. In the extremely rare event that despite chewing very well and taking only very small portions, you are still having trouble holding down solid food, it may also be helpful to reintroduce a small amount of carbohydrate in the form of half of a small potato boiled in plain water. Again, eat this very slowly and chew very well.

Day 2:

To the menu for the first day add a little yogurt and cottage cheese. It is best to make your own yogurt and cottage cheese so you can be sure there are no additives that might make you sick. See Chapter 12 for recipes.

If you happen to have a food sensitivity to dairy (or additives that might be in the yogurt or cottage cheese) you will feel worse within 24 to 48 hours. If so, immediately withdraw the yogurt and cottage cheese from your menu. Go back to the menu for the first day until you feel good again. When you feel good again, instead of dairy, introduce an easy-to-digest protein such as tofu. If you have a food sensitivity reaction, you will feel worse within 24 to 48 hours. In this case you are reacting either to soy or an additive in the tofu. As with the triggering of any other sensitivity, fall back to those foods you know to be safe, until you feel good again.

Hopefully you will not have food sensitivities to both cow's milk (and cow's milk products) and soy, but if you do, other protein sources to try include lentils, goat's milk, sheep's milk, and meat from organically raised animals. You may need to go to a health food store or wild-game meat supplier for the latter items. See the resource section in Chapter 10 for a list of mail-order suppliers.

Day 3:

Increase the portions from the second day. Add a carbohydrate such as a plain, baked potato, plain cooked millet, or other plain, cooked grain.

Day 4:

As long as you are not feeling worse, continue to introduce a new food each day, preferably a food consisting of a single ingredient. For example, instead of eating bread, try wheat berries cooked in pure water. A complex food such as bread actually contains many different ingredients, any one of which might cause an adverse reaction.

Although beginning the fourth day you can eat "normally, You should continue to follow these practices:
1. Chew well (until the food is liquefied).
2. Don't overeat. (If you are not hungry, you should not eat, no matter how good something might look or smell, no matter if it is your normal mealtime and no matter if you were previously accustomed to eating much more at a sitting.)
3. Reintroduce no more than one new food item per 24-hour period. If you find that you respond slowly to food challenges, reintroduce no more than one new food item per 48 to 72 hours.
4. If you take a turn for the worse, immediately remove any suspect foods from your diet. Suspect foods are any new foods you have reintroduced within the last 48 to 72 hours. Avoid a given suspect food for at least seven days.
5. Only test food items when you are already feeling good. Otherwise, eat only foods from your safe list.
6. If you have problems within 24-36 hours of testing a food for a second time, remove that food from your diet for one year.

Long-Term Benefits

There are at least three long-term benefits of fasting.

First, just like a house benefits from spring cleaning, your body benefits from time devoted to cleaning out fat, toxins, and any other waste material that is mucking up your system. Afterwards, you are leaner, lighter and function better.

Second, fasting activates your body's natural ability to heal. Energy normally taken up by digestion jump-starts the healing process. As long as you break a fast properly, this healing will continue long after the fast is over.

Third, selective reintroduction of food after fasting is one of the most reliable ways of detecting and precisely identifying food sensitivities. Knowing if you have food sensitivities and exactly what they are is powerful information that can mean the difference between perpetual illness and rapid healing. Chapters 5-11 explain how to use this information to heal.

Resource

Paavo O. Airola, N.D., *There is a Cure for Arthritis* (West Nyack, N.Y.: Parker Publishing Company, Inc., 1968).

Chapter 5: Food Sensitivities— How to Avoid Offending Foods and Food Additives in a World of Vague, Incomplete and Confusing Food Labels

Highlights:

- ❑ How to identify the presence of problematic ingredients using a combination of label-reading and other knowledge.
- ❑ Three ways to reduce exposure to toxins.
- ❑ How to find safe products.
- ❑ Why to avoid genetically engineered food.

Effort Involved:

- ❑ **The effort involved in learning to identify from food labels whether a given product is free of hidden allergens is variable.** The effort depends on the number and exact identity of your food sensitivities. It involves familiarizing yourself with names used on food labels and knowing what types of products are likely to contain problem ingredients.
- ❑ **Reducing exposure to toxins involves purchasing organically grown produce, using safe storage containers, avoiding skin contact with, and inhalation of, problem foods, and buying from reliable sources.**

Payoff:

- ❑ The ability to identify and avoid foods and other products that contain any of your problem ingredients. By avoiding substances that trigger your food sensitivities, the damaging reactions that used to be triggered in your body cease. Your digestive track and your arthritis finally get a chance to heal.

Using Labels to Identify Allergens—2 Problems

You might naively think that once you have identified your problem foods it will be simple to eliminate them from your diet. Indeed, if you cook all your own food from fresh produce and other natural, organically grown ingredients that contain no additives, eliminating offending foods is relatively simple. The problem is that most of us want the convenience of eating commercially processed food. Unfortunately, such food often contains additives that can make people with food sensitivities sick. To avoid triggering your sensitivities, you must read labels very carefully.

In addition to reading labels, you must also know how to overcome two problems. These are:

1. Loopholes that allow unlisted ingredients.
2. Alternative names that can obscure the identity or the source of an ingredient.

Problem No. 1—Loopholes that Allow Unlisted Ingredients

The first loophole involves "standard recipes." The second loophole involves "incidental additives."

The "Standard Recipes" Loophole

In the United States more than 300 types of processed foods are exempt from labeling requirements as long as they are prepared according to a "standard recipe." Foods normally produced according to standard recipes include dairy products, pasta, baked goods, mayonnaise, canned fruits and vegetables, margarine, peanut butter, soft drinks and jelly. Ingredient listings may appear on these labels, but the listing is at the discretion of the manufacturer. These listings are not required to be complete. This makes it impossible for the consumer to know if the absence of additives on a label means that no additives are present, or only that the food is covered by a standard recipe and contains numerous additives.

Ice cream, considered a standard food, can have up to 30 additives that do not have to be indicated on the label. Monosodium glutamate (MSG) must appear on the label of canned vegetables since this use is not part of a standard recipe, but MSG may be added to mayonnaise and salad dressings without being listed, if a standard recipe is followed.

The "Incidental Additives" Loophole

In the United States, manufacturers are not required to list "incidental additives" on food labels. Incidental additives are substances that become part of a food without intentionally being added during the production process. They include approved food additives already present in one foodstuff that is then used in the manufacture of another food product.

The Limited Times When You Can Rely on Food Labels to Offer Full Disclosure

Food labels only reliably reveal what is added to a product if the product is both a single "food" and also not one of the "standard recipe" foods mentioned above. For example, the label on a box of Nutrasweet® lists cornstarch or dextrose as an ingredient. In contrast, a can of diet soft drink lists a nonnutritive sweetener such as Nutrasweet® but does not list cornstarch or dextrose (both can trigger corn sensitivities), even though it is a major component by weight of Nutrasweet®. Another example is that chocolate may contain many ingredients, and the label on chocolate is required by law to list these ingredients. However, only the word "chocolate" and not its "incidental additives" are required on the label of a product that contains chocolate. The labels for mole sauce and chocolate cake are therefore only required to disclose "chocolate" and not ingredients such as possible corn syrup (which can trigger corn sensitivities) or lecithin (which can trigger soy, egg or corn sensitivities, depending on the source of the lecithin).

The Solution—How to Protect Yourself From Undisclosed Ingredients

Reading labels is not enough. To be safe a person with food allergies must also know all the possible "standard recipe" ingredients and all the possible incidental additives that might be present in a given product.

Of course this assumes you are eating processed food. The very best way of protecting yourself against hidden allergens is not to eat any commercially processed food. If your food sensitivities are severe, this might be necessary for recovery. Unfortunately, this is not convenient. Unless you cook all your own food, it is also nearly impossible.

The second best way to protect yourself is to know if anything to which you are sensitive is likely to be used in a product. This can require some detective work. For instance, for years I was highly sensitive to dextrose, a product derived from corn that is added to table salt to keep it from clumping. Dextrose in table salt is considered an incidental additive and need not be listed on the label of salted products. Because most processed

81

food contains table salt and therefore dextrose, most processed food was off-limits to me. It was up to me to check for salt and to know that if salt was present, it usually meant dextrose was as well.

This kind of reading between the lines gets even more complex. For instance, cheese is a "standard recipe" product. Most cheese is salted with table salt even though it doesn't have to say so on the label. Before I knew this, I sometimes reacted poorly to cheese without knowing why. This problem went away once I started eating cheese only if its label stated that it was made with sea salt (sea salt usually has no dextrose added) or stated that it was completely free of salt.

To learn if anything you are sensitive to is likely to be used in a product, first familiarize yourself with the lists of names used on food labels that can indicate hidden allergens. These lists are found in Chapter 6.

Second, familiarize yourself with the lists of products that can contain various hidden allergens. These lists are found in Chapter 7. For the lists in both Chapters 6 and 7, you only need to look those that correspond to your own problem foods.

Third, familiarize yourself with other additives that you should avoid. These are listed in Chapter 8.

Finally, learn all the possible ingredients that can be contained in the types of food you eat. To do this, read recipes. Also read labels from many brands of a given product. Some manufacturers provide a full listing of ingredients. For "standard recipe" products, this can alert you to the possibility of problematic, but unlisted ingredients in other brands with more limited disclosure.

Problem No. 2—Use of Alternative Names to Hide Additives

Alternative names are sometimes used to "hide" additives in processed foods. For example, monosodium glutamate is a flavor enhancer that is added to many foods. Monosodium glutamate, or MSG, makes many people sick, often with migraine headaches, and sometimes with a wide range of other symptoms that can include arthritis. Because many people will not knowingly eat products that contain MSG, a powerful lobby of food manufacturers that use the additive has influenced legislation to allow for dozens of alternative names for MSG. Of course, this makes it much more difficult for consumers to know if a food contains MSG.

Names that can signal the presence of MSG include: monosodium glutamate, monoammonium glutamate, monopotassium glutamate, glutamic acid, hydrolyzed protein, Accent, Ajinomoto, Zest, Vetsin, Gourmet powder, subu, Chinese seasoning, glutavene, glutacyl, RL-50, hydrolyzed vegetable protein (12 to 20 percent MSG), hydrolyzed plant protein, natural flavorings (can be HVP), flavorings, kombu extract, carrageenan, caseinate, Mei-jing, Wei-jing, vegetable powder, vegetable broth, chicken broth and beef broth.

For more information, look under MSG in the section "More Additives to Avoid" near the end of Chapter 8.

Even when there is no desire to deceive, alternative names can still hide the source of an ingredient. For instance, gelatin used commercially is made from one of two processes. One process uses cattle hides and bones. Allergic reactions to gelatin derived from cattle bones have been reported in people sensitive to beef. This means that whenever a product contains gelatin, it is potentially unsafe for people with beef sensitivities. Because of the very real risk that the gelatin in any given product was made from cows, whenever a person with beef sensitivities reads the name gelatin on a label, he or she needs to consider it to be an alternative name for beef allergens.

To complicate things further, gelatin is used to make many products, including Jell-O, wine and yogurt. This means that the presence of Jell-O®, wine, and yogurt also signal the possible presence of beef allergens. In the same way, since gelatin used commercially is also made from pork skins, anyone with pork sensitivities needs to consider gelatin and products made with gelatin as unsafe, since they may contain pork allergens.

The Solution—How to Learn the Alternative Names

The problem of additives being hidden by using alternative names on labels is annoying. The only solution I know of, short of waging a war to change labeling laws, is to learn all the alternative names that can be used to hide your problem ingredients. The lists in Chapters 6-8 are an excellent place to start. In fact, if your list of problem foods is similar to my old list, these chapters may very well contain everything you need to know. If not, these chapters plus the current chapter will still give you a good idea of how to figure out this information for your own unique situation.

Other Hidden Dangers—How to Avoid Triggering Sensitivities through Contact and Inhalation

In addition to causing adverse reaction by ingestion, corn and wheat and possibly other problem foods can also cause adverse reactions through contact and through inhalation.

Contact sources for corn include baby powder, underarm deodorants, shaving cream, after-shaves, bath oils, deep-heating rubs, skin lotions, shampoo, soap, hair styling mouse and gels, adhesives, starched clothing and pet food, including fish food, bird food, rabbit and guinea pig food, cat food and dog food. Corn can be inhaled from a number of sources, including cooking odors, spray laundry starch, baby powder and dust from pet food.

Contact sources for wheat include bath oils, massage oils, adhesives and the pet foods listed above. Sources of inhalation include cooking odors, airborne flour in bakeries and kitchens, from sanding drywall (seaming paste can contain wheat) and dust from pet food.

Besides containing corn and wheat, pet foods commonly contain many other ingredients to which people are frequently sensitive. Fish food can contain wheat, rice, corn, oats, soybeans, potatoes and yeast. Bird food can contain corn, millet, oats, soybeans, molasses from cane, gelatin, peanuts, wheat, apples, whey, yeast, egg, safflower, barley, rice, sweet potatoes, buckwheat and bell pepper. Rabbit and guinea pig food can contain alfalfa, oats, wheat, soybeans, corn, cane molasses, whey, milo, peanuts, rice, almonds, cashews and tomatoes. Cat food can contain fish, chicken, rice, corn, egg, beet, yeast, wheat and soy. Dog food can contain chicken, beef, egg, cheese, yam, pork, wheat, sunflower, corn, citrus, onion, garlic, beet, yeast and cane molasses.

Systematically eliminate exposure to your problem foods through contact and inhalation. Use the lists in this section and in Chapters 6-8 combined with avid reading of product labels to identify the products you need to eliminate.

3 Steps to Reduce Exposure to Hidden Toxins

1. Eat Organically Grown Food Whenever Possible

A small but significant amount of all food tested by the FDA contains pesticides exceeding allowable tolerances, and less than one percent of all food shipments are tested. The FDA's testing methods are able to detect only about half the pesticides registered with the EPA. Many of the pesticides that escape detection, moreover, pose moderate to high threats to health. Produce grown in direct contact with the ground, such as celery, potatoes and carrots, tend to have the highest concentrations of pesticides. Fruits and vegetables such as strawberries, peaches and bell peppers that consumers expect to be unblemished also tend to have high concentrations of pesticides. Foreign-grown produce is much more likely to be contaminated than domestic produce.

The lesson here is that it is difficult to know the level of pesticide residue in foods grown by our modern system of agribusiness. If you are ill, it's a good idea to protect yourself by purchasing organically grown produce whenever possible. It is especially important to substitute organic produce for those types of produce that tend to carry the highest levels of contamination when grown nonorganically.

2. Be Careful About Food Storage Containers

Another source of contamination is food packaging. Lead can leach into food from the leaded solder used in certain cans. Plastics are troublesome because they can leach harmful chemicals into foods. Even paper cartons can be problematic because they may contain residues of dangerous manufacturing chemicals like PCBs, dioxin and formaldehyde. Chemicals in "microwave ready" packages are also worrisome because microwave ovens can raise temperatures enough to vaporize some harmful chemicals.

Whenever possible, buy fresh, organically grown produce. Don't store it in plastic—glass or cloth or paper manufactured without toxic chemicals. Heat food in the oven or on the stove in good-quality metal, glass or enamel cookware. Avoid heating food in plastic containers in a microwave oven.

3. Reduce Overall Toxic Chemical Exposure

Many people with food allergies also have chemical sensitivities. Unfortunately, it is impossible in today's world to fully escape exposure to the many toxic chemicals so prevalent in modern life. However, you can greatly minimize exposure and may need to in order to recover from illness. Though it is beyond the scope of this book to serve as a guide in this matter, if you suspect you have chemical sensitivities, consult books that explain in depth how to overcome such sensitivities. Two good books to use are *The Complete Guide to Food Allergy and Intolerance* by Jonathan Brostoff and Linda Gamlin and *Home Safe Home: Protecting Yourself and Your Family from Everyday Toxics and Harmful Household Products* by Debra Lynn Dadd.

Toxic chemicals that can make food sensitivities worse are found in many food additives, pesticide residues, tobacco smoke, coal smoke and exhaust fumes, gasoline vapors, perfumes, scented toiletries, paint, varnish, mothballs, and gases given off by plastics, coated paper, newsprint, new fabric and carpets.

One reason for limiting exposure to even "safe" levels of common chemicals is that these levels have been determined by testing single substances in the absence of other toxic substances. Under real life conditions, however, we are often exposed to many toxic substances simultaneously. The cumulative toxic effect can be much greater than the effect of any given substance alone. For instance, Debra Lynn Dadd in the food section of her book *Nontoxic and Natural* cites a study by Dr. Benjamin Ershoff at the Institute for Nutritional Studies in California. In this study, rats were given different combinations of three common food additives: sodium cyclamate, food dye Red No. 2 and polyoxyethylene sorbitan monostearate. At first rats were fed only one of the three additives and nothing happened. When the test animals were given sodium cyclamate and Red No. 2, they stopped growing, lost their hair and developed diarrhea. When the rats were given all three additives, they lost weight rapidly and all died within two weeks.

How to Get Safe Products

How to Find Safe and Reliable Sources

Many sources of contamination are not reflected on product labels. Labels are printed in advance and are sometimes used despite the fact that they do not reflect last-minute changes in ingredients. Products sold in open bins may have been contaminated by the scoops having been exchanged between bins. For instance, if the scoop from a cornmeal bin is inadvertently placed in a buckwheat bin, a person allergic to corn and buying buckwheat is in trouble. Contamination may also be present in a batch of rye flour made from rye grown in a field that in the previous year grew corn. Corn from a few volunteer corn plants may have gotten mixed in with the rye. Millers who don't realize how sensitive some of us can be to even small amounts of some products contaminate flour by grinding several kinds of grains on the same stones. Food can also be contaminated in transit.

A large tanker truck carrying a load of corn oil may carry soy oil as its next load without adequate cleaning between loads. A corn sensitive person may then become sick from contaminated soy oil. It is hard to say how often these types of contamination happen, but they do happen.

The lesson is, whenever possible, to eat food prepared from fresh, pure ingredients that you know to be safe. Patronize reputable companies and farmers that take steps to ensure purity and accurate labeling. Organic farms, farmers markets and health food stores are good places to seek out quality produce and dealers. Let your suppliers know of your particular need for pure, uncontaminated food. Individuals and companies are more likely to take the extra effort to keep foodstuffs free of residue from other types of food if they understand the dire consequences for some of us if they don't.

Even when you find certain products and brands that you tolerate well, make sure you continue to check labels and talk to suppliers. Companies sometimes change product ingredients. As a preemptive move, you might even let suppliers know about your food allergies and how happy you are with their products. Let them know that they are doing a good thing by not changing ingredients or becoming sloppy in their production practices.

How to Find Safe Alternative Formulations

Familiarize yourself with the hidden allergen lists given in this chapter. Then read labels carefully to find items that are safe for you to use. If you cannot find a suitable formulation of a given product yourself, ask for help. I have found pharmacists and the employees at health food stores to be particularly helpful.

Health food stores often carry products with alternative formulations that are useful for people with food and contact sensitivities. For instance, skin lotions often contain ingredients that are problematic for people with corn, soy and wheat allergies. Health food stores often carry cocoa butter (from the beans used to make chocolate), coconut butter, lanolin (oil from the wool of sheep), jojoba oil (oil from the nut of desert shrubs native to Arizona, California and northern Mexico), and shea butter (from the Shea butter nut from a tree that grows in Africa, particularly in Ivory Coast), all of which are good for moisturizing dry skin. A wide variety of soaps and shampoos made from many alternative formulations are also available. When I still had my food sensitivities, to avoid any corn and wheat products in my shampoo, I used a liquid castile soap. It didn't lather quite as nicely as products sold as shampoo, but it did get my hair clean. If you have dry skin or a dry scalp, you may wish to avoid soaps made with coconut oil, which many people find to be particularly drying.

A Dangerous Gamble—Genetically Engineered Food

A documented case of genetic engineering transferring an allergen from one crop into another has already occurred.[33]   Hoping to improve the nutritional value of a protein supplement for hogs and poultry, scientists at Pioneer HiBred International spliced a gene from Brazil nuts into soybeans. Studies financed by Pioneer, and carried out by Steve L. Taylor of the University of Nebraska in Lincoln, showed that the transferred protein is one of the major allergens in Brazil nuts. If ingested by susceptible people, it could trigger life-threatening reactions.   Ironically, while the Pioneer study was under way, other scientists published animal data suggesting this same protein is not a major allergen. Taylor stated, "This just emphasizes why we cannot rely exclusively on animal-based tests for these determinations."

Life-threatening classical food allergies like many nut allergies are relatively easy to detect with laboratory tests. That is why Dr. Taylor's studies could show that the Brazil nut gene that scientists at Pioneer HiBred International spliced into soybeans coded for a major allergen capable of triggering life-threatening reactions.   However, there is no reliable laboratory test to detect the presence of allergens that trigger delayed food intolerance reactions. This means that scientists have no way of testing whether genes transferred by genetic engineering also transfer major food-sensitivity-triggering allergens. Without this testing, the transfer of genes from one type of plant or animal to another makes food produced from these genetically engineered organisms unsafe for people with food sensitivities.

Soybeans aren't the only genetically engineered crop to cause an uproar. In 2000 there was a major recall in the United States of products containing genetically modified StarLink corn.   Some consumers filed lawsuits claiming they had allergic reaction to this corn.   Scientists have also documented the presence of genetically engineered genes in old maize varieties.[34] The scary fact is that the jumping of genetically altered genes from modified corn into old varieties is "relatively common," something that ten years ago scientists were claiming would not happen at all.

The introduction by genetic engineering of even desirable qualities, such as disease resistance, will likely create ongoing problems for people with food

---

[33] "Allergies to this Soy would be Nutty," *Science News*, 149 (1996):164.

[34] "Transgenes Migrate into Old Races of Maize," *Science News*, 160(2001)342.

sensitivities. This has already happened with plants produced by traditional plant breeding methods. Modern varieties of wheat are allergenic for many people because of disease-resistance genes. Older, heirloom varieties of wheat such as spelt and kamut do not have these disease-resistance genes and thus can be tolerated by many people who otherwise react adversely to wheat.

Genetically altering crops to be pesticide resistant allows these crops to be sprayed with higher levels of pesticides. That means higher levels of toxic pesticide residue in food, something that makes the food supply unsafe for everyone, but especially food-sensitive individuals who tend to be more sensitive to toxic chemicals.

The day of genetically engineered crops being common in our food supply is here. Large companies like Monsanto have already added new traits to old staples. Monsanto has genetically engineered soybeans, canola, tomatoes, potatoes, sugar beats and corn to be pesticide resistant and disease resistant. Other crops like alfalfa, apple, walnut, cantaloupe, squash, rice and sunflower have also been genetically engineered. In the United States these genetically engineered varieties can be included in food products without any labeling to indicate their genetic engineering. Because the testing required by the FDA for new, genetically engineered foods does not reliably detect allergens that trigger food sensitivities, I do not consider genetically engineered crops to be safe for people with food sensitivities.

People with food sensitivities need complete and accurate information on food labels. To this end, foods from genetically engineered crops should be clearly labeled as such. Let our government officials, food companies, etc. know how important it is to clearly label all instances of food from genetically engineered sources. Write letters to the USDA and to the editor of your local paper to help raise awareness. When I had food sensitivities, my diet was already quite restricted. I had adverse reactions to a great many foods. The last thing I wanted was for foods like soy that had been safe for me to become off-limits because of genetic engineering that was not acknowledged on food labels.

The Value of Detective Work—My Experience with Corn Sensitivity

Part I

To ferret out all your hidden food sensitivities you must learn to pay attention to your body instead of to what so-called experts might tell you is possible. You might also have to do a bit of detective work. After two years of repeated therapeutic fasts and diligently paying attention to how my body reacted to different foods, I thought that I had gone about as far as I could go in terms of modifying my diet to regain my health. However, it still seemed that the arthritis was in my body ready to flare up, and I was still experiencing some fatigue. On trips I would slowly feel more and more tired over the course of several days. When I finally realized that the dextrose in table salt was causing my fatigue, it was a great revelation to me. The part of me trained as a chemist didn't think that dextrose, which is a sugar, could even act as an allergen. What was missing from the story is the fact that dextrose, like most commercially used food additives, is not a chemically pure substance. It retains impurities from its source material.

Once I cut out table salt from my diet, I stopped getting rundown on trips. At home I needed about one hour less sleep a night. Previously, at home I usually cooked everything from scratch and used sea salt. Only occasionally did I have anything with table salt (identified as just "salt" on most labels). But that was enough to keep the low-level fatigue going. On trips I often ate food prepared by others. Consequently I often consumed dextrose and had much more difficulty keeping the fatigue under control. For the longest time it never occurred to me that the dextrose used commercially might be produced from a substance to which I reacted adversely.

I was very sensitive to corn products. Discovering in a book on food additives that dextrose is made from corn syrup solved the mystery for me of why I react so poorly to it. However, the same food additives book in which I learned the corn origin of dextrose also states, "Studies have shown that corn syrup and corn sugar (dextrose) are free of allergenic properties, even for patients who are sensitive to cornstarch." All I can do is laugh about that statement, because I did my own detailed observations on how I was affected by dextrose. My studies proved to me, beyond any shadow of a doubt, that I reacted quite adversely to dextrose.

Part II

After I discovered my allergy to table salt and eliminated that source of corn allergen from my diet, I was generally doing well. This higher background state of health then allowed me to notice that whenever I had my normal brand of grape juice or apple juice I felt bad for a day or two. I was inexplicably tired and a bit cranky, signs I had long practice in recognizing as the first signs of a developing arthritis flare-up. Usually this feeling would pass without getting worse, so it was a while before I paid sufficient attention. The only ingredient besides grape and apple in these juices was vitamin C. I found brands that had no added vitamin C and those brands did not make me tired or cranky. I retested the vitamin-C-fortified brands and I again reacted with tiredness and crankiness.

90

It finally dawned on me that for months I had been hearing an advertisement on the radio that stated that a certain company was a supplier of vitamin C produced by a corn-based fermentation process. At that point I understood why I react poorly to vitamin-C-fortified products, but not fruits and vegetables that naturally contain high levels of vitamin C, such as strawberries, red bell peppers and citrus fruit. I wasn't reacting to the vitamin C itself, but to impurities left over from the commercial production (using corn) of vitamin C or to some other aspect of commercial vitamin C production. I later learned that vitamin C is produced using corn syrup as a source of glucose that is subjected to several chemical reactions to produce synthetic ascorbic acid that is similar but not identical to vitamin C found naturally in foods.

One vitamin company that I contacted (Kal®, maker of Nutra brand vitamins) uses vitamin C produced in this manner and claims that it is impossible for its products to trigger corn allergies because there is no corn protein left after chemical synthesis of ascorbic acid. This company claims that any allergic reaction to its vitamin C product is due to an allergy to its new synthetic molecule of ascorbic acid, not due to a corn allergy. Kal® also claim that legitimate corn allergies are sometimes triggered by vitamin C made by the exact same chemical process that it uses, because the raw material supplier has already combined the vitamin C with excipients such as cornstarch. (Excipient is the company's word for an incidental additive that need not be declared on food labels.)

Unfortunately, the consumer usually has no way of knowing if any given ascorbic acid has a pre-added excipient. The only choice is to rely on the few companies, such as Kal®, that are sensitive to issues of added excipients. The way labeling laws are set up, if we want to use these kinds of products, we have no choice other than to let these hopefully vigilant companies be our watchdogs and ensure that no allergenic excipients are added. Inquiring at health food stores is a good way to locate such companies.

Kal® also mentioned that some of its vitamin capsules are coated with zein, a type of corn protein coating. It claims that zein has a low allergenic potential, but anyone allergic to corn would do well to be tested specifically for an allergic reaction to zein, since it is so widely used as a coating in the nutritional supplement and pharmaceutical industries. If a zein allergy is suspected, Kal® suggests using only its uncoated tablets.

While I had my food sensitivities, I never felt the possible benefits justified the risk of testing this company's vitamin C tablets to see if I could tolerate them. However, other corn sensitive individuals who have a stronger desire to take vitamin C tablets might find products from such companies a very useful option.

No matter what the actual details concerning the products from this vitamin company, without strong assurances to the contrary, ascorbic acid or vitamin C listed on a label is a likely indication that people as sensitive as I was to corn will react poorly. This is because of the high likelihood that excipient cornstarch is included in the ascorbic acid or vitamin C.

Part III
In researching this book I discovered many chemical names that I hadn't previously known could indicate the presence of corn allergens in a product. In using these new names to check products, I noticed that my toothpaste contained four suspect ingredients. As an experiment, I started using baking soda to brush my teeth. After a month I definitely felt more energetic. I needed less sleep and had more enthusiasm and endurance during the day. I wouldn't have described myself as feeling bad or tired before I eliminated my toothpaste, but afterward I felt more energetic than I had in years.

The Lesson
To fully eliminate offending foods from your diet, you need to become your own researcher. Don't let yourself be talked out of your findings by some "expert" who has never taken your unique situation into account. Even if no one else in the whole world has ever had or will ever have the same adverse reactions to certain foods, that doesn't matter. What matters is that you will have discovered exactly what you need to do (or in this case not eat, touch or inhale) to give yourself the gift of better health.

Checklist—Steps to Take to Avoid Offending Substances

Identify the Source of the Problem:
❏   Study the allergen lists in Chapters 6 and 7.
❏   Familiarize yourself with the names of the additives to avoid that are discussed in Chapter 8.
❏ Carefully read the labels on foods that you commonly consume to identify problematic ingredients.
❏ Compare labels on different brands at the grocery store to familiarize yourself with additives that may be present but not listed on "standard recipe" foods.

❑ Read recipes from many different cookbooks to familiarize yourself with the range of ingredients that can be used in your favorite dishes. This will aid you when questioning waiters and waitresses about possible problematic ingredients.

Reduce Overall Toxic Exposure:

❑ Buy safe food storage containers.
❑ Use safe containers for heating food, especially in the microwave.
❑ Use nontoxic cleaning supplies in your home.
❑ Avoid cigarette smoke and exhaust fumes.

Find Safe Products:

Visit one or more health food stores in order to:
❑ Buy from suppliers that take food quality seriously.
❑ Locate sources of organically grown food.
❑ Find alternative formulations for products with problematic ingredients.
❑ Find alternative foods to replace foods to which you are sensitive.

Start Cooking from Scratch Using Fresh, Wholesome Ingredients:

❑ Find a recipe that sounds good to you.
❑ Modify the recipe as necessary to eliminate all traces of foods to which you are intolerant (see Chapter 10 for help with modifying recipes).
❑ Purchase the necessary ingredients.
❑ Have fun cooking and eating.
❑ Develop a repertoire of quick and easy recipes so you can still eat well even when you have little time for cooking (see Chapter 12 for ideas).

Political Action to Ensure a Safe Food Supply:

❑ Write to your grocery store, local paper, the USDA, etc. to spread the word about the danger of genetically engineered food to people with food sensitivities..
❑ Write to thank companies that currently make products that you can enjoy and let them know how important it is to you that the ingredients they use continue to remain uncontaminated by other foods to which you react poorly.
❑ Call airlines and conference food providers ahead of time and educate them on your specific food needs, including the exact name of products that you can eat and specific information on how they can purchase these products.

Long-Term Benefits

Learning to glean the information you need from food labels plus the type of detective work that has also been described lead to big payoffs. The value is not only feeling better within a few days, but often eventual desensitization to problem foods. Very small amounts of offending substances, such as corn products in table salt, vitamin C and toothpaste, are often tolerated in the sense that they do not produce overt clinical symptoms. However, these small amounts can keep the body in a state of hypersensitivity so that you don't fully well.

After total elimination of an offending substance for four to six months, many people find that they can occasionally tolerate substances at dosages to which they were formerly sensitive. For many of us that means a much greater latitude in eating out and in being able to tolerate "inert" ingredients in medicines that are not needed on an ongoing basis. For some that means occasionally being able to deliberately eat certain previously off-limit foods with no ill effects. In the very best of cases, food sensitivities permanently and completely disappear after complete elimination for a period of six months to two years. See Chapter 13 for more details.

Resources

Jonathan Brostoff and Linda Gamlin, *The Complete Guide to Food Allergy and Intolerance* (New York: Crown Publishers, Inc., 1989).

Debra Lynn Dadd, *Home Safe Home: Protecting Yourself and Your Family from Everyday Toxics and Harmful Household Products* (New York: Jeremy P. Tarcher/Putnam Books, 1997).

Chapter 6: Super-Important Information–Names on Food Labels that Can Indicate Hidden Allergens

Highlights:

❑ Extensive lists of names used on food labels that can indicate the presence of hidden allergens. These lists are provided for 12 frequently allergenic foods.

Effort Involved:

❑ Familiarize yourself with the lists that correspond to your problem foods.

Payoff:

❑ Learning names that can indicate the presence of your problem foods allows you to avoid triggering your food sensitivities. This is an important step in the process of healing from food sensitivities and arthritis.

How to Use this Chapter

The lists in this chapter contain names that identify potential hidden allergens and are organized by the type of hidden food.

Once you have identified your particular problem foods (see Chapters 2-4), study the lists that correspond to your problem foods. Familiarize yourself with the names that correspond to your problem foods. Then read the label on anything you are considering eating. If one of these names appears, don't eat it. The risk is not worth it.

The information in Chapter 5 on reading food labels makes it even easier to avoid hidden allergens. In completely clearing your life of problem foods, you will probably also find the additional information in Chapter 7 on hidden allergens and in Chapter 8 on additives to avoid to be quite useful.

How My Food Sensitivities Affect the Completeness of the Allergen Lists

For more than ten years I was sensitive to the following substances: wheat, corn products such as corn oil, cornstarch, cornmeal (but not fresh corn on the cob—evidently I reacted to field corn but not sweet corn), rice, beef and food additives such as the dye that makes cheese orange. The hidden allergen foods lists that involve my particular food sensitivities are the most extensive and the ones with which I have personal experience. In particular, corn products are used extensively as additives. As a highly corn sensitive individual it took me years to identify and eliminate all the sources of corn products that were triggering problems for me. I wish that I had my advice on how to avoid corn products years ago, because it would have saved me years of pain and fatigue. Although I have tried to compile useful lists for other common allergenic foods through library research and label reading, your own personal experience and that of others with a given allergy that I did not happen to have are likely to uncover further hidden sources.

If you discover other sources of hidden allergens, please share this information by e-mailing it to me at Barbara@ConqueringArthritis.com. I will continue to update the hidden-allergen list and make it available on my Web site.

Names Used on Food Labels that can Indicate Hidden Allergens

The following pages contain lists of names used on food labels. These names are red flags indicating the presence or possible presence of certain allergens.

Beef Allergens:

- beef broth
- bouillon
- consommé
- gelatin (Commercial gelatin can be produced by two different processes. One process uses pigskins and the other cattle hides and bones. Allergic reactions to gelatin derived from bone have been reported in human patients sensitive to beef, but the same patients did not have this response to gelatin from a pork source. Unfortunately it is impossible to know from most labeling if gelatin is derived from beef or pork sources.)
- glycerides:
    monoglycerides
    (glyceryl monostearate,

monostearin,
monoglyceryl stearate)
diglycerides
triglycerides
acetylated glycerides
glyceryl triacetate
(triacetin)
diacetyl tartaric esters of
mono- and diglycerides
ethoxylated mono- and
diglycerides
(polyglycerates;
polyoxyethylene
stearates)
- glyceryl-lacto esters of
fatty acids (glyceryl
lactopalmitate,
lactopalmitate)
- lactated fatty acid esters of
glycerol and propylene
glycol (lacto esters of
propylene glycol)

propylene glycol monostearate
(propylene glycol mono- and
diesters)
- oxystearin
- polyglycerol esters of fatty
acids
- succinylated mono- and
diglycerides
- succistearin
- hamburger
- liver
- Jell-O® (gelatin)
- meat broth
- meat sauce
- Ovaltine®
- roast
- rennet
- steak
- tallow
- wine (gelatin can be used in
wine production)
- yogurt (gelatin)

Chickpea Allergens:

- besan
- gram flour

- ground split grams

Citrus Allergens:

- grapefruit
- lemon
- lime

- orange
- pectin

Corn Allergens:

(Note: some people react only to processed corn products or only corn on
the cob and corn kernels; others react to all corn products).

- alcohol
- ale
- beer
- bourbon
- brandy
- gin
- grain :

- vodka
- whiskey
- wine
- other alcohols
- aspirin
- baking powder
- bleached flour

- butter (unless specifically unsalted)
- caramel
- cheese (unless specifically made with sea salt or unsalted)
- chewing gum base
- chocolate (unless specifically made with cane sugar instead of corn syrup or corn sweetener)
- coffee (to enhance flavor some coffee beans are coated before roasting with polysaccharides, which can come from corn sources)
- cysteine
- disodium 5'-ribonucleotides
- corn
  - corn flour
  - cornmeal
  - corn solids
- cereal
- cereal binder
- cereal filler
- cereal protein
- malted cereal extract
- dextrin
- maltodextrin
- flavoring
  - artificial flavors
  - imitation flavors
  - natural flavors
- gelatin capsules
- glycerides:
  - monoglycerides (glyceryl monostearate, monostearin, monoglyceryl stearate)
  - diglycerides
  - triglycerides
  - acetylated glycerides
- glyceryl triacetate (triacetin)
- diacetyl tartaric esters of mono- and diglycerides
- ethoxylated mono- and diglycerides (polyglycerates; polyoxyethylene stearates)
- glyceryl-lacto esters of fatty acids (glyceryl lactoplamitate, lactopalmitate)
- lactated fatty acid esters of glycerol and propylene glycol (lacto esters of propylene glycol)
- propylene glycol monostearate (propylene glycol mono- and diesters)
- oxystearin
- polyglycerol esters of fatty acids
- succinylated mono- and diglycerides
- succistearin
- glycerin
- glycerol
- gluten
  - corn gluten
  - vital gluten
  - high gluten flour
- grain
- ham (cured, tenderized)
- honey (is sometimes adulterated with corn syrup)
- hydrolyzed plant protein (HPP)
- hydrolyzed vegetable protein (HVP)
- hydrolyzed cereal solids
- lactic acid
- lecithin (usually isolated from soybeans, but is also

isolated from corn and eggs;
cannot tell the source from
most labeling)
- lysine
- mannitol
- maize
- maple syrup (glucose derived
from corn is sometimes used
as an "extender", maple
syrup blends may also
contain corn products)
- milk (in paper cartons)
- mull-soy
- MSG (monosodium
glutamate)
  - glutamic acid
glutamic acid hydrochloride
  - monoammonium
    glutamate
  - monopotassium
    glutamate
  - monosodium glutamate
- oil
  - corn oil
  - vegetable oil
  - partially hydrogenated
    oil
  - hydrogenated oil
- olives (unless specifically
made with sea salt
- other natural ingredients
- polydextrose
- pablum
- rice (coated)
- salt
  - sodium-free salt
    substitutes
  - seasoning salts
  - table salt
- sirimi (an imitation seafood
created with a starch binder,
in some cases cornstarch, in
other wheat starch. Be aware

that restaurants tend to mix
imitation with real seafood in
salads and other dishes.)
- sorbitol
- sorbitan derivatives:
  - polysorbate 60
    (polyoxyethylene-20-
    sorbitan monostearate)
  - polysorbate 65
  - polysorbate 80
  - sorbitan monostearate
- soy milk
- spices
- starch
  - cornstarch
  - food starch
  - modified food starch
  - modified starch
  - gelatinized starch
  - edible starch
- sweeteners
  - aspartame
  - confectioner's sugar
  - corn sugar
  - corn syrup
  - dextrose
  - Equal® sweetener
  - fructose
  - fruit sugar
  - glucose
  - glucose syrup
  - high fructose corn syrup
  - Honey Sweet®
  - invert sugar
  - invert syrup
  - levulose
  - Nutrasweet®
  - NutraTaste®
  - other brands of artificial
    sweeteners
  - powdered sugar
  - saccharin
  - sodium saccharin

- Splenda®
- sugar
- Sugar Twin®
- Sweet 'N Low®
- Weight Watchers® Low Calorie Sweetener
- textured vegetable protein (TVP)
- vinegar
- vitamin B-12 (cobalamine, cyanocobalamin)
- vitamin C
- vitamin E
- vanilla
- vanillin
- xanthan gum
- xylitol
- yeast (can be grown on corn mash or with corn sweetener)
- yogurt (modified cornstarch, high fructose corn syrup, aspartame)
- zein (corn protein)
- Z-Trim

Egg Allergens:

- albumin
- egg albumin
- egg whites
- lecithin
- hydrolyzed lecithin
- livetin
- ovomucin
- ovomucoid
- vitellin
- wine (can be made with albumin)

Milk Allergens:

- albumin
- buttermilk solids
- caramel
- carob
- casein
  - ammonium caseinate
  - calcium caseinate
  - magnesium caseinate
  - potassium caseinate
  - sodium caseinate
- cheese
- chocolate
- cream
- flavors
  - artificial flavors
  - imitation flavors
  - natural flavors
- hydrolyzed casein
- hydrolyzed milk protein
- high-protein flour
- kefir
- lactate
- lactose
- lactalbumin
- lactalbumin phosphate
- margarine
- milk derivatives
- milk protein
- milk solids
- sour milk solids
- sour cream solids
- whey protein concentrate
- whey
  - delactosed whey
  - demineralized whey
- wine (can be made with casein and/or milk powder)
- yogurt

Peanut Allergens:

- artificial walnuts
- hydrolyzed plant protein (HPP)
- hydrolyzed vegetable protein (HVP)
- hydrogenated vegetable oil
- partially hydrogenated vegetable oil
- peanut oil
- vegetable oil

Pork Allergens:

- baked beans
- bacon
- brains
- chips
- chops
- cracklings or chitterlings
- gelatin
- glycerin
- ham
- hot dogs
- kidneys
- lard
- liver
- ribs
- roast
- sausage
- shortening
- souse (head cheese)
- wieners
- wine (gelatin made from pigskins can be used in wine production)

Rice Allergens:

- basmati
- beer
- bran
- miso
- multigrain
- rice
- saki
- soy sauce
- tamari
- tempeh

Soy Allergens:

- choline bitartrate
- choline chloride
- glycerides:
  - monoglycerides (glyceryl monostearate, monostearin, monoglyceryl stearate)
  - diglycerides
  - triglycerides
  - acetylated glycerides
- glyceryl triacetate (triacetin)
- diacetyl tartaric esters of mono- and diglycerides
- ethoxylated mono- and diglycerides (polyglycerates; polyoxyethylene stearates)
- glyceryl-lacto esters of fatty acids (glyceryl

lactoplamitate, lactopalmitate)
- lactated fatty acid esters of glycerol and propylene glycol (lacto esters of propylene glycol)
- propylene glycol monostearate (propylene glycol mono-and diesters)
- oxystearin
- polyglycerol esters of fatty acids
- succinylated mono- and diglycerides
- succistearin
- glycerin
- guar gum (extracted from the seed of the guar plant, a legume resembling the soybean plant that may cause problems in some soy sensitive people)
- lecithin
- soy lecithin
- hydroxylated lecithin
- natural flavorings
- MSG (monosodium glutamate)
  - glutamic acid
  - glutamic acid hydrochloride

- monoammonium glutamate
- monopotassium glutamate
- monosodium glutamate
- hydrolyzed plant protein (HPP)
- hydrolyzed vegetable protein (HVP)
- soy oil
- soy protein isolate
- soy protein concentrate
- soy sauce
- fermented soy sauce
- hydrolyzed soy sauce
- shoyu
- tamari
- textured vegetable protein (TVP)
- textured soy protein
- vegetable oil
  - hydrogenated vegetable oil
  - partially hydrogenated vegetable oil
- vitamins
- wine (soy flour can be used in wine production)

Wheat Allergens:

- alcohol
- barley malt
- batter
- biscuit
- beer
- bouillon
- bran
- bread
- bulgur
- bulking agent

- cereal binder
- cereal filler
- cereal protein
- chocolate
- couscous
- cracker
- cream of ...
- croutons
- crust
- dextrin

- durum
- extracts
- farina
- fiber
- flavorings
- flour
- gluten
  - vital gluten
  - high gluten flour
- graham flour
- grain
- macaroni
- malted cereal extract
- matzos
- MSG (monosodium glutamate)
  - monoammonium glutamate
  - monopotassium glutamate
  - monosodium glutamate
  - glutamic acid
  - glutamic acid hydrochloride
  - hydrolyzed vegetable protein (HVP)
  - hydrolyzed plant protein (HPP)
  - hydrolyzed cereal solids
- pumpernickel
- roux
- rye bread
- self-rising flour
- semolina
- soy sauce
- fermented soy sauce
- hydrolyzed soy sauce
- shoyu
- tamari
- tempeh (wheat is often used to buffer the starter culture used in making tempeh)
- starch
  - gelatinized starch
  - modified starch
  - modified food starch
  - edible starch
  - food starch
- seitan
- sirimi (imitation seafood is created with a starch binder, in some cases cornstarch, in others wheat starch. Also be aware that restaurants tend to mix imitation with real seafood in salads and other dishes.)
- vinegar
- distilled vinegar
- wheat
- wheat germ
- wheat germ oil
- wheat gluten
- wheat flour
- white flour
- white sauce
- yeasts (some)
- vitamin E

Yeast Allergens:

- alcohol
- bread and breading
- cheese
- citric acid (almost always a yeast derivative)
- coffee
- enriched flour of any type (vitamins used for enrichment made from yeast)
- fruit juice
- fortified products (such as milk fortified with vitamins)
- mushrooms
- MSG (monosodium glutamate)
  - glutamic acid
  - glutamic acid hydrochloride
  - monoammonium glutamate
  - monopotassium glutamate
  - monosodium glutamate
- nuts
- peanuts
- pistachios
- tea
- torula (a type of yeast used in health foods)
- tomato sauce
- vinegar
- vinegar may also be used in the following foods and may not be included on the label:
  - baby cereals
  - barbecue sauce
  - barley cereal
  - chili and peppers
  - horseradish
  - ketchup
  - mayonnaise
  - mincemeat
  - mustard
  - olives
  - pickles
  - salad dressings
  - sauerkraut
  - spices (cinnamon, pepper)
  - tomato sauce
- yeast

Write Me

The lists in this chapter are works in progress. If you discover other names that should be added, please send them to me at Barbara@ConqueringArthritis.com

The updates you submit will make it that much easier for those who follow us to get well.

Long-Term Benefits

Knowledge is power. In particular, knowing how to identify the possible presence of your problem foods allows you to make empowering distinctions. This knowledge allows you to avoid foods that cause you harm. It allows you to select foods that are safe for you to eat. You gain the power to stop the damage caused by triggering food sensitivities before it ever starts.

The key to making these empowering distinctions is knowing which names used on food labels can indicate the presence of a problem food. The lists in this chapter give you this information.

References

Nicholas Freydberg and Willis A. Gortner, *The Food Additives Book* (New York: Bantam Books, 1982).

Phyllis Saifer, *Detox: a Successful and Supportive Program for Freeing your Body from the Physical and Psychological Effects of Chemical Pollutants at Home and Work, Junk Food Additives, Sugar, Nicotine, Drugs, Alcohol, Caffeine, Prescription and Nonprescription Medication, and other Environmental Toxins* (Los Angeles: Jeremy P. Tarcher, Inc., 1984).

George R. Schwartz, M.D., *In Bad Taste: The MSG Syndrome* (Santa Fe, NM: Health Press, 1988).

Jonathan Brostoff and Linda Gamlin, *The Complete Guide to Food Allergy and Intolerance* (New York: Crown Publishers, Inc., 1989).

Marilyn Gioannini, *The Complete Food Allergy Cookbook: the Foods You've Always Loved Without the Ingredients You Can't Have*, (Rocklin, CA: Prima Publishing, 1997).
The author of this excellent book has sensitivities to wheat, corn, all dairy products, beef, fruits, tomatoes, peppers and potatoes. I highly recommend this book if your list of food sensitivities is similar.

Bette Hagman, *More from the Gluten-Free Gourmet: Delicious Dining Without Wheat* (New York: Henry Holt and Company, Inc., 1993).
Bette Hagman is gluten intolerant and has written several excellent books that focus on eliminating gluten from the diet and still eating well. These books are useful for those who are gluten intolerant or wheat intolerant, but rely heavily on corn and rice products. The recipe sections are thus of little value to those of us like me with wheat, corn and rice intolerances.

Robert Goodman, *A Quick Guide to Food Additives* (San Diego, CA: Silvercat Publications, 1990).

Chapter 7: Food Sensitivities—
Products that Can Contain Hidden
Allergens

Highlights:

❑   Hidden allergens are found in many places you might not suspect. This
    chapter provides lists that will alert you to products that may be
    keeping you sick.

Effort Involved:

❑   Familiarize yourself with the lists that correspond to your problem
    foods.
❑   Avoid products that are a problem.

Payoff:

❑   Avoiding products that contain your problem foods allows you to avoid
    triggering your food sensitivities. This is an important step in the
    process of healing from food sensitivities and arthritis.

How to Use this Chapter

The following lists contain products that may have hidden allergens. They
are organized by the type of hidden problem foods they may contain.

Once you have identified your particular problem foods (see Chapters 2-4),
learn how to recognize the presence of your problem foods in prepared food
and other products. The lists of names used on product labeling given in
Chapter 6 are a good place to start. The lists of products in this chapter are
a further aid. These lists are a wake-up call to the many possible sources of
contamination in your life. You are likely to stay at least mildly sick until
you eliminate all sources of contamination in your life.

Products that Can Contain Hidden Allergens

Products that Can Contain Beef:

- baby foods (some)
- drugs processed from beef or containing beef fractions:
  - adrenal cortical extract
  - heparin
  - insulin
- gelatin products:
  - cakes
  - candies
  - capsules (including medicine and nutritional supplements in capsules)
  - ice cream
  - Jell-O®
  - pastries
  - puddings
  - pies
- sherbets
- glandulars and enzymes (read labels carefully or contact the manufacturer):
  - adrenal
  - heart
  - liver
  - pancreas
  - pancreatin
  - pituitary
  - spleen
  - thyroid
- glue
- gravies and sauces
- meats
- vitamins containing liver

Products that Can Contain Chickpeas:

- Indian and Pakistani food
- hummus

Products that Can Contain Citrus:

- baked goods
- drinks
- dog food
- yogurt (pectin)
- jams and jellies (pectin)

Short List of Products that Can Contain Corn:

- anything with Nutrasweet® or other artificial sweeteners in it
- anything with vitamin C added (vitamin C is made commercially using a corn-based fermentation process)
- baking powder
- biodegradable plastic
- cornstarch
- corn solids
- corn syrup
- frozen fruit
- fruit juices
- jellies
- "pure" vanilla extract
- other extract-type flavorings

- many instant beverages such as coffee and hot chocolate drink
- many gravies
- many medicines
- many pies
- many reduced-calorie foods such as yogurt, sour cream, etc.
- most Chinese foods
- most frozen and canned vegetables
- most prepared food
- most medicine in tablet form
- soft drinks
- salted butter
- soy sauce
- table salt (contains dextrose made from corn)
- vitamin pills

Longer List of Products that Can Contain Corn:

- Any food that is salted with table salt (contains dextrose), seasoning salts (contain MSG), or sodium-free salt substitutes (contain MSG)
- Any food that contains an artificial sweetener. (When added in dry form these sweeteners are often less than 5 percent sweetener and more than 95 percent dextrose, maltodextrin, and/or modified cornstarch, all of which are corn products; it is possible to purchase many of these sweeteners in a liquid form that is free of dextrose, maltodextrin and modified cornstarch and presumably free of other corn products as well.)
- Any food containing sweetener made from corn, such as dextrose, fructose, fruit sugar, glucose, glucose syrup, corn sugar, corn syrup, high-fructose corn syrup, levulose, invert sugar or invert syrup. Also beware of confectioner's sugar and powdered sugar because they usually contain about 3 percent cornstarch. Almost any food that contains added sweetener can potentially contain one of these sweeteners, including fruit juices, soft drinks, syrups, chocolate, baked goods, yogurt, peanut butter, etc.
- Any food thickened with cornstarch, food starch or modified food starch, such as many puddings, gravies, sauces, and in particular, the sauces on most Chinese foods
- Any food containing flavorings such as vanilla extract, almond extract, etc. (many extracts contain corn syrup and/or alcohol derived from corn)
- Any food containing MSG (many names can be used to list MSG, including monosodium glutamate, glutamic acid, glutamic acid, hydrochloride, monoammonium glutamate, monopotassium glutamate, monosodium glutamate, hydrolyzed protein, and protein hydroxylates)
- Any food that is deep-fried, since corn oil is often used for this
- Any food containing alcohol (such as beer, bourbon, gin, vodka and whisky, etc. Ale, beer, brandy, gin, whiskey, and vodka manufactured in North America are usually fortified with corn. Most domestic wines

contain corn, except California wines with 13 percent alcohol or less. Imported wines and brandies are usually corn-free.)

- Any food containing ground or processed meat (including lunchmeat, ham, bacon, fish products and sausage) since syrups (including corn syrups) are often added to ground meat to help minimize shrinkage and improve flavor, juiciness and texture
- Baby foods (most)
- Baby formulas
  - Prosobee®
  - Similac®
  - Nutramigen®
- Baked goods that contain baking powder, salt, corn sweetener or yeast (commercially produced yeast often contain traces of corn)
- Candy and candy bars
- Canned and frozen vegetables, since corn sweeteners and/or salt (contains dextrose) are usually added
- Chewing gum
- Cheese (unless the label states no-salt or sea salt on label)
- Chocolate (corn syrup, lecithin, etc.)
- Condiments such as ketchup, prepared mustard, some mayonnaise
- Grits
- "Reduced-calorie" or "reduced-fat" products (cornstarch, maltodextrin, dextrin, modified food starch, etc. are often substituted for fat)
- Salad dressings
- Syrups (may contain corn syrup or other corn sweeteners)
- Many "cream of ..." products
- Meat products (cereal binder, cereal filler, cereal protein, corn syrup, modified food starch, hydrolyzed corn protein, salt)
- Nondairy creamers
- Sour cream (modified food starch, dextrose)
- Soy sauce
- Tamari
- Worcestershire sauce
- White or distilled vinegar (and products containing vinegar such as salad dressings, pickles, mustard, mayonnaise, relishes, olives and sauerkraut are all suspect unless you know that the vinegar was specifically not made using corn.)
- Yogurt (corn sweeteners or artificial sweeteners in flavored varieties)

Drinks that Can Contain Corn Products:

- alcohol (such as beer, bourbon, gin, vodka and whisky, etc.)

- coffee (coffee beans can be roasted with a coating of hydrolyzed cornstarch; corn products can be added as part of sweeteners, whiteners and flavoring agents)
- fruit juices (vitamin C, corn syrup)
- instant coffee
- instant tea
- soft drinks (regular drinks have corn syrup and diet drinks have the dextrose, maltodextrin and/or modified cornstarch found in artificial sweeteners)

Personal Hygiene Products that Can Contain Corn:

- baby powder
- laxatives (can contain corn products labeled as starch, cornstarch, citric acid, maltodextrin, etc.)
- mouthwashes (can contain corn products in the form of alcohol, caramel, glycerin, sorbitol, saccharin, flavor, etc.)
- skin lotions (can contain corn products in the form of glycerin, glyceryl stearate, glycol stearate, lecithin, sorbitol, xanthan gum, fragrance, citric acid, vitamin E, etc.)
- shampoo and hair styling products (can contain corn products in the form of glycol distearate, alcohol, citric acid, propylene glycol, sorbitol, vitamin E, etc.)
- shaving cream (can contain corn products in the form of polysorbates, sorbitol, fatty acid esters, "other ingredients," vitamin E, etc.)
- soap (can contain corn products in the form of glycerin, fragrance, etc. Glycerin can come from many sources besides corn oil, but the source can be impossible to determine from the label. When in doubt, contact the manufacturer or buy only products that reveal source materials on the label.)
- toothpaste (most toothpastes have one more of the following suspect items: flavor, glycerin, sorbitol, propylene glycol, sodium saccharin and xanthan gum. Your best bet is to shop for toothpaste at a health food store and find several brands with a minimum of suspect additives, such as only glycerin. Then contact those companies regarding the source of the glycerin. If enough of us make our needs known, perhaps safe products will become available to us. Until you find a suitable commercial toothpaste, you can always use plain baking soda.)

Medicines that Can Contain Corn Products:

- A wide range of medicines, including cough syrups, aspirin and most anti-inflammatory drugs contain corn products (as "inert ingredients" such as cornstarch often identified only as starch, and corn syrup, dextrose, dextrin, maltodextrin, ascorbic acid, citric acid, vitamin C, zein, etc. Zein is the name of a corn protein that is widely used as a coating on vitamins and medicines. Beware, therefore, of "pharmaceutical glaze" and any type of coated tablets even if zein is not a list ingredient.)

- Medicines in the form of capsules, lozenges, ointments, suppositories, tablets and vitamins often contain corn products. Gelatin capsules are often dusted with cornstarch.

- Dextrose, which is derived from corn, is the most common sugar used for intravenous feeding. Many corn-sensitive patients react to these IVs with problems that are commonly attributed to "surgical complications." If you are corn-sensitive and in the hospital, you will need friends and family to provide safe food and be on guard 24 hours a day to prevent the hospital staff from further worsening your condition by triggering corn sensitivities with IVs, oral medications, sterile gloves dusted with talc-containing cornstarch, etc.

Other Sources of Corn Allergens:

- Adhesives in shoes
- Glue on envelopes, stamps, labels, stickers, tape, etc.
- Pet food, including cat, dog, fish, bird, rabbit and guinea pig food
- Starch on clothing, linens and handicraft items (Linit is another name indicating cornstarch.)
- Cornstarch used to keep photographic film, paper cups and plates, waxed and plastic containers, plastic bags, and other items from sticking together
- Starch (often cornstarch) is used to make biodegradable foam packaging that is coated with wax and may soon be used to package food
- Sterile gloves coated with talc which contains cornstarch
- Some cigarettes are blended with corn sugar
- Grain fed to animals shortly before slaughter can cause sensitivity reactions to the grain in people eating the meat

Products that Can Contain Eggs:

- baby foods
- baked goods
- baking powder
- batters for fried food
- breakfast cereals
- cake flours
- candies
- custards
- diet supplements
- eggnog
- egg substitutes
- frostings
- fruit drinks
- ice cream
- laxatives
- macaroni

- meat products
- noodles
- Ovaltine®
- Ovomal®
- pancakes
- pastas
- pet food, including birdfeed, dog and cat food
- puddings
- salad dressings
- sodas (root beer)
- sweet sauces
- soups
- syrups
- tartar sauce
- wine

Products that Can Contain Milk:

- au gratin dishes
- baby food
- baked goods
- breakfast cereals
- butter
- creamed soups
- candies
- caramel
- cheese
- cocoa drinks
- diet supplements
- fruit drinks
- frostings
- gravies
- hot dogs
- kefir
- meat products
- nondairy creamers
- omelets
- pet food, including bird, rabbit and guinea pig food
- sauces
- sour cream
- wine (casein or casinates can be used as clarifying agents)
- yogurt

Products that Can Contain Pork:

- candy bars
- Chinese, Mexican and Polynesian foods
- cocktail dips
- drugs:
  - calcium and magnesium stearates
  - capsules
  - heparin
  - tonics and pills for anemia (hog stomach contains an intrinsic factor)
- fried foods
- glandulars and enzymes (read labels carefully or contact the manufacturer):
  - adrenal
  - mixed enzyme products
  - pancreas
  - pancreatin
  - pituitary
  - thymus
  - thyroid
- glue
- ice cream
- instant foods (such as mashed potatoes)
- Jell-O®

- margarine
- mayonnaise
- nondairy creamer
- potato chips
- processed cheeses (in jars and carbons)
- puddings
- salad dressings
- soaps and cosmetics (glycerine)
- soups with pork
- vegetables flavored with pork
- vegetable stock

Products that Can Contain Peanuts:

- anything made with or fried in peanut oil
- anything containing textured vegetable protein (TVP)
- baked goods
- chili
- mixed nuts
- peanut butter
- pet food, such as birdfeed and rabbit and guinea pig food
- sauces

Products that Can Contain Potatoes:

- "clamshells" used to package fast food (can contain potato starch)

Products that Can Contain Rice:

- beer
- miso
- rice vinegar
- rice bran
- rice cakes
- rice noodles
- rice wine (saki)
- meat products (cereal binder, cereal filler, cereal protein, MSG, etc.)
- miso
- pet food, including cat, dog, fish, bird, rabbit and guinea pig food.
- soy sauce
- shoyu
- starch
  - gelatinized starch
  - modified starch
  - modified food starch
- tamari
- tempeh
- some vitamins derived from rice bran
- Z-Trim

Foods that Can Contain Soy:

- artificial meats and nuts
- baby formulas
- baked goods
- candy
- cereals
- coffee substitutes

- drinks such as Gatorade®
  (partially hydrogenated
  soybean oil)
- fried foods
  - corn chips
  - potato chips
  - tortilla chips
- ice cream
- margarine and butter
  substitutes
- meats
  - canned meats and fish
  - hamburgers (fast food)
  - luncheon meats
  - pork-link sausages
- milk substitutes
  - infant formulas
  - nondairy creamers
  - soy milk
- nuts:
  - any nuts roasted in soy
    oil
  - soy (formed to look like
    other nuts)

- soybeans (toasted, salted
  and used as nuts)
- pasta
- peanut butter (some)
- sauces
  - soy sauce
  - steak sauce
  - tamari
  - teriyaki sauce
  - Worcestershire sauce
- tempeh
- nondairy creamer (lecithin)
- mayonnaise
- meat products
- milk substitutes
- miso
- seasoning salts
- sodium-free salt substitutes
- soups
- vegetable sprays (lecithin)
- vitamin E
- other vitamins

Other Products that Can Contain Soy:

- adhesives
- automobile parts
- biodegradable plastic
- blankets
- candles
- cat, dog and fish food
- celluloid (movie film, slides,
  etc.)
- cloth
- clothing
- cosmetics
- enamels
- fertilizer
- illuminating oil
- linoleum
- lubricating oil

- massage creams
- pet food, including cat, dog,
  fish, bird, rabbit and guinea
  pig food
- plastics, especially in Ford
  cars
- nitroglycerine
- paints
- paper finishes
- paper sizing
- plywood glues
- printing ink
- shampoo (hydrolyzed soy
  protein)
- skin lotion (lecithin)
- soap
- telephones

- textile finishings
- toys
- varnish

Products that Can Contain Wheat:

- alcohol, including beer, gin and whiskey
- baby foods (some)
- baked goods
- biodegradable packaging (can contain wheat starch and wheat straw, feels like dense Styrofoam and can be made into disposable coffee cups, plates, supermarket meat trays and carryout boxes)
- biodegradable plastic
- any thing with "bread" or "flour" in it such as mole sauce, gravies, white sauces
- breakfast cereal
- candy (companies are not required to list any product that they may use to dust the block the candy is rolled on for shaping. Some companies use wheat flour for dusting.)
- candy bars
- chocolate
- cocoa
- cooking sprays
- fixatives for false teeth
- garlic capsules
- hand cream and lotion
- ice cream (thickening agents)
- ketchup
- lip gloss
- nondairy creamers
- makeup (many contain wheat germ oil)
- meat products (cereal binder, cereal filler, cereal protein, MSG, hydrolyzed wheat protein, etc.)
- matzos
- mayonnaise
- mixed spices
- mustard
- Ovaltine®
- packaging materials, especially biodegradable packaging materials
- pastes and glues on stamps and envelopes
- pet food, including cat, dog, fish, bird, rabbit and guinea pig food
- Postum®
- shoyu (a sauce similar to soy sauce)
- salad dressings
- soups and bouillons
- shampoos
- soy sauce
- tamari
- tempeh (wheat is often used to buffer the starter culture used in making tempeh)
- vinegar
- vitamin E
- vitamins

Products that Can Contain Yeast:

- any type of alcoholic product
- antibiotics (can be derived from yeast)
  - chloromycetin
  - Lincocin
  - -mycin drugs such as streptomycin
  - penicillin
  - tetracyclines
- barbecue sauce
- black tea
- bread and breading
- buttermilk
- cakes and cake mixes
- canned refrigerated biscuits and rolls
- cheese (all types, including cottage cheese)
- citric acid (almost always a yeast derivative)
- coffee (regular and instant)
- cookies
- crackers
- doughnuts
- dried fruits of all kinds (dates, figs, prunes, raisins)
- dried roasted nuts
- enriched farina, cornmeal, and corn grits
- flour (enriched with vitamins made from yeast)
- fruit juices of all types (only homemade are yeast-free)
- grapes (the mold on grapes is sometimes cross-reactive with yeast sensitivities)
- herb teas
- ketchup
- malted products (candy, cereals, malted milk drinks)
- melons (the mold on melons, especially cantaloupes, is sometimes cross-reactive with yeast sensitivities)
- pet food, including cat, dog, fish, bird, rabbit and guinea pig food.
- vitamins (unless otherwise stated on label)
- all B-vitamin capsules

Write Me

The lists in this chapter are works in progress. If you discover other names that should be added, please send them to me at Barbara@ConqueringArthritis.com

Long-Term Benefits

As mentioned in Chapter 6, knowledge is power. In particular, knowing which products may contain your allergens, allows you to be on guard against accidental exposure.

References

Nicholas Freydberg and Willis A. Gortner, *The Food Additives Book* (New York: Bantam Books, 1982).

Phyllis Saifer, *Detox: a Successful and Supportive Program for Freeing your Body from the Physical and Psychological Effects of Chemical Pollutants at Home and Work, Junk Food Additives, Sugar, Nicotine, Drugs, Alcohol, Caffeine, Prescription and Nonprescription Medication, and other Environmental Toxins* (Los Angeles: Jeremy P. Tarcher, Inc., 1984).

George R. Schwartz, M.D., *In Bad Taste: The MSG Syndrome* (Santa Fe, NM: Health Press, 1988).

Jonathan Brostoff and Linda Gamlin, *The Complete Guide to Food Allergy and Intolerance* (New York: Crown Publishers, Inc., 1989).

Marilyn Gioannini, *The Complete Food Allergy Cookbook: the foods You've Always Loved Without the Ingredients You Can't Have* (Rocklin, CA: Prima Publishing, 1997).
The author of this excellent book has sensitivities to wheat, corn, all dairy products, beef, citrus fruits, tomatoes, peppers and potatoes. I highly recommend this book if your list of food sensitivities is similar.

Bette Hagman, *More from the Gluten-Free Gourmet: Delicious Dining Without Wheat* (New York: Henry Holt and Company, Inc., 1993).
Bette Hagman is gluten intolerant and has written several excellent books that focus on eliminating gluten from the diet and still eating well. These books are useful for those who are gluten intolerant or wheat intolerant, but rely heavily on corn and rice products. The recipe sections are thus of little value to those of us like me with wheat, corn and rice intolerances.

Robert Goodman, *A Quick Guide to Food Additives* (San Diego, CA: Silvercat Publications, 1990).

Chapter 8: Additives to Avoid

Highlights:

- ❑ Ten additives to avoid.
- ❑ Twenty-nine names that can indicate the presence of MSG.
- ❑ Nineteen suspect food additives.
- ❑ Checklist for avoiding hidden allergens.

Effort Involved:

- ❑ Familiarize yourself with the lists that correspond to problem additives.
- ❑ Avoid products that contain these additives.

Payoff:

- ❑ Avoiding products that contain your problem additives allows you to avoid triggering your food sensitivities, helps strengthen your general health, and helps avoid developing new food sensitivities.

10 Additives to Avoid

1-3. BHA, Calcium and Sodium Propioate

Butylated hydroxyanisole (BHA) used to retard rancidity and calcium and sodium propionate used to inhibit mold are known to provoke reactions in allergic persons.

4. Artificial Colors

FD&C Yellow No. 5 (Tartrazine) has been found to cause allergic reactions. Most people allergic to it are also allergic to aspirin. It is used in candy, desserts, cereals and dairy products.

5. Food Flavorings

Approximately 1700 flavoring agents are added to various types of food. Because it is not required by law, the individual chemical components that constitute a flavoring are rarely identified on food labels. For this reason any product labeled with "artificial flavors," "imitation flavors" or even "natural flavors" is suspect for anyone with food sensitivities.

6. Papain

Papain is an enzyme derived from papaya fruit. It is used in meat tenderizers, condiments, seasonings, gravies and as a digestive aid to increase the digestibility of protein.

If inhaled papain can cause an allergic reaction and allergic sensitization may occur from ingestion.

7. Pectin

Commercially, pectin is derived from citrus peels and apple pomace (the residue from apple pressings). For this reason, people with food sensitivities to citrus or apples should avoid processed foods that contain pectin. Pectin is often added to ice cream and ices, processed fruit and juices, fruit jellies, jams and preserves and to soft candies.

8. Chewing-gum base

The Food and Drugs section of the code of Federal Regulations for chewing-gum base specifies hundreds of substances that are permitted to be used separately or in combinations in chewing-gum base. Because the regulation requires that only chewing-gum base be listed on the label, there is no way for a consumer to identify what a product actually contained.

9. Gums

The following gums should be avoided by people prone to food sensitivities because they not only cause allergic reactions themselves, they broaden the spectrum of sensitivities and allergies to other foods:

Gum arabic (acacia gum) which is obtained from the sap of a number of species of acacia, a Middle Eastern tree.

Gum tragacanth, the dried sap obtained from several species of Astragalus, a wild shrub in the Middle East.

Sterculia gum (gum kadaya, gum karaya, India gum, Indian tragacanth), the dried sap of various species of Sterculia, a tree native to central and eastern India, and also found in Africa, Australia, China and Indochina.

10. MSG

MSG (monosodium glutamate) is a flavor enhancer often used in Chinese restaurants. It is famous for causing headaches and other symptoms, including arthritis-like symptoms. According to Dr. George R. Schwartz, M.D., MSG is a toxic substance whose effect is dose-related. The intensity of symptoms produced by MSG and the number of people reacting will increase as the dose is increased. More susceptible people just react at a lower dose. Because it is known to cause a variety of physical problems, it makes sense for people with arthritis to avoid MSG.

Because MSG is on the GRAS (Generally Recognized as Safe) list of the Food and Drug Administration, it is not considered a food additive, but an unregulated seasoning classed by the FDA as a flavor enhancer. It is very difficult to know for sure if MSG is present, because so many different names can indicate its presence. Certain "standard recipe" foods, such as mayonnaise, salad dressings and beer, can also legally contain MSG without listing MSG on the label.

Some foods are advertised as containing "No MSG", even when it has been added. Apparently some food producers are not aware that hydrolyzed vegetable protein (HVP) contains MSG. Products containing HVP (and thus MSG) are also frequently advertised as "all natural," and often HVP is designated simply as "natural flavorings."

Foods that contain MSG include seasoning salts, bouillon, hydrolyzed vegetable protein, meat tenderizers, most prepared spaghetti sauces, most sausages, some bacons, and some ethnic foods such as gefilte fish and matzo balls. MSG is a standard ingredient in most canned soups, soy sauces, bouillon cubes, soup stocks, frozen dinners and much fast food.

28 Names that can Indicate the Presence of MSG:

1. Accent®
2. ajinomoto
3. beef broth
4. carrageenan
5. caseinate
6. chicken broth
7. Chinese seasoning
8. glutacyl
9. glutamic acid
10. glutavene
11. gourmet powder
12. flavorings
13. kombu extract
14. hydrolyzed protein
15. hydrolyzed vegetable protein (12 to 20 percent MSG)
16. monosodium glutamate
17. monoammonium glutamate
18. monopotassium glutamate
19. natural flavorings (can be HVP)
20. protein hydrolysate
21. RL-50
22. subu
23. mei-jing
24. wei-jing
25. vetsin
26. vegetable powder
27. vegetable broth
28. zest

19 Other Suspect Food Additives

Some food additives are produced from whole foods. Others are produced commercially using microorganisms. Still others are produced commercially by chemical synthesis. In each case it is possible to have a food sensitivity not to the named additive but to impurities left over from the commercial production process or from other unlisted materials added to it.

For example, I have never had a food sensitivity to vitamin C itself, but for years I reacted adversely to vitamin C that had been added to food products. Commercially produced vitamin C is made using a corn-based fermentation process and often has other ingredients such as cornstarch added to it. I was sensitive enough to corn products that a single glass of apple juice fortified with vitamin C was enough to bring on crankiness and fatigue for a day or two. I did fine with apple juice that was free of additives.

When my research has been able to identify starting materials for commercially produced food additives, I have listed the additive name in the hidden allergen lists in Chapter 6. These lists are arranged by the name of the problematic food that is involved.

The following lists are food additives that are commercially produced from starting materials I have not been able to identify. Because their starting materials are unknown, these additive should be considered suspect by anyone with food sensitivities.

4 Food Additives Produced from Unknown Starting Materials by Fermentation with Microorganisms:

1. cysteine
2. disodium 5'-ribonucleotides
3. lysine
4. vitamin B-12 (cobalamine, cyanocobalamin)

15 Food Additives Produced from Unknown Starting Materials by Chemical Synthesis:

1. biotin
2. carotene
3. disodium 5'-ribonucleotide
4. folic acid
5. glycine
6. methionine
7. natural colors
8. propionic acid
9. propyl gallate
10. sorbic acid
11. potassium sorbate
12. vitamin A
13. vitamin B-1 (thiamin)
14. vitamin B-2 (riboflavin)
15. vitamin B-6 (pyridoxine)

Checklist: Avoiding Hidden Allergens

- ❑ Familiarize yourself with the lists for hidden allergens for your particular food sensitivities. These lists are found in Chapters 6 and 7.
- ❑ Familiarize yourself with the "10 Additives to Avoid" and "18 Other Suspect Food Additives" listed in this chapter.
- ❑ Systematically remove products that may contain problem ingredients. Remove these from your:
  - ❑ refrigerator
  - ❑ pantry
  - ❑ toiletries
  - ❑ medicines
  - ❑ vitamins
  - ❑ pet food
  - ❑ cleaning products
- ❑ Find alternative formulations for products that contain suspect ingredients:
  - ❑ Avidly read labels at stores.
  - ❑ Ask the staff at health food stores for suggestions.
  - ❑ Ask your pharmacist to suggest alternative formulations of over-the-counter products and to research the availability of alternative formulations for your prescription medications.
  - ❑ Look in cookbooks, books like Debra Lynn Dadd's book *Nontoxic and Natural*, and alternative health care books to find easy instructions for easy-to-make alternative formulations of foods, medicines, toiletries and cleaning supplies.

Long-Term Benefits

Removing foods and other products that contain ingredients that trigger your food sensitivities is a great support in getting well again. The information in Chapters 5-8 gives you the power to remove hidden allergens and problem food additives, and replace them with healthier alternative formulations.

As mentioned in Chapter 5, removing all the sources of hidden allergens has big benefits. Not only will you feel better within a few days, but often you will eventually be able to tolerate previous problem foods.

Total elimination is important because very small amounts of offending substances, such as the corn products in table salt, vitamin C and toothpaste, are often tolerated in the sense that they do not produce overt clinical symptoms. However, these small amounts can keep the body in a state of hypersensitivity and leave you feeling less than fully well.

After total elimination of an offending substance for four to six months, many people find that they can occasionally tolerate substances at dosages to which they were formerly sensitive. For many of us that means a much greater latitude in eating out and in being able to tolerate inert ingredients in medicines that are not needed on an ongoing basis. For some that means occasionally being able to deliberately eat certain previously off-limit foods with no ill effects. In the very best of cases, food sensitivities permanently and completely disappear after complete elimination for a period of six months to two years. See Chapter 13 for more details.

References

Nicholas Freydberg and Willis A. Gortner, *The Food Additives Book* (New York: Bantam Books, 1982).

Lynn Lawson, *Staying Well in a Toxic World: Understanding Environmental Illness, Multiple Chemical Sensitivities, Chemical Injuries, and Sick Building Syndrome* (Chicago, IL: Noble Press, 1993).

Debra Lynn Dadd, *Nontoxic & Natural: How to avoid Dangerous Everyday Products and Buy or Make Safe Ones* (Los Angeles: J.P. Tarcher, 1984).

Debra Lynn Dadd, *Home Safe Home: Protecting Yourself and Your Family from Everyday Toxics and Harmful Household Products* (New York: Jeremy P. Tarcher/Putnam Books, 1997).

Phyllis Saifer, *Detox: a Successful and Supportive Program for Freeing your Body from the Physical and Psychological Effects of Chemical Pollutants at Home and Work, Junk Food Additives, Sugar, Nicotine, Drugs, Alcohol, Caffeine, Prescription and Nonprescription Medication, and other Environmental Toxins* (Los Angeles: Jeremy P. Tarcher, Inc., 1984).

George R. Schwartz, M.D., *In Bad Taste: The MSG Syndrome* (Santa Fe, NM: Health Press, 1988).

Jonathan Brostoff and Linda Gamlin, *The Complete Guide to Food Allergy and Intolerance* (New York: Crown Publishers, Inc., 1989).

Robert Goodman, *A Quick Guide to Food Additives* (San Diego, CA: Silvercat Publications, 1990).

Chapter 9: Strategies for Restocking Your Kitchen with Safe Food

Highlights:

❑ How to restock your kitchen for with safe food.

Effort Involved:

❑ **To use this chapter you must have already identified your food sensitivities and learned to recognize the presence of problem ingredients.** Chapters 3 and 4 describe how to test for food sensitivities. Chapters 5-8 teach what you need to know to avoid problem ingredients.

❑ **Remove unsafe food and restock your kitchen with safe food.** The effort involved here depends on the extent of your food sensitivities. If almost everything you had been eating is now off-limits, considerable effort will be involved in getting rid of old food and finding new types of food that are safe and appealing. If much of what you have been eating is OK, much less effort will be involved.

Payoff:

❑ Easy access to a wide variety of foods you enjoy.

Setting Yourself Up for Great Meals—6 Hints for Restocking your Kitchen

When you discover your food sensitivities it may initially seem like most of your favorite foods are off-limits, especially if you have multiple food sensitivities. However, with some creative substitutions you can create many tasty versions of your favorite foods that contain no offending ingredients. The key to this new way of cooking is restocking your kitchen with some basic alternative ingredients that replace the old allergenic ingredients.

1. Make a List of What Needs to Be Replaced

Familiarize yourself with Chapters 5 and 6 on hidden allergens before undertaking this task.

The following are examples of some of the many things that need to be replaced if you are corn intolerant:

Instead of:	Use instead:
Baking powder	Any of the 12 alternative leavenings listed in Chapter 10, including grain-free baking powder
Cornstarch	Any of the 34 alternative thickeners or binders listed in Chapter 10 including arrowroot powder, potato starch, kudzu powder, tapioca and taro powder
Corn syrup	Any of the 16 alternative sweeteners listed in Chapter 10, including honey, pure maple syrup, rice syrup and barley syrup
Cornmeal	Millet or millet flour
Corn oil	Canola oil or olive oil
Table salt	Sea salt
Salted butter	Unsalted butter
Soft drinks	Fruit juices without corn syrup or added vitamin C; teas, including herbal teas
Vanilla extract	Extracts made without corn syrup or alcohol derived from corn
Soy sauce	Barley miso
White vinegar	Apple cider vinegar, rice vinegar
Anything with added salt unless the label specifies sea salt	Salt-free products, products made with sea salt
Anything made with nondairy creamers	Products made with milk or cream

2. Locate Safe Alternatives

Make a trip to a health food store (the kind that sells food, not just pills) or study a health food catalog. I recommend looking in the yellow pages of your phone book to locate a good store. Look for ones that mention organic food and produce, special diet foods, and special allergy items in their ads. The resource section at the end of this chapter lists two companies that have excellent health food catalogs.

Familiarize yourself with the wide variety of alternative food types and products available. The staff at a good health food store tends to be very knowledgeable and can help guide you to suitable alternatives. Ethnic grocery stores, farmers markets and organic farms are other good sources of alternative ingredients that you might want to add to your diet.

3. Buy Some of These Alternative Ingredients

Buy some of the new, alternative ingredients you are likely to use and enjoy.

4. Try New Recipes and Practice Modifying Old Favorites

Try out some of the recipes in this book, use the substitution guide to modify your favorite recipes and/or look through cookbooks for new recipes that you can easily modify. Once you have a repertoire of safe foods that you enjoy, then ...

5. Remove Unsafe Food from Your Kitchen

Go through your kitchen and remove anything that contains ingredients you should not have. You may wish to donate this food to family, friends or a food bank. You may wish to clean out the kitchen one shelf at a time or all at once. You may even wish to leave some allergenic food in the house out of consideration of other household members. Just make sure you and the other members of your household are aware of all the ways in which those allergenic foods have the potential to make you sick.

Food odors, handling of allergenic food, and contamination of otherwise safe food with allergens from sloppy food-handling techniques can cause symptoms. For instance, the smell of baking bread makes some gluten-intolerant people sick. When there is enough odor in the air to smell the baking bread, there is also enough gluten in the air to have an adverse effect.

If you prepare food for others using items that cause problems for you, you might also get sick. For instance, if you are intolerant of cornstarch but cook for others with cornstarch, you may inadvertently create problems for yourself by accidentally inhaling some of the starch that finds its way into the air. Some cornstarch might accidentally stick to your hands and later touch your lips. You might accidentally nick yourself with a knife and have the cornstarch get directly into your bloodstream through the nick. You might also wipe up some spilled cornstarch with a sponge that is later used to wash dishes. This could possibly lead to the dishes you cook with or eat from being contaminated with traces of cornstarch.

Your safe food can be contaminated with allergens through sloppy food handling. In the scenario above, if you don't wipe the counter well, it could result in everything you set on the counter being contaminated with cornstarch. Another example is that someone might spread butter on a piece of toast and then get toast particles in the stick of butter by either returning excess butter from the toast or using a contaminated knife to get more butter. If toast is a problem food for you, the remaining butter is now unsafe.

Sloppy food handling can also be a problem when food is being served. Perhaps you are at a potluck dinner party and have brought along a special vegetable dish that is safe for you. For everyone else the host has made rice, but since you are allergic to rice, you have also brought along a special bowl of millet for you. Problems can arise if someone serving himself or herself rice accidentally drops some of it in your millet or in the vegetable dish. It is not uncommon for someone who does not happen to be thinking of your special food needs to even use the serving spoon for the rice to dish out the vegetable dish or a little taste of the millet, thus contaminating all or part of your dinner. In an attempt to be helpful, without even thinking of it or remembering it later, someone might also walk into your kitchen and use the rice spoon to stir the vegetable dish or transfer the millet, thus contaminating what had once been your safe food.

As mentioned earlier, dirty counters are another possible source of contamination. Perhaps someone in your household accidentally left a very fine dusting of flour, cornstarch, table salt, toast particles, or something else you cannot tolerate on the counter. You then set down something you are about to eat, perhaps an apple or a piece of cheese, directly on the counter. Contamination from the counter sticking to your snack may very well make you sick, without you ever knowing why.

If you are going to stay well, you need the cooperation of others in your household. Don't expose yourself needlessly to your allergens through SMELL, TOUCH, SLOPPY FOOD HANDLING or GIVING IN to the temptation of eating something you shouldn't just because it was convenient. You want your kitchen to be a haven filled with good things that you like to eat, not a danger zone filled with allergenic booby traps.

6. Use Quality Cookware

Invest in quality cooking equipment. Quality cookware makes cooking a pleasure. Inferior cookware can make even the best of chefs look bad. Start with a good set of sharp knives and some good pots and pans. Then consider a blender or food processor for smoothies (fruit purees similar to a milkshake), soups and grinding soft grains such as oatmeal into flour. In addition, microwave ovens, toasters, cookie sheets, etc. should be thoroughly cleaned to remove any allergenic food particles. An assortment of clean, allergen-free food storage containers is also useful.

A final purchase you might consider is a small grain grinder, available from health food stores and garden supply catalogs. Freshly ground grain tastes far superior to flour purchased at a store and is healthier.

Long-Term Benefits

Getting enough good-tasting, well-balanced food can be a problem when you have food sensitivities. You may find cooking at home to be your best source of safe food. Removing food from your kitchen that is unsafe for you and stocking it with safe foods that you enjoy is the first step in enjoying safe home-cooked meals.

Resources

Special Foods!
9207 Shotgun Court
Springfield, VA 22153
703-644-0991
703-644-1006 fax
e-mail: kslimak@ix.netcom.com
Web: www.specialfoods.com
This company offers a wide variety of unusual and appealing foods for people with food sensitivities. Products are made from many sources, including white sweet potatoes, malanga, cassava, true yams, lotus roots, Jerusalem artichoke tubers, amaranth, quinoa, milo, water chestnut, buckwheat, papaya, mangos and star fruit.

Gold Mine™ Natural Food Co.
7805 Arfons Drive
San Diego, CA 92126-4368
800-475-3663
This company offers many of the products available in a good health food store, including cookware, grain mills, and a wide variety of organic foods.

Great Plains Foods
308 Walnut
P.O. Box 368
Brighton, CO 80601
800-BUY-WILD
This company sells exotic game meats.

Allergy Research Group
A Division of NutriCology, Inc.
P.O. Box 489
400 Preda Street
San Leandro, CA 94577-0489
800-782-4274
This company offers a wide variety of hypoallergenic vitamins and supplements, including unbuffered and buffered forms of vitamin C from beets.

Chapter 10: How to Modify Your Favorite Recipes

Highlights:

- Strategies for making favorite foods using alternative ingredients.
- Discussion of alternative leavenings, binders, moisturizers, grains, flours, oils, milks, meats and sweeteners.
- Examples of how to modify a recipe.

Effort Involved:

- **To use this chapter you must have already identified your food sensitivities and learned to recognize the presence of problem ingredients.** Chapters 3 and 4 describe how to test for food sensitivities. Chapters 5-8 teach what you need to know to avoid problem ingredients.
- **Remove unsafe food and restock your kitchen with safe food.** Chapter 9 guides you through this process.
- **Try out new recipes and learn to modify old recipes so they are once again safe.** The effort involved here will depend on the extent of your food sensitivities and also on your prior cooking experience. If almost everything you had been eating is now off-limits, it will take some effort to find and create enough new and safe recipes to keep you happy and well-fed. By the same token, if you have little cooking experience, it will take more effort to learn to modify recipes than if you cook frequently and routinely modify recipes as a matter of course. Either way, this chapter will walk you through the process.

Payoff:

- Easy access to a wide variety of foods you enjoy.
- Ability to re-create the taste and texture of foods you desire.

Safe Versions of Your Favorite Foods—How to Modify Your Favorite Recipes

Everyone has favorite foods. What should you do if your favorite foods are suddenly off-limits? The answer: modify the recipe to create a safe and tasty alternative.

This section will show you how to do just that. Your choice of alternative ingredients is vast. First, alternative leavening, binding, thickening, moistening and sweetening agents are discussed. Next, substitutions that you can use for grains, flours, oils, milk and meats are listed. Finally, using these substitutions, the process of modifying a recipe is explained.

The 4 Steps for Modifying a Recipe

1. Identify offending ingredients.
2. Identify the role each offending ingredient plays with respect to leavening, binding, thickening, moistening and sweetening. Be aware of how these ingredients affect texture and taste.
3. Use the substitution guide and your own knowledge of what taste and texture you are looking for to select suitable substitutions.
4. Write down your substitutions and evaluate the finished product. How was the taste and texture? Did it need more or less leavening, binding, thickening, moistening or sweetening? What is your best guess of exact amounts or different ingredients that would make the recipe even better? Write down your answer, so you will have it as an easy reference next time.

For inspiration, browse through a variety of cookbooks to get a feel for ingredients, relative proportions and creative substitutions.

Substitution Guide

11 Leavening Options

Some leavenings contain hidden allergens such as cornstarch, wheat, yeast and eggs. If these allergens are a problem for you, read this section to learn about leavenings and/or mechanical leavening strategies that are safe for you.

1. Baking Powder

Commercial baking powder usually contains cornstarch. To make your own corn-free version, mix 1 part baking soda, 2 parts cream of tartar and 2 parts arrowroot powder, potato starch or flour of your choice. The arrowroot powder, potato starch or flour is to help keep the acid (cream of tartar) and alkali (baking soda) components from reacting with each other during storage, to keep the mixture free-flowing, and to make the leavening power of your mixture equivalent to an equal measure of commercial baking powder.

This mixture does not hold its leavening power well over time, so only make enough at a time to last you a few weeks. This mixture is "single acting" and most of the carbon dioxide gas bubbles that create the leavening effect are released as soon as the baking powder contacts liquid. Therefore, mix wet and dry ingredients separately and combine at the last moment with a minimum of stirring. Then transfer quickly into a baking container and preheated oven.

2. Baking Soda

Baking soda used alone has no leavening properties. However, used in combination with acid ingredients, such as sour milk or lemon juice, it yields a very tender crumb texture. The proportion of baking soda to sour milk or buttermilk is usually 1 tsp. soda to 1 cup sour milk or 3 tsp. lemon or 3 tsp. vinegar. Hypoallergenic, unbuffered vitamin C (available made from various plant sources) or rhubarb concentrate are two more possibilities for acid ingredients that can be used with baking soda. Use 1/4 tsp. unbuffered vitamin C or 3 tsp. rhubarb concentrate per 1 tsp. baking soda.

3. Cream of Tartar

Cream of tartar, which is made from grapes and is a byproduct of winemaking, has no leavening properties when used alone. However, used in combination with an alkali ingredient, such as baking soda or bicarbonate of soda powder (sodium bicarbonate), and a liquid, it quickly releases carbon dioxide bubbles. Its use is explained above in the discussion of baking powder.

4. Baker's yeast

Baker's yeast added to dough provides leavening in the form of carbon dioxide bubbles produced as the yeast grows. Food-intolerant individuals need to be aware that commercial baker's yeast may contain traces of various substances such as corn or wheat that can trigger sensitivity reactions. At least one brand, Red Star™ is available free of grains and preservatives.

5. Sourdough

Sourdough cultures are cultures of wild yeast captured from the air that produce not only leavening but also organic acids and fragrant compounds that give sourdough products their distinctive sour aroma. Commercial sourdough starter cultures are available but are likely to contain wheat flour and possibly other allergens that can be hard to identify. To be on the safe side it is probably better to start your own culture from wild yeast in the air in your kitchen.

To capture wild yeast, place a raw, grated potato (or other starch source that you can tolerate, such as cooked rice or cooked millet) in a jar with a spoonful of honey or maple syrup or other sweetener that you can tolerate. Add some water and stir to make a soft mixture. Cover with cheesecloth and leave at room temperature for a few days. Look at the sourdough each day and stir it. When it smells sour and fermented, it is ready to refrigerate. If it turns green or moldy, discard and try again. A gray liquid smelling of alcohol on the top of the starter is normal.

To use, turn sourdough out into a large bowl. Add flour and water according to your recipe. Be sure to return some of your sourdough to the refrigerator for future use. It is best to use your sourdough at least once every two to three weeks, that is, add fresh water and flour and let it sit at room temperature for a while to keep the yeast lively. Even if you are not baking, you can let the sourdough culture "grow" for a few hours or overnight at room temperature. If you have not used your culture for a while you might want to let it "grow" overnight the night before using it, to reinvigorate it and cut down on long rising times.

Sourdough tends to leaven more slowly than commercial yeast or baking soda, but in the process imparts its distinctive taste and aroma.

6. Eggs
Eggs and especially whipped egg whites provide leavening in baked goods.

7-11. 5 Mechanical Measures for Providing Leavening
The first five leavening agents provide leavening by releasing carbon dioxide gas bubbles that are trapped in a batter or dough, thereby causing it to rise.

The following five mechanical measures provide leavening by trapping air or steam in the batter or dough:

1. Use a blender or wire whip to beat air bubbles into batter (especially good for pancakes and waffles just before putting on a grill).
2. Use a preheated oven (more water vapor is trapped when the outside of the batter or dough bakes quickly).
3. Cream fat and sugar together before adding to dough (provides a softer and lighter texture).

4. Beat eggs till frothy and beat egg whites to state of "stiff but not dry" before adding to the rest of the recipe.
5. Fold and mix batters. (The objective is not to lose any of the air that has been beaten into the components, while still mixing the components. This is especially noticeable in the case of adding stiffly beaten egg whites to other ingredients.)

One advantage of using these measures for providing leavening is that trapping air and water vapor require no special ingredients and are in no danger of introducing allergens or upsetting a strict rotation diet schedule. (See Chapter 13 for information on rotation diets.) Another advantage is that many alternative and whole-grain flours such as rye tend to produce very heavy, dense baked goods, and this tendency can be mitigated to some degree by the proper mechanical methods.

8 Alternatives to Eggs for Baking

Eggs provide leavening and binding in many products such as breads, pancakes, muffins, waffles and, of course, soufflés. Some commercial egg substitutes will reproduce both these functions but still contain eggs. If you react poorly to eggs, carefully read the ingredient listing. Ingredient names like albumin, lecithin, livetin, ovomucin, and others given in Chapter 6 often indicate the presence of egg.

The following chart lists egg substitutes for baking along with attributes of each.

8 Egg Substitutes for Baking

Substitute	Binding	Adds moisture	Leavening	Other Comments
1. Arrowroot powder	Yes	No	No	Adds no particular taste
2. Psyllium seed husk powder	Yes	No	No	Adds fiber but no particular taste
3. Flaxseed	Yes	No	No	Adds fiber, essential fatty acids, texture, but no particular taste
4. Tofu	Yes	Yes	No	Nutritious, but made from soy, a common allergen
5. Tapioca flour	Yes	No	No	Adds no particular taste
6. Bananas 7. Prune puree 8. Butternut squash puree	Yes	Yes	Yes	Add distinctive tastes

As the chart above shows, arrowroot powder, psyllium seed husk powder, flaxseed (must be boiled or ground before using. Details are given below) and tapioca flour make good binders in baked goods, but do not add taste or moistness. Tofu adds moistness and binding power. Bananas, prune puree and butternut squash puree bind, and add moistness, sweetness and a distinctive taste. Details on the use of these alternatives are given below.

1. Arrowroot
Use 1 tsp. arrowroot powder per cup of nonglutenous flour. Gluten is a binding constituent found in wheat, spelt, kamut, rye, oats and barley. Gluten is not found in corn, rice, quinoa and millet.

2. Psyllium Seed Husk Powder

For each cup of nonglutenous flour in a recipe, combine 1 Tbsp. psyllium seed husk powder with 3 Tbsp. water and let the mixture sit for a few minutes. Then add it to your baking mixture. Alternatively, add psyllium to dry ingredients, and add 2 to 3 Tbsp. extra liquid.

3. Flaxseed

For each cup of nonglutenous flour in a recipe, boil 1 Tbsp. flaxseed in 1 cup water for 15 minutes. Let cook down to 1/2 to 1/4 cup. Cool and add to baked goods, substituting for part of liquid ingredients. Alternatively, add 1 Tbsp. of ground flaxseed to dry ingredients and 2 to 3 Tbsp. of extra liquid.

4. Tofu

In baking, 1/4 cup tofu can be substituted for each egg as a binder. Silken tofu works better than firm tofu.

5. Tapioca flour

Use 1 Tbsp. tapioca flour per 1 cup flour.

6-8. Bananas, prune puree and butternut squash puree

Bananas work well as a substitute for eggs in baked goods such as banana bread and muffins. Prune puree is a particularly tasty substitute in gingerbread and brownies. Butternut squash puree works well in corn bread. Because each of these substitutions acts as a moisturizer, they also reduce the amount of oil needed in baked goods.

23 Alternatives for Thickening and Binding

White (bleached wheat) flour is used in pies, soups, gravies, and sauces as a thickener and a binder. The following are equivalent to the thickening and binding power of 1 tsp. white (bleached wheat) flour:

1. 1/3 tsp. kudzu (kuzu)
2. 1/2 tsp. arrowroot
3. 1/2 tsp. potato starch
4. 1/2 tsp. rice starch
5. 1/2 tsp. taro starch
6. 1/2 tsp. malanga flour
7. 1 tsp. cornstarch
8. 2 tsp. quick-cooking tapioca (for sauces not to be frozen)
9. 1/2 tsp. quick-cooking tapioca (for sauces to be frozen, per 1/2 cup liquid)
10. 1 tsp. white or brown rice flour
11. 1 tsp. soy flour
12. 1 tsp. oat flour
13. 1 tsp. barley flour
14. 1 tsp. rye flour
15. 1 tsp. spelt flour
16. 1 tsp. kamut flour
17. 1 tsp. buckwheat flour
18. 1 tsp. millet flour
19. 1 tsp. quinoa flour
20. 1 tsp. sorghum flour (milo maize)

21. 1 tsp. white sweet potato flour
22. 1 tsp. cassava flour
23. 2 tsp. sago pearls

1. Kudzu

Kudzu powder, made from the roots of the same plant that has overgrown much of the deep South, is widely used in Japanese cookery for many of the same purposes for which we in the West use arrowroot, cornstarch or gelatin. Its delicate flavor, translucency and medicinal properties make it especially valued in sauces, soups and desserts.

In Japan, the strongly alkaline biochemical action of kudzu powder and kudzu root is used to restore good health by alkalizing the bloodstream. Partially refined kudzu powder has a history of healing chronic intestinal ailments. It is sometimes used in Japan as a nourishing health food for invalids and the elderly. In Japanese hospitals the powder is often prescribed for patients on a liquid diet, since it is soothing, nutritious and easy to digest.

To use, crush the chunky powder with the back of a spoon. Combine powder and cold liquid in a small bowl. Stir well, then mash any remaining lumps with fingertips. Pour through a small, fine-mesh strainer into cooking liquid. For clear soups use ½ to ¾ tsp. per cup liquid. For thick sauces use 1½ to 2¼ Tbsp. per 1 cup liquid. For jelled liquids and glazes use 2 Tbsp. per 1 cup liquid. Acidic liquids such as lemon juice require 10 to 15 percent more kudzu powder for thickening or jelling than water or alkaline liquids such as apple juice. This 10 to 15 percent more translates into not quite an extra ½ tsp. kudzu powder for each Tbsp. kudzu that one would normally use.

2. Arrowroot

Arrowroot flour or starch was mentioned above in the section on binders for baking. It also makes a good thickener. Produced from a plant that grows in the West Indies, arrowroot is a popular base for cream sauces and clear and delicate glazes. In recipes calling for sugar, avoid lumping by mixing arrowroot flour and sugar together and then adding gradually to cold liquid. Otherwise, make a paste of 1 tsp. arrowroot powder to 1 cup liquid called for in the recipe. Introduce this paste gradually into hot but not boiling liquid. Bring the liquid to a boil. To prevent lumps gently stir for about 10 minutes or until the mixture gelatinizes.

3-4. Potato Starch and Rice Starch

Potato starch and rice starch do not yield as finely textured a product as kudzu and arrowroot powders, so they are better suited for thickening more robust soups and sauces, not fine confections and glazes.

Use 1 tsp. potato starch or rice starch to moderately thicken 1 cup liquid. Do not heat the liquid very close to the boiling point, since these thickeners lose their thickening power when heated too much. The thickening power of potato starch also does not last long, so if using potato starch, serve immediately.

5. Taro Powder or Dasheen

Taro powder or dasheen is used as a base for puddings and confections, in the dough for Chinese pastries and to make poi, a cooked paste common in Polynesian countries. Taro tubers cooked like boiled potatoes, mashed, and then strained through cheesecloth can also be used to make the dishes mentioned above. See Chinese and Polynesian cookbooks for recipes.

6. Malanga Flour

Malanga flour is made from a root closely related to taro root. It is one of the most hypoallergenic foods in the world because its starch grains are the smallest and most easily digested of all known complex carbohydrates.

Special Foods!, a company specializing in unusual foods for people with food sensitivities, has many malanga flour products available. Special Foods! is listed in the resources section at the end of this chapter.

7-9. Cornstarch

Cornstarch, tapioca and arrowroot are all recommended for thickening very acid fruits because they do not lose thickening power as quickly as flour does in the presence of acid. However, cornstarch does lose its thickening power very quickly if overcooked or, strangely enough, if too much cornstarch is used. Follow cooking directions given for arrowroot powder.

8-9. Tapioca

Tapioca, made from cassava root, is popular for sauces and fruit fillings that are to be frozen. These sauces thaw without breaking down or becoming watery. Tapioca is also popular for making very clear glazes. Cook the tapioca and fruit juice or water only to the point of boiling and remove from heat. Beware of overcooking, as the tapioca will become stringy. After 10 minutes of cooling the glaze should be thick enough to apply to the food you are glazing.

10-22. Alternative Flours

White or brown rice flour, soy flour, oat flour, barley flour, rye flour, spelt flour, kamut flour, buckwheat flour, quinoa flour, millet flour, sorghum flour (also called milo maize), white sweet potato flour and cassava flour can be used as thickeners, similar to the way white (wheat flour) can be used in pies, soups, gravies and sauces. Because most of these flours are not usually as highly refined as white flour, the thickened product tends to be a bit grittier. Each flour has a slightly different taste and texture, so experiment and see what works best for you. Sorghum flour is used primarily for thickening soups.

23. Sago Pearls

Sago pearls, made from palm, must be soaked for at least one hour before use. Use 1/4 cup pearls per 1/2 cup water. If the water is not completely absorbed, the pearls are too old to use. Follow the cooking directions for tapioca.

9 Additional Thickeners and Binders

1. eggs
2. egg substitutes
3. gelatin
4. agar (kanten or agar-agar)
5. Irish moss or carrageenan
6. pectin
7. sweet potato starch
8. bracken starch (warabi denpun)
9. xanthum gum (xanthan gum)

1. Eggs

Eggs can be used as thickeners in many dishes. These include soups such as egg drop soup, casseroles and baked goods.

2. Egg Substitutes

All eight of the egg substitutes for baking listed in the chart earlier in this can also serve as thickeners and binders in other types of foods. This includes sauces, puddings and soups.

3. Gelatin

Gelatin is derived from collagen, commercially from hides, sinews or crushed bones of cows or pigs. Gelatin melts at room temperature and will not gel acidic liquids having a pH of less than 4.5. In practical terms this means gelatin does not do a good job jelling acid fruit juices such as pineapple juice, rhubarb juice or strawberry juice. Use 1 Tbsp. per 2 cups liquid.

4. Agar, Kanten and Agar-Agar

Agar (also called kanten or agar-agar) is made from the sea vegetables *Gelidium* and *Gracilaria*. Sold as flakes, bars or powder, it keeps jelled foods firm yet delicate in the very hottest weather and jells even acidic pineapple juice. Agar makes excellent jams and jellies without the addition of sugar or honey (unlike commercially available pectin, which requires considerable sweetening). Use 1 tsp. agar per 1 cup liquid. Soften first by soaking in 1/4 cup cold liquid, then dissolve in ¾ cup hot liquid.

5. Irish Moss or Carrageenan

Irish moss or carrageenan is made from seaweed and is used as an emulsifier, stabilizer and thickener in a variety of foods. Allow from 2 to 4 tsp. powder per 1 cup liquid, depending on how stiff a gel is desired. To use, follow the directions given for agar. It needs to be heated to 140°F to dissolve and becomes thin in the presence of acid.

6. Pectin

Pectin, derived commercially from citrus and apple pulp, requires high levels of sugar to jell. However, high-pectin fruits such as apples, crab apples, quinces, red currants, gooseberries, plums and cranberries can be used alone or with low-pectin fruits to make excellent jellies, jams, fruit butters and pastes with little or no added sugar. See a cookbook such as *The Joy of Cooking* by Irma Rombauer and Marion Rombauer Becker for detailed instructions. To use commercial pectin, follow the directions given on the package.

7. Sweet Potato Starch

Sweet potato starch (kansho denpun or satsuma denpun) is widely used in Japan and may be available in some Asian food stores.

8. Bracken Starch

Bracken starch (warabi denpun) is extracted from the root of the bracken fern. It is used in Japan mostly to make a popular confection called Warabi Mochi. To use, follow the directions for kudzu powder given earlier in this chapter.

9. Xanthum Gum

Xanthum gum, also known as xanthan gum, is derived from the bacteria *Xanthomonas compestris*. It is an ingredient used along with eggs in many gluten-free bread recipes to provide the binding power that is usually provided by the gluten in wheat, kamut, spelt, rye and other gluten-containing flours. Usually 1 tsp. xanthum gum and 1 egg are used per each cup of gluten-free flour such as corn or rice flour.

Although the xanthum gum itself is not usually allergenic, corn-sensitive individuals may find it allergenic since the growth medium for the bacteria often contains corn. Unless the growth medium is identified on the label as corn-free, or the product itself is identified as corn-free, corn-sensitive individuals will want to avoid xanthum gum.

24 Grain and Flour Options

The following flours, and the grains and tubers from which they are made, are commercially available:

1. cornmeal	14. amaranth flour
2. white or brown rice flour	15. sorghum flour (milo maize)
3. soy flour	16. white sweet potato flour
4. oat flour	17. cassava flour (gari)
5. oat bran	18. yam flour (ebulo)
6. barley flour	19. malanga flour
7. rye flour	20. lotus flour
8. spelt flour (an heirloom variety of wheat)	21. water chestnut flour
	22. artichoke flour
9. kamut flour (an heirloom variety of wheat)	23. bean flours (urad dal flour, chickpea flour or besan, white bean flour, etc.)
10. teff flour (distantly related to wheat)	24. nut meals (pecan meal, walnut meal, almond meal, chestnut flour, etc.)
11. buckwheat flour	
12. millet flour	
13. quinoa flour	

All of the flours and meals listed above can be used for making bread, muffins, cookies, crackers, pancakes, waffles, dumplings, etc. Those flours that contain the most gluten (**wheat, spelt, kamut, rye, oats, barley**) or soluble fiber (**bean flours, yam flour, buckwheat**) hold together the best when baking. Of these, **buckwheat** and **rye** tend to yield a heavy, dense product. **Barley** tends to produce a cakelike texture.

An additional binder can be useful to aid cohesion of baked goods made primarily with one of the flours that does not have good binding properties. Options for these binders are listed above in the section on thickeners and binders. These options include eggs, kudzu (kuzu) powder, arrowroot powder, potato starch, rice starch, taro starch, malanga flour, cornstarch, sweet potato starch, bracken starch, sago pearls, tapioca flour and xanthum gum.

Millet flour, especially coarsely ground, makes an excellent substitute for cornmeal in corn bread. **Oatmeal, oat bran, cornmeal** and **cassava flour** (gari) can be used to make quick, hot breakfast cereals. **Yam flour** (ebulo) is traditionally stirred into boiling water by Africans and stirred until a thick, lumpy paste is formed that is served with chili, vegetable stew or beef stew. **Bean flours** are widely used in India to produce steamed savory breads that are so flavorful and delicious it is hard to believe they are made from such healthy ingredients. Bean flours are also especially suitable for making crepes.

In addition, the grains, beans and tubers that are the source of these flours can also be cooked in their whole-food form to add a wide variety of tastes and textures to any meal while supplying quality carbohydrates and protein.

Nut flours such as pecan meal, walnut meal, almond meal and chestnut flour can be used to make exquisite tortes and other desserts. See Chapter 12 for "Oma's Pecan Square Recipe," a recipe for a cakelike dessert that uses pecan meal instead of flour.

Water/Cooking Times for Grains

Grain (4-6 servings)	Water	Salt	Cooking Time
1 cup kamut	3 cups	1/4 tsp.	2 hours
1 cup spelt	3 cups	1/4 tsp.	1 1/2 to 2 1/2 hours
1 cup whole barley	3 cups	1/4 tsp.	1 1/2 to 1 3/4 hours
1 cup pearled barley	3 cups	1/4 tsp.	45 to 55 minutes
1 cup milo	3 1/2 cups	1/4 tsp.	1 to 1 1/4 hours
1 cup amaranth	2 1/2 cups	1/4 tsp.	30 to 35 minutes
1 cup quinoa	2 cups	1/4 tsp.	20 minutes
1 cup teff	3 cups	1/4 tsp.	15 to 20 minutes
1 cup millet	3 cups	1/4 tsp.	25 to 30 minutes
1 cup rye	4 cups	1/4 tsp.	1 1/2 to 2 hours
1 cup white or raw buckwheat	3 cups	1/4 tsp.	20 to 25 minutes
1 cup roasted buckwheat	2 1/2 cups	1/4 tsp.	20 to 30 minutes
1 cup oat groats	3 cups	1/4 tsp.	2 to 2 1/2 hours
1 cup white rice	2 cups	1/4 tsp.	20 minutes
1 cup wild rice	4 cups	1/4 tsp.	60 minutes
1 cup brown rice	2 1/2 cups	1/4 tsp.	45 to 50 minutes

Cooking Grains

Grains other than **white rice** and **buckwheat** benefit from rinsing before cooking. **Quinoa** in particular must be rinsed well to remove its naturally soapy and somewhat bitter coating.

The longer-cooking grains also benefit from soaking overnight. This improves their ease of digestion, makes them creamier and reduces cooking time.

All grains other than buckwheat can be combined in a pan with the proper amount of water and salt, soaked several hours to overnight in the refrigerator, brought to a boil on the stove and then simmered. If you presoak, cooking time will be slightly less than the time given in the chart.

For fluffier grains, add the grains after the water has come to a boil, then simmer for the time specified.

Buckwheat Recipe

For buckwheat groats (kasha), heat a little oil in the bottom of the pan. If desired, sauté an onion and/or some mushrooms in the oil. Then add 1 cup buckwheat and stir to coat the grains with oil. Preheat the proper amount of water (see chart above) to the boiling point. Add the boiling water to the mix and simmer for the specified time. Avoid unnecessary stirring.

This method ensures that the buckwheat grains hold their texture. If buckwheat is pre-soaked or even just heated together with the water, it tends to turn into unappealing mush.

16 Alternative Sweeteners

Some people are allergic to cane sugar, the commonly used sugar in the United States. Alternative sweeteners include:

1. pureed vegetables
2. pureed fruit
3. fruit juice concentrates
4. dried fruit
5. dates
6. commercial fruit sugar concentrates
7. date sugar
8. beet sugar
9. maple syrup
10. rice syrup
11. barley malt
12. barley syrup
13. stevia
14. honey
15. blackstrap molasses
16. sorghum molasses

If you are used to eating food that is highly sweetened with refined sugar, initially food that is only moderately sweetened with natural alternatives will not taste sweet. With time, however, your palate will adapt to the rich flavors and natural sweetness of less highly refined food and the other will lose most of its appeal. Eating slowly and chewing thoroughly brings out the natural sweetness in food and speeds the adaptation to a more natural diet.

Natural sweetening ingredients include **pureed vegetables, pureed fruits** and **fruit juice concentrates.** For instance, many baked goods benefit from the addition of **pureed or mashed vegetables** such as butternut squash, pumpkin, sweet potato, white potato, zucchini, carrot, onion, etc. A popular addition to cakes to cut oil and sugar but retain moisture and sweetness is applesauce. Other fruit purees, such as prune puree, also work well in baked goods. In drinks and many desserts you can use frozen apple, grape, orange and pineapple juice concentrates for sweetening. **Dried fruits** and **dates** add sweetness and texture to cookies. There are also several more **concentrated sweeteners** based on concentrated fruit sugars that are on the market that are so sweet they produce desserts very similar to those containing cane sugar.

More options for refined, noncane sugar include: **date sugar, beet sugar, maple syrup, rice syrup, barley malt and barley syrup.** Health food stores are a good source of these sweeteners.

Yet another option is **stevia,** an herb that is very sweet. Unlike most artificial sweeteners, you can bake and cook with stevia at any temperature and for any length of time without it breaking down. It has a slight licorice aftertaste. Because stevia is so sweet, in its pure form only miniscule amounts are needed to give substantial sweetening power. Its use is complicated because it is sold diluted with powdered stretchers to make it easier to measure or dissolve in a liquid. Check ingredient listings to make sure that any stretchers or other additives are not on your "off-limits" list.

Honey is a good sweetener for beverages such as tea. It also lends moistness to baked goods. Many health food and natural food cookbooks have traditional recipes modified to contain honey instead of sugar.

Blackstrap molasses is a byproduct of the sugar manufacturing process and is very high in minerals, especially iron. It is not particularly sweet, but it adds a distinctive favor to foods such as gingerbread. If you are sensitive to cane sugar, avoid blackstrap molasses.

146

Sorghum molasses is sweeter and made from milo. Sorghum molasses can be used in place of light molasses if you are sensitive to cane sugar or "regular" molasses, which is made from cane.

2 Options for Moisteners

In most baked goods, oil serves primarily as a moistener. **Pureed fruit** (banana, apple, pear, prune, peach, etc.) or **pureed vegetables** (butternut squash, pumpkin, sweet potato, potato, zucchini, carrot, onion, etc.) can be substituted for most of the butter, oil or margarine in appropriate recipes, such as muffins or other quick breads. For each cup of oil that is left out, use 1 to 5 times the amount of puree. For example, if you leave out ½ cup of oil, use ½ to 2½ cups puree, depending on how moist you want the end product to be. For best results, leave a small amount of oil in the recipe and use nonstick baking containers.

11 Options for Fats and Oils

The fats and oils listed below are some of the many commercially available:

1. olive
2. flax
3. avocado
4. canola
5. peanut
6. sesame
7. safflower
8. sunflower
9. almond
10. butter
11. ghee

Of the oils listed, **olive oil, flaxseed oil** and **avocado oil** are the most healthful. **Flaxseed oil** and **avocado oil** should not be heated, but instead used in dressings and vinaigrettes. **Olive oil** is very tasty in dressings and vinaigrettes and can stand up to light sautéing as well.

Canola oil is the healthiest choice for more sustained heating but is not heat-resistant enough for deep-frying. **Peanut oil** can be used for deep-frying, but the same properties that make it or any other oil heat-resistant also make it a much less healthy oil in general.

Sesame oil used in small amounts adds variety with its distinctive taste. For the sake of food rotation schedules, small amounts of **safflower, sunflower, peanut** and **almond** oils are also acceptable.

If you want the texture or buttery flavor available only from **butter** or **ghee** (clarified butter), go ahead and use it in small amounts. Do not use shortening or margarine because the hydrogenation process used to create these products produces unhealthy trans-fatty acids.

20 Alternatives to Cow's Milk

Depending on the recipe, you can substitute:

1. water
2. vegetable broth
3. fruit juice
4. vegetable puree (Blending a portion of the vegetables in a soup in a blender and then returning them to the soup will often create a creamy texture.)
5. sheep's milk
6. coconut milk
7. soy milk
8. rice milk
9. almond milk
10. pecan milk
11. cashew milk
12. Brazil nut milk
13. filbert milk
14. walnut milk
15. pine nut milk
16. toasted quinoa milk
17. sunflower seed milk
18. pumpkin seed milk
19. sesame seed milk
20. goat's milk

Goat, sheep, soy and **rice milk** are available in health food stores. **Coconut milk** is available in Asian grocery stores. A **recipe for nut and seed milks** is given in Chapter 12.

Alternative Meats

Some people believe that a vegetarian diet is the healthiest and most humane type of diet. Other people believe that they need to eat at least some meat to stay healthy.

If you have food sensitivities, your choice of safe protein sources may be severely limited. It is certainly prudent to discover a wide variety of foods, including a wide variety of protein sources that are safe for you. A rotation diet that lets you eat any particular food no more often than once every fifth day is one way to prevent developing additional sensitivities to those foods that are currently safe.

Many people are sensitive to one or more of the commonly available meats, such as beef, pork, chicken and turkey. Sometimes this is due to something intrinsic to the type of meat itself. Sometimes it is due to the nature of "factory farm" rearing. For instance, some people cannot tolerate the antibiotic residues or corn allergen residues in animals raised on factory farms. Sometimes sensitivity problems are triggered by something added during meat processing, such as table salt, nitrates, MSG, casein, food dyes, or any other preservatives, flavor enhancers or additives of any type.

If you have problems with one or more of these types of meat, you may want to try meat from animals that are raised organically on a natural diet, with free access to a healthy outdoor environment, instead of on highly processed feed without free access to the out-of-doors. Health food stores are one source. Of course, you will want to get this meat as free as possible of any additives.

Game meats provide another healthy alternative. Commercial sources, such as Dale's Exotic Game Meats, sell many kinds of game and sometimes offer discounts to allergy patients. Because wild animals tend to get a lot of exercise and be leaner than domestic animals, their meat is best prepared by a tenderizing cooking method such as long, slow cooking with liquid. Stewing and crockpot cooking work well.

Modifying A Corn Bread Recipe—2 Examples

Its simple to modify a corn bread recipe to be free of corn allergens, yet still have a pleasing texture and taste.

The Original Standard Corn Bread Recipe

The following recipe is taken from a cookbook called *The Political Palate* by the Bloodroot Collective:

Plain Corn Bread

1. Butter an 8 x 8 x 2 Pyrex baking dish. Preheat oven to 400°. Melt ¼ **cup sweet butter**.
2. Whisk together **1¼ cups unbleached white flour, 1 Tbsp. baking powder, 1 tsp. salt, 1 cup cornmeal** and **2 Tbsp. sugar**.
3. In a small bowl, beat **2 eggs** well. Stir in **1¼ cups buttermilk** and the melted butter.
4. Combine wet and dry mixtures until just blended. Do not overmix. Turn into pan and bake until lightly browned (about 20-25 minutes).

Serves 6-8

How to Make the Modifications

First, identify the ingredients that must be removed. For a corn-sensitive individual, the following items are off-limits:

- most **commercial baking powder** (contains cornstarch)
- **table salt** (contains commercial dextrose, which is a corn product)
- **cornmeal**
- **buttermilk** (contains modified food starch, which is a form of cornstarch) and

- **salted butter** (dextrose in the salt)

Second, identify the role each offending ingredient plays with respect to leavening, binding, thickening, moistening and sweetening. Be aware of how these ingredients affect texture and taste.

In the recipe above, baking powder provides leavening, table salt provides saltiness, cornmeal provides a gritty texture, buttermilk provides a tangy, acid taste and salted butter provides fat.

Third, use the substitution guide and your own knowledge of what taste and texture you are looking for to select suitable substitutions.

To get a corn-allergen-free bread very much like the original corn bread, I recommend the following substitutions:

Use a **grain-free baking powder,** such as those at health food stores, or make your own from 1 part baking soda, 2 parts cream of tartar and 2 parts arrowroot powder, potato starch or flour of your choice.

In place of table salt, use **½ tsp. sea salt** that contains no additives. When using sea salt, use only half the amount of salt called for in regular recipes. Sea salt is twice as strong as regular salt because sea salt is 100 percent salt. Regular salt is diluted 1:1 with dextrose.

In place of cornmeal, use **coarsely ground millet**. You can buy millet at a health food store and then put it through a grain-grinding mill set to a coarse texture. You can also "grind" it in a blender or food processor. Millet is soft, so it is very easy to grind. The millet flour for sale in health food stores is generally ground too finely to produce the somewhat coarse texture of good corn bread. If this coarse texture is what you are after, it is definitely worth it to coarsely grind your own millet.

In place of the buttermilk, use **3½ tsp. lemon juice OR 3½ tsp. apple cider vinegar** and **1¼ cups milk**. Add the lemon or vinegar after the other wet ingredients have already been mixed. When added directly to the milk, the milk tends to curdle.

Because of the acid in the recipe, **plain baking soda** could be used in place of baking powder.

In place of **salted butter**, use **unsalted butter**.

Modification No. 1—Plain Millet Bread

1. Butter an 8 x 8 x 2-inch Pyrex baking dish. Preheat oven to 400°. Melt **¼ cup unsalted butter**.
2. Whisk together **1¼ cups unbleached white flour, 1 Tbsp. grain-free baking powder, ½ tsp. sea salt, 1 cup coarsely ground millet** and **2 Tbsp. sugar**.
3. In a small bowl, beat **2 eggs** well. Stir in **1¼ cups milk** and the melted butter. Then add **3½ tsp. lemon juice OR apple cider vinegar**.
4. Combine wet and dry mixtures until just blended. Do not overmix. Turn into pan and bake until lightly browned (about 20-25 minutes).

Serves 6-8

Other Possible Substitutions

- ❑ Substitute olive oil or canola oil for the butter.
- ❑ Substitute winter squash for most of the butter, for the binding power of the eggs and for the sweetness of the sugar.
- ❑ Substitute maple sugar, rice syrup or barley syrup for the sugar.
- ❑ Substitute soy milk, rice milk, or a nut milk plus lemon juice or vinegar for buttermilk.
- ❑ Substitute spelt or kamut or rye flour for the white flour.
- ❑ Add hot peppers and pepitas (squash seeds) for spice and texture.

Most of these substitutions are used in the corn bread recipe below, which was inspired by a spicy corn bread recipe in the cookbook, *The Perennial Political Palate.*

Modification No. 2—Spicy, Moist Millet Bread

1. Preheat oven to 400°. Steam **2¼ cups winter squash**. Set aside.
2. Dice **2 or 3 frying peppers** and a **jalapeno pepper**. (Frying peppers are "mild" hot peppers.) Sauté in **1 to 2 Tbsp. oil** until golden brown. Remove from heat and set aside. Lightly oil a 12 x 12 x 2-inch pan.
3. Whisk together: **2 cups coarsely ground millet, 1½ tsp. baking soda, 1½ tsp. grain-free baking powder, ½ tsp. sea salt** and **2⅓ cups rye flour**.
4. Use a food processor to puree squash with **½ cup maple syrup, ¼ cup oil**, and **1⅓ cup soy milk**.
5. Turn wet ingredients into the dry, add peppers, and stir quickly together. Turn into prepared pan. Sprinkle **¼ cup pepitas** (squash seeds) over the top of the millet bread.
6. Place in oven. When the bread puffs, turn heat down to 350° and bake until done, about 40 minutes.

Serves 9

Checklist—Modifying a Recipe

❑ Identify offending ingredients. Knowing your food sensitivities (Chapter 3), and knowing how to avoid hidden allergens (Chapters 5-8) are necessary for successfully carrying out this step.

❑ Identify the role, if any, that each offending ingredient plays with respect to leavening, binding, thickening, moistening and sweetening. The sections in this chapter on each of these qualities can help you identify which of these roles each ingredient might play. For instance, eggs can provide leavening, binding, thickening AND moistening. Also be aware of how each ingredient affects the overall texture and taste.

❑ Use the substitution guide in this chapter and your own knowledge of what taste and texture you are looking for to select suitable substitutions. If you consistently pay attention to the taste and texture of food you like and strive to recreate it in your experiments in the kitchen, this step will become second nature.

❑ Write down your substitutions and evaluate the finished product. How was the taste and texture? Did it need more or less leavening, binding, thickening, moistening or sweetening? What is your best guess of exact amounts or different ingredients that would make the recipe even better? Write down your answer, so you will have it as an easy reference next time.

❑ For additional ideas about proportions and ingredients, browse through recipes from several cookbooks. Especially useful are cookbooks written for someone with your particular food sensitivities, cookbooks that reflect a style of cooking that mostly uses types of food that agree with you, and cookbooks that have many versions of a type of food for which you have a hankering.

Long-Term Benefits

Getting enough good-tasting, well-balanced food can be a problem when you have food sensitivities. This chapter is a good guide to the many alternative foods available that you may be able to eat. It can get you started cooking with these ingredients. It can get you started successfully recreating the taste and texture of some of your favorite foods that you may be missing.

The long-term benefits are that you will have the skills you need to successfully supply yourself with a wide variety of foods you enjoy. You will be able to guide others (friends, chefs) who wish to make special dishes for you. Apply the lessons in this chapter and reap the benefits of good food. These include feelings of safety, comfort, and joy, the physical sensations of palate gratification, and the overall blessings of good health.

Resources

Special Foods!
9207 Shotgun Court
Springfield, VA 22153
703-644-0991
703-644-1006 fax
e-mail: kslimak@ix.netcom.com
Web: www.specialfoods.com
This company offers a wide variety of unusual and appealing foods for people with food sensitivities. Products are made from many sources, including white sweet potatoes, malanga, cassava, true yams, lotus roots, Jerusalem artichoke tubers, amaranth, quinoa, milo, water chestnut, buckwheat, papaya, mangos and star fruit.

Gold Mine™ Natural Food Co.
7805 Arfons Drive
San Diego, CA 92126-4368
800-475-3663
This company offers many of the products available in a good health food store, including cookware, grain mills, and a wide variety of organic foods of interest to those of us with food sensitivities.

Great Plains Foods
308 Walnut
P.O. Box 368
Brighton, CO 80601
800-BUY-WILD
This company sells exotic game meats.

Irma S. Rombauer and Marion Rombauer Becker, *The Joy of Cooking* (New York: The Bobbs-Merrill Company, Inc., 1975).
There are many more recent editions of this book, but I find that older editions as well as older cookbooks in general are more useful. The recipes in older editions use fewer pre-processed ingredients, use a broader range of ingredients, and give better descriptions of how to make things from scratch.

Nicolette M. Dumke, *5 Years without Food: The Food Allergy Survival Guide* (Louisville, CO: Adapt Books, 1997).

William Shurtleff and Akiko Aoyagi, *The Book of Kudzu: A Culinary and Healing Guide* (Wayne, NJ: Avery Publishing Group Inc., 1985).

The Bloodroot Collective, *The Political Palate: A Feminist Vegetarian Cookbook* (Bridgeport, CT: Sanguinaria Publishing, 1980).

The Bloodroot Collective, *The Perennial Political Palate: A Feminist Vegetarian Cookbook* (Bridgeport, CT: Sanguinaria Publishing, 1993).

Bette Hagman, *The Gluten-free Gourmet Cooks Fast and Healthy* (New York: Henry Holt and Company, Inc., 1996).
I recommend you find this or another other gluten-free cookbook if you find that you cannot tolerate gluten. Bette Hagman and others have written many gluten-free cookbooks. Any of these will provide you with a treasury of already modified recipes.

Linda Edwards, *Baking for Health* (Garden City Park, NY: Avery Publishing Group, 1988).
This book explains the basic principles and gives many recipes for baking using whole foods and minimally processed ingredients. It is a useful guide.

Chapter 11: Strategies for Eating Out and for Traveling

Highlights:

- Five steps for getting a good meal at a restaurant.
- Ten hints for eating well on an extended trip.

Effort Involved:

- Start with a list of your food sensitivities. Chapters 3 and 4 describe how to test for food sensitivities. You also need to read Chapters 5-8 with a particular emphasis on learning the tricks you need to know to avoid ingredients that are a problem for you.
- Read labels and recipes to learn about problem ingredients that might show up in restaurant versions of foods you like to order.
- Identify certain types of restaurants that usually make food you can eat.
- Make a restaurant kit to supplement and improve food you order.
- Work with restaurant staff.
    - Call ahead during nonrush hours.
    - Have waiters identify the ingredients in food you are considering eating.
    - Prepare and carry a list of what you like and can have and a list of ingredients to which you are intolerant.
    - Collaborate with staff to get not just a safe meal, but a tasty and satisfying meal.
- Take safe food along on trips and learn how to pick up additional safe food along the way.
- Take along items that will allow you to conveniently store, prepare and eat the food you take.

Payoff:

- Ability to eat well at restaurants and while traveling, despite food sensitivities.

How to Get a Good Meal at a Restaurant—5 Important Steps

You can do many things to make eating out both possible and enjoyable.

1. Know Your Food

Become so knowledgeable about possible sources of allergens in your diet that by quizzing your waiter or waitress and possibly the cook, you can make sure that the food you eat is safe for you. This is best done by familiarizing yourself with the list of hidden allergens in Chapters 5-7 and by becoming an avid label and recipe reader.

If you don't protect yourself, no one else is likely to either. If you don't trust what the restaurant staff is telling you or can't determine if something is safe to eat, don't eat there. Calling ahead at a nonpeak time is a good way to screen out restaurants that cannot meet your needs and to find ones that can.

2. Find Compatible Cuisines

Identify certain kinds of restaurants that usually make food you can eat. I found that eating out at Thai, Indian and Pakistani restaurants gave me many entree choices. They tend not to salt their food, tend to not use starch or wheat, and are usually willing to serve dishes without rice or with rice on the side. Health food and vegetarian-oriented restaurants often had at least one entree on the menu that I could eat or were willing to fix something special for me. Shirley and Angie Crenshaw, profiled in Chapter 1, tend to do well eating Chinese, Japanese and other Asian-style food, because it usually doesn't to contain wheat or dairy products. This style of food did not work well for me, however, because of its reliance on cornstarch and rice. Other types of cuisine were problematic for me, but sometimes still workable. There is a local Italian restaurant that serves unlimited refills of a wonderful salad that agreed quite well with me. It was the only thing on the menu that I could eat, but with a salad that good, I was still a frequent visitor.

3. Have a Last-Resort List

Have in mind what you might like to eat that the restaurant might be able to supply. Even if there is nothing on the menu you can eat, the restaurant might be able to supply something like plain, steamed vegetables and a plain potato, or perhaps plain oatmeal and a boiled egg.

4. Bring Your Own Condiments ("My Condiments to the Chef")

Make a restaurant kit. Include items that you can use to transform plain food into something special.

When food sensitivities were still an issue for me, my kit contained sea salt, nutritional yeast, rosehip tea bags, unsalted butter and my own salad dressing. I didn't particularly enjoy plain salads, plain vegetables and plain potatoes, especially when I was eating out and wanted the meal to be especially good. However, with my restaurant kit, my potato was delicious with a safe form of butter, sea salt and nutritional yeast, and my salad and vegetables much better with the addition of my own salad dressing. (See Chapter 6 or 13 for an explanation of why corn-sensitive individuals need to avoid table salt.)

For extended trips when refrigeration is an issue, you might want to use olive oil and vinegar in place of butter and perishable salad dressings. Unsalted peanut butter is another example of something that I could tolerate that doesn't need refrigeration, and that can turn plain vegetables into something special.

Also consider taking along special items that restaurants are not likely to have on hand, but that they could use to cook something special for you. Depending on your sensitivities, this might include special pasta or grains, quick-cooking beans or lentils, or unsalted peanut butter or nuts for making sauces.

5. Chat up the Staff/Carry Along Two Lists

Collaborate with waiters and chefs to get meals that are not listed on the menu. As an aid, 1) prepare a list of foods that includes your intolerance, what you are allowed and like, and a few quick recipes for what you like, and 2) prepare a exhaustive list of ingredients that you are not allowed.

The first list is for the waiter and chef. The second list is a reference for you so that if the chef suggests using a food whose contents are not immediately familiar to you, you can check the ingredients listing on the label against your list of disqualifying ingredient names.

When I visited Yellowstone National Park in the mid-1990s, the company that ran the restaurants in the park was very aware of special food needs. I had excellent experiences collaborating with the waiters and cooks to come up with tasty, special meals that were safe for me to eat. In many good restaurants, the staff is willing to go out of its way to help you get a safe meal.

If possible, call ahead during a nonrush period at the restaurant to make your needs known and ascertain to what extent it is able to accommodate you. Consider bringing along certain key ingredients that they might not have on hand.

The key to being a good collaborator is twofold: 1) providing suggestions to get the chef's imagination going, and 2) being informed about what is in various foods to know if the chef's suggestions are really safe for you. Ask the waiter to bring out the food labels of suspect ingredients if you are not 100 percent sure they are safe.

Example of First List

Below is an example of a list I made to show waiters and chefs:

Special Dietary Needs for Barbara Allan:

Foods to which I am allergic:
wheat (including white flour)
corn products such as corn oil, cornstarch, modified food starch, cornmeal, corn syrup and maltodextrin, but not
       fresh corn on the cob (evidently, I was allergic to field corn but not sweet corn.)
rice
food additives such as the dye that makes cheese orange
dextrose in table salt
commercially produced vitamin C (whenever it is listed as an ingredient)
beef

Suggested Foods that I CAN eat:
- unsalted oatmeal or oatmeal salted with sea salt
- milk
- plain yogurt (no added cornstarch, corn syrup, dextrose, etc., just cultured milk and pectin)
- plain fruit juices with no added vitamin C or sweeteners
- plain fruit
- plain steamed vegetables (no table salt or salted butter)
- plain potatoes (no table salt or salted butter)
- tempeh that was made only with soy and starter mold but not any sort of additional grains
- stir-fried tofu and vegetables (no table salt, tamari, soy sauce, flour)
- tofu baked with apple cider vinegar and/or sesame oil
- tofu and vegetables with peanut sauce, parsley-almond sauce, or tahini sauce

- peanut sauce or parsley-almond sauce (I can provide the unsalted peanut butter or the raw almonds):

Peanut Sauce Recipe 1
¼ cup chopped fresh cilantro
¾ cup unsalted peanut butter (I can provide)
2 Tbsp. chopped fresh mint
¼ tsp. hot chili pepper flakes
1 cup water
4 Tbsp. fresh lime juice

Wash the cilantro and pat dry. Add all the ingredients to a food processor and blend until smooth. Makes 1 ¾ cup sauce.

Peanut Sauce Recipe 2
1 small onion, chopped medium fine
1 inch of fresh ginger root, peeled and chopped fine
       or
1 tsp. powdered ginger
       or
1 tsp. curry powder
       or
1 ½ tsp. coriander seeds **and** 1 ½ tsp. cumin or fennel seeds
canola oil
¾ cup unsalted peanut butter (I can provide)
1 cup hot water
½ tsp. sea salt

Sauté onion and ginger or other spices over high heat in a bit of canola oil. When onions are translucent, add the last three ingredients, mixing to form a sauce. Cook over low heat one minute. Makes 1 ¾ cups sauce.

Peanut Sauce Recipe 3
¾ cup unsalted peanut butter (I can provide)
1 cup hot water
OPTIONAL:
½ tsp. sea salt

Place ingredients in blender. Blend until smooth. Makes 1 ¾ cups sauce.

Parsley-Almond Sauce
3 Tbsp. raw almond butter or raw almonds (I can provide)
1 tsp. barley miso

½ cup hot water
1 cup fresh parsley
OPTIONAL:
1 clove minced garlic

Place ingredients in blender. Blend until smooth. Makes 1 cup sauce.

Tahini Sauce
1 cup unsalted tahini
½ cup water
OPTIONAL:
2 Tbsp. Fresh lemon juice
1/4 to ½ cup plain yogurt
3 cloves minced garlic

Place ingredients in blender. Blend until smooth. Makes 1 1/2 cups sauce.

Fresh Salsa
1 bunch cilantro
1 small onion, chopped
2 large red, ripe tomatoes, chopped
OPTIONAL:
1 hot chili pepper, chopped

Place ingredients in blender. Blend until smooth. Makes 1-2 cups.

More foods I CAN eat:
- pinto beans cooked without salt, served with an avocado and/or fresh salsa made without salt (see salsa recipe above)
- lentils cooked without salt and served with fresh salsa (see salsa recipe above).
- tossed salad WITHOUT added croutons, cheese, meat, bacon bits, dressing or salt
- salad dressing of olive oil and apple cider vinegar (beware, not all cider vinegar is made only with apples; if it was made with grain or wheat it will make me sick)
- fresh, ripe avocado instead of salad dressing
- sour cream that does not contain salt, starch, dextrose, etc. (suggested brand: Prairie Farms)
- kasha (I can provide buckwheat groats) and vegetables

Kasha with Onions
3 Tbsp. canola oil
3 medium onions, chopped
1 cup buckwheat groats (I can provide)
2 cups boiling water
OPTIONAL:
1 tsp. sea salt
1 cup chopped fresh mushrooms
1 dollop unsalted butter

Sauté onions and optional mushrooms in oil until onions are translucent. Add buckwheat groats and sauté while stirring until the groats are coated with oil and cooking juice. Add boiling water and let simmer on low heat for about 15 minutes. Serve with optional sea salt and optional unsalted butter. Serves four to six.

Please make the entire recipe. I want leftovers to take along with me when I leave.

How to Make the Second List

Use Chapters 5-7 to compile a second list of no-no ingredients. Make a photocopy of those pages in these chapters that are relevant to you.

This second list is for you to take along for your own reference. Don't expect busy restaurant staff to take the time to read and understand this list, especially if it is a long one. This list is your master list of ingredient names that can indicate that a product might cause problems for you. It should also list products that often contain ingredients that you do not tolerate, as a reminder why you shouldn't try certain tempting items.

Checklist for Eating Well at Restaurants:

❑ Learn about possible sources of problem ingredients in your diet. To do this:
  ❑ Read Chapters 5-7.
  ❑ Read labels and recipes.
❑ Identify types of restaurants, such as Thai, Japanese, Italian, Mexican, vegetarian or health food, that usually have menu items that are safe for you.
❑ Identify certain types of safe foods that restaurants are likely to be able to provide, even if they are not listed on the menu.
❑ Make a restaurant kit to supplement and improve food you order.

- Nonperishable condiments: Depending on your food sensitivities and personal preference, include items such as sea salt, nutritional yeast, apple cider vinegar, herbal tea bags, etc.
- Perishable condiments: If you are out for just a few hours, you could include perishable items such as unsalted butter.
- Main ingredients: Food items for the chef to cook or otherwise use in the preparation of your meal.
- Work with restaurant staff.
  - Call ahead during nonrush hours to check if a given restaurant is willing and able to accommodate your special needs.
  - Have waiters identify the ingredients in food you are considering eating, including bringing out labels if there is any question of safety.
  - Prepare and carry two lists:
    - List one includes your basic intolerances along with what you like and can have (you might include a few recipes).
    - List two includes ingredient names that can indicate the presence of something to which you are intolerant and types of products you should avoid.
  - Collaborate with staff to get not just a safe meal, but a tasty and satisfying meal.
    - Use the first list to help inspire the chef to come up with creative suggestions.
    - Use the second list to make sure that the chef's suggestions are safe.

The Challenges of An Extended Trip—10 Hints for Eating Well While Traveling

When traveling to unfamiliar places, it is often difficult for people with food sensitivities to predict when and whether they will be able to purchase suitable, safe, appealing food. Therefore, travel with an adequate supply of safe food, so that no matter what happens, you need not go hungry or experience the crankiness of everyone but you getting something really good to eat.

1. Pack Food

If you travel by car, pack an ice chest and a box of nonperishables.

2. Treat Yourself

Take along food that is both a special treat and is easy to eat while traveling.

For a trip one September, I made hummus with strips of red, yellow and green bell peppers for dippers. I still have vivid memories of the crisp fall weather, the Illinois countryside and how delicious the food tasted that day.

3. First Things First

Eat perishables first. I like to pack cooked meals that taste good cold, for example, millet bread and black-eyed peas, stir-fried vegetables with tofu, or hummus with vegetable dippers.

By the time the ice in the cooler has melted, I am ready to focus on less perishable food.

4. Treat Yourself Again

Stash away some not-so-perishable treats. They will provide comfort and security for those times when you want something good, but nothing else around is safe or appealing. For a two-week trip out west, I made oatmeal cookies that contained flaxseeds. I made them because they are healthy and taste good. Since I hid them, they lasted well into the second week of our trip when the more perishable food I had prepared was all eaten. An added benefit, that I only realized after being slyly kidded, is that flaxseeds are very effective in correcting constipation, which many people experience when traveling.

Homemade "zone" bar cookies are also an excellent travel food. Because the protein and carbohydrate content are balanced, they often seem like the perfect snack when I need a boost. (See the next chapter for the recipe.)

Some other examples of food that I frequently pack or pick up along the way are: oatmeal, fresh fruit, dried fruit, fruit juice, crackers, bread, peanut butter, nuts, canned tuna, sea salt, nutritional yeast, olive oil, vinegar and herbal tea bags (rosehips, ginger, Roast-O-Roma™, Vata Tea™, Echinacea, alfalfa and mint).

One of my emergency foods is oatmeal. One-minute oatmeal or oatmeal that has been partially pulverized in a blender does not need to be cooked. Just let it soak in water, milk or fruit juice for a few minutes. I like to add dried fruit and nuts for a more interesting taste and texture.

Juice packs are another convenience. They do not need refrigeration and are easy to carry along when you're on foot.

5. Pick Up Supplements Along the Way

As you travel, supplement the food you have packed with milk, fruit, fruit juice and other safe items available at grocery stores, health food stores, farmers markets and convenience stores.

A phone book and a city map can help you find health food stores in an unfamiliar city. If you need help, call the store and let them give you directions.

6. Heating Coil

Take along a ceramic mug and a heating coil that fits in a mug. This can be used for making tea or simple cooking such as boiling eggs in a mug.

A hot cup of my favorite tea while relaxing in a hotel room is often a luxury that helps smooth over the difficulties of the day. Knowing that I can always add variety to my diet by boiling some eggs for breakfast or for later in the day is also empowering.

7. Camp Stove

Take along a camp stove and some easy recipes, and use roadside rest areas to cook up a quick hot meal.

8. Bring Condiments

Take along a traveler's kit for eating in restaurants (described in step No. 3 of How to Get a Good Meal at a Restaurant). Use this to supplement and enhance the food available to you at restaurants.

For me, taking along unsalted butter, sea salt, vinegar and nutritional yeast often meant the difference between unsalted, boring, plain, steamed vegetables, an undressed salad with a dry baked potato, or the same but with an interesting and tasty dressing and/or butter and salt.

Consider taking along special items that restaurants are not likely to have on hand, but that they could use to cook something special for you. Depending on your sensitivities, this might include special pasta or grains, quick-cooking beans or lentils, or unsalted peanut butter or nuts for making sauces. (See Step No. 4 under How to Get a Good Meal at a Restaurant)

9. Doggie Bags

Make the most of restaurant leftovers. When you find a place that makes food that is safe and that you like, order extra to take along for later.

10. Cook in Exotic Locations

Stay, at least occasionally, in accommodations that include access to a kitchen or kitchenette. This will allow you to cook for yourself and replenish your supplies of safe, cooked food. On extended trips this is often a welcome break from locating a suitable restaurant and negotiating with restaurant staff. Cooking for yourself is also considerably less expensive than eating out.

Hotels, motels, bed and breakfasts, cabins, rooms for rent and houses for rent often have a kitchen or kitchenette available. Such accommodations are not necessarily any more expensive than a plain motel room. For example, in the mid-1990s, on the Florida Gulf coast in mid-March, just outside of St. Joe State Park, I rented a two-bedroom house with a fully appointed kitchen for just $40 a night.

One trick for locating this type of accommodation is to call ahead to the local chamber of commerce, especially in a small community. Explain what you would like. You can often find very nice, relatively inexpensive, locally owned businesses in this manner.

Long-Term Benefits

Ours is a mobile society. Being unable to get safe food at restaurants and while traveling places a huge restriction on where we can go and what we can do. Learning how to acquire safe food while away from home allows us to travel without the burden of always carrying enough food for the entire length of our trip.

Chapter 12: No Need to Feel Deprived—46 Quick and Delicious Recipes for Healthy, Allergen-Free Food

Highlights:

❑ Discussion of the arthritis-healing effects of the foods used in the recipes in this chapter.

❑ Forty-six recipes for quick, delicious, allergen-free food.

❑ Resources for more allergen-free, healing recipes.

Effort Involved:

❑ To prepare allergen-free food you must first have a list of your problem foods. Chapters 3 and 4 explain how to test for food sensitivities.

❑ You must be able to recognize if a given product contains your allergens. Chapters 5-8 explain how to do this.

❑ If your food sensitivities are to corn, wheat, rice, beef or food additives, you can use the recipes in this chapter exactly the way they are. Those were my food sensitivities. The recipes do not contain any of these common problem allergens.

❑ If your food sensitivities are to other types of foods, use the options built into many of these recipes plus the information in Chapter 10 to modify the recipes so they are safe for you.

Payoff:

❑ Tasty, healthy, healing food.

The Arthritis-Healing Effects of the Foods used in These Recipes

The idea of using food as a pharmacy is an ancient one that in the last decade has become quite trendy again. The recipes in this chapter incorporate foods that are known to have a beneficial effect on arthritis. Some of these health-promoting effects are listed below.

Indian Spices

Many Indian spices have been found to be useful in promoting health. Fresh and dried ginger, garlic, turmeric, cloves and bay leaves used in cooking have all been shown to be anti-inflammatory in many scientific tests. Many spices, including turmeric, chili pepper, ginger, cumin, asafetida, fennel and coriander have long been used to improve digestion. Scientific studies have confirmed that these spices stimulate the secretion of various digestive enzymes. Fresh and dried ginger additionally have more than 100 other beneficial effects including helping to heal stomach ulcers, reducing and preventing nausea, acting as an antidepressant and improving peripheral circulation. Licorice and cardamom help heal ulcers. Fenugreek and cinnamon are well-known for helping the body regulate blood-sugar levels, and fenugreek also helps prevent intestinal gas.

A good Indian cookbook will provide you with many great recipes that include these spices.

Dal

Dal is a general name used in Indian cooking to indicate more than 100 types of lentils and peas. Dal also refers to indicate a soup or gravy made from lentils or peas. These soups and gravies are an excellent way to get the benefits of the Indian spices with which they are made. They are also a tasty protein source that is easy to prepare and goes well with a variety of vegetables and grains.

Soy products

Much has been written on the healthy aspects of soy products in the diet. They lower the level of cholesterol in the bloodstream and reduce the risk of cancer, especially breast cancer. Many postmenopausal women find that the boost in estrogen levels from eating soy eases the discomfort that is often associated with the changes brought about by menopause.

Soy products include tofu, tempeh, food-grade soybeans and TVP (textured vegetable protein).

Caution: Textured vegetable protein can include many ingredients besides soy, such as corn, wheat and other grains. Tempeh can also include other ingredients, including rice and wheat. Don't eat either of these products unless you know it to be safe for you.

167

Sea Salt

Regular table salt is mixed about half and half with dextrose, which in its commercial form is a corn product. That means that table salt can be a big problem for corn-intolerant individuals.

Pure sea salt (iodized versions are available) does not contain dextrose, just beneficial trace minerals. Be sure to read labels, however, because occasionally sea salt is sold mixed with dextrose.

Because pure sea salt is pure salt, use only half as much as you would if using table salt.

Fresh Fruits, Vegetables, Beans, Bean Flour and Whole-Grain Flour

These items all contain dietary fiber, which is important for at least two reasons.

First, people with arthritis tend to have sluggish circulation and elimination. Fiber increases the effectiveness and efficiency of digestive-tract elimination, thus helping to reverse one of the factors that creates a predisposition to arthritis in the first place.

Second, soluble fiber, which is found in abundance in apples, beans and bean flour, lowers the glycemic index of anything in your digestive tract. In simple terms this means that your body doesn't have to work as hard to keep your blood-sugar levels on an even keel. The less you stress your body with every meal, the more energy your body has left over for healing.

Yogurt, Miso, and Sauerkraut

Many people with arthritis and food intolerances have an unhealthy array of microorganisms growing in their digestive tracts. Correcting this problem will often result in a lessening or complete reversal of the arthritis and food intolerances.

Yogurt, miso and fresh sauerkraut all contain friendly microorganisms that help restore a healthy balance in your digestive tract. Just eating these foods is not usually enough to restore a healthy balance, but combined with measures described in Chapter 2, they are part of an effective treatment program.

Cabbage Juice

Cabbage juice and to a lesser extent cabbage are high in proteins called mucins. These proteins induce the stomach wall to secrete a protective coating that protects it from stomach acid. This allows a stomach with ulcers and other problems to heal. Spring and summer cabbages that are as fresh as possible from the field have the greatest ulcer-healing ability.

Since digestive tract problems—especially a condition called leaky gut syndrome (see Chapter 2)—are major contributing factors to arthritis and food intolerances, anything that helps heal the stomach is important in treating not just the symptoms but the underlying cause of the problem.

Flaxseed Oil

Flaxseed oil is high in anti-inflammatory omega-3 fatty acids.

Each day your body has about a 1 percent turnover of the fatty acids in your cell membranes. If you eat a diet high in flaxseed oil and low in other types of oil every day for six to eight weeks, at the end of that time you will have converted enough of the fatty acids in your cell membranes into anti-inflammatory omega-3's for you to start to notice a reduction in the painfulness and tenderness in your joints.

About these Recipes

The recipes in this chapter are divided into nine sections: beverages, yogurt, salads and dressings, lentil dishes, chickpea dishes, sauces, vegetable dishes, breads, snacks and desserts. At the end of these recipes is a section listing the location of recipes found elsewhere in this book.

Beverages

Beverages can be both delicious and health-promoting. As the recipes below show, there is a wide array of choices beyond the world of coffee, soda and black tea.

1. Freshly Made Carrot-Cabbage-Celery Juice

This juice is great for restoring health. It is an important part of therapeutic fasting, but is good anytime. Cabbage juice is particularly good for healing the stomach. Carrot juice is chock-full of nutrients and makes the cabbage part of the juice taste **much** better. Celery is good for lowering high blood pressure. All three have anti-cancer effects.

For this recipe you will need an electric juicer. Cheap ones start at about $30. High-quality ones run about $200. You get what you pay for, but either type will work for making juice. Once you have the juicer, the rest is easy.

1/2 lb. organic carrots
1/8 of a small cabbage
OPTIONAL:
1 celery stalk

Wash and trim the vegetables. Cut into pieces. Put through a juicer. Adjust the amount of cabbage used to suit your taste.

Yield: 1 cup

2. Vegetable Broth

Like freshly made vegetable juice, vegetable broth is great for restoring health. It is also an important part of therapeutic fasting, but is good anytime. Its alkalizing effect balances the body's tendency to become overly acidic during fasting or illness. It is also mineral-rich.

Broth is a great energizing drink in the morning with a little miso. Miso is a fermented soybean paste that is highly prized in Japan and available in the United States at health food stores. Use broth with miso as a hot drink in the morning to replace coffee.

2 potatoes, chopped into half-inch pieces
1 cup carrots, sliced
1 cup celery, sliced
OPTIONAL:
1 cup any other available vegetables, such as beet greens, turnip greens, parsley, or a little of everything.

Place vegetable in a stainless steel stockpot. Add 1½ quarts of water. Cover, bring to a boil, then simmer on low for about 30 minutes. Strain and serve warm. If not used immediately store in refrigerator. Always serve warm.

3. Excelsior

The author of *There is a Cure for Arthritis*, Dr. Paavo Airola, recommends excelsior as a way for those with constipation to restore normal bowel movement. Correcting constipation is important for any long-term healing of arthritis.

1 cup vegetable broth
1 Tbsp. whole flaxseed
1 Tbsp. wheat bran

Soak flaxseed and wheat bran in vegetable broth overnight. In the morning, warm up, stir well and drink, seeds and all. Do not chew the flaxseeds—drink them whole.

If you have a wheat sensitivity, skip the wheat bran.

4. Herbal Tea

Clover, nettle and especially alfalfa tea are all very good for helping to heal arthritis. However, it you have lupus, avoid alfalfa.

I recommend buying these herbs loose from a health food store and enjoying them one at a time or as a mixture made to suit your own taste. I like to add a little loose mint to my tea to enhance the taste.

To brew, add 1 to 2 Tbsp. of the loose leaves to a 2-cup tea pot. Add boiling water. Let steep with the lid on for 10-15 minutes. Pour through a strainer and enjoy.

5. Ginger-Turmeric Milk

This drink is good for calming inflammation and is one of the most stomach-soothing ways I have found to take ginger. Drink this twice a day, early in the morning and just before bedtime. If pressed for time, double the recipe, drink one serving and reheat the second.

Bring ½ cup of water to a boil and add:

> ½ tsp. turmeric
> ½ Tbsp. freshly shredded ginger root
> 4 to 6 green cardamom pods, ground, or about ½ tsp. cardamom powder

Let the mixture simmer for a minute or two, then add:
> 1 cup milk

Boil 3 minutes, then strain and serve.
If you like, stir in honey or maple syrup to taste.

Yield: 1 serving

6. Ginger Ale

> 2 inches of fresh ginger, peeled and thinly sliced
> 4 to 6 cups water
> 4 limes
> Honey to taste
> OPTIONAL:
> seltzer water

Boil ginger in water for 20-30 minutes. Let cool. Juice limes and add to ginger water. Add honey to taste. Depending on your preference, you can discard the ginger or snack on it while drinking the ginger ale. This ale tastes excellent without a fizz, but if you like carbonation, add some seltzer water.

> Yield: approximately 4-6 cups

7. Nut and Seed Milk

Nut and seed milks are very tasty. They are good on cereal and in cooking.

> ½ cup nuts or seeds (for example, pecans, almonds, filberts, walnuts, cashews, Brazil nuts, sunflower seeds, pumpkin seeds, sesame seeds, toasted quinoa seeds, etc.)
> 2 cups water
> OPTIONAL:
> 1 to 2 dates, 1 fig or a small handful of raisins

Place nuts or seeds and optional ingredients in a blender. Blend until finely ground. Add ½ cup water and blend at low speed for a few seconds. Then blend on high for a couple of minutes. Gradually add 1½ cups water and blend well, using a spatula to scrape the sides of the blender as needed.

Some milks, such as those made from almonds or sesame seeds, need to be strained for best results. Taste the milk after it has been blended. If it is already smooth, it is ready to use. If it has small pieces in it, strain it through cheesecloth or a fine sieve.

Will keep 4 or 5 days under refrigeration.

> Yield: 2 cups

8. Banana Smoothie

I like this recipe better than ice cream. Vary the amount of milk to control consistency. Smoothies can be thick like ice cream or thin like shakes.

1 cup milk
1 or 2 small frozen bananas
10 almonds or other seeds or nuts

Place ingredients in blender. Blend on low for a few seconds, then switch
to high for about a minute.

Yield: about 2 cups

9. Fruit Smoothie

This is basically the same recipe as above, except you substitute any fruit
for the bananas and substitute water for the milk.

¼ cup nuts or seeds
1 cup water
About 1 cup fresh or frozen fruit, any variety

Place ingredients in blender. Blend on low for a few seconds, then switch
to high for about a minute.

Yield: about 2 cups

10. Refreshing Lassi

This is a great drink on a hot day. It is especially good if you use
homemade yogurt.

½ cup fresh plain yogurt
1½ to 2 cups pure water
⅛ to ¼ tsp. turmeric
½ tsp. fresh ginger, grated
1 tsp. fresh lemon juice
1 Tbsp. raw honey

Blend the ingredients together. This is a thin drink—much thinner than the
normal thickness of smoothies. It supports digestion, especially when taken
at the end of a meal.

Yield: 2 to 2 ½ cups

Yogurt and Cottage Cheese

No store-bought yogurt can match the taste and creamy texture of freshly
made homemade yogurt. As an added benefit, you know and control

exactly what goes into the yogurt. Of course, the live bacteria in yogurt support good health, especially after a round of antibiotics or when gut bacteria are in a state of imbalance, by reseeding the gut with healthy intestinal flora.

Cottage cheese can be made from homemade yogurt. A recipe is included for this as well.

11. Homemade Yogurt

To control temperature during the incubation time, you can use a homemade yogurt maker that has a temperature-controlled chamber, you can pour your heated mixture into a wide-mouthed thermos bottle, or you can make an incubation chamber with a cheap Styrofoam cooler and a light bulb. The cooler is placed upside down with the light bulb inside, and the cooler is then propped open just enough to keep a constant 99°F incubation temperature. If you like baking with sourdough or commercial yeast cultures, this same set-up can be used to provide optimal rising conditions for your dough.

Do not bake with yeast and make yogurt on the same day. Too much yeast in the air tends to contaminate yogurt cultures, rendering them unpalatable.

> 1 quart pasteurized skim milk
> > OR
> 3 ¾ cups water and 1½ cups nonfat dry milk powder
>
> 2 to 3 Tbsp. live culture yogurt from grocery store or health food store

Heat milk to just above body temperature, just over 99°F—but do not boil. Add the yogurt and stir well. Place in cups or a bottle for incubation. Let it stand 5 to 8 hours or overnight at a constant incubation temperature of 99°F, using one of the incubation strategies mentioned above. In 5 to 8 hours the culture should be solid and ready to serve. Discard any cultures that are discolored or smell funny.

Save 2 or 3 spoonfuls of your fresh, homemade yogurt to use as a starter culture for your next batch.

Yield: 1 quart yogurt

12. Cottage Cheese

Make yogurt using the recipe above. Place the yogurt in warm water, approximately 115°F, for 1 to 2 hours, until curdled. Place cheesecloth or a clean linen canvas over a strainer or drainer. Pour the curdled yogurt over it. Allow all the whey (the clear yellowish liquid) to pass through. The solids that remain are cottage cheese. If the curds of cheese are too hard, add a little sweet cream and stir. Using whole milk instead of low-fat or nonfat milk makes for a softer cheese as well.

Salads and Dressings

Salads are an important source of fresh vegetables, and an important part of any healthy diet. The dressings below add variety and extra appeal to salads and use oils and spices that have an anti-inflammatory and health-restoring effect.

13. Green Salad

Use any available vegetables: lettuce, spinach, beet greens, watercress, green onions, parsley, grated carrots, tomatoes, celery, cucumbers, green or red bell peppers, avocado, green cabbage, red cabbage, radish, artichokes, Swiss chard, broccoli, cauliflower, kohlrabi, etc.

Wash vegetables. Break leaves into bite-sized pieces. Cut, chop or shred other vegetables. Place in a big salad bowl. Add a couple of spoonfuls of olive oil, flaxseed oil or one of the dressings listed below. Toss until the vegetables are coated with oil or dressing.

If using oil, add the juice of half a lemon or 2 tsp. apple cider vinegar. Also feel free to add your favorite spices and herbs, such as basil, dill, cilantro, chives, mint, garlic, kelp, paprika or anise. Nutritional yeast, chopped nuts, or flaxseeds are also good sprinkled on salads.

Toss once more and serve immediately. This salad can be served alone, with cottage cheese or with a cooked vegetable such as baked potatoes or baked sweet potatoes.

14. Anti-inflammatory Oil and Vinegar Dressing

This is a great way to get the anti-inflammatory effects of the omega-3 oil in flaxseed oil.

1 cup flaxseed oil (available at health food stores)

2 tsp. apple cider vinegar
OPTIONAL:
1 or more cloves of garlic, minced
Your favorite herbs or spices.

Combine the ingredients. Let sit overnight if using garlic to let the taste infuse into the oil.

Yield: about 1 cup

15. Avocado Dressing

This dressing is a fancy way to use avocados. If you are in a hurry, just slice or mash an avocado and add it to a salad, as is.

Juice of ¼ of a lemon or a lime
1 small avocado, peeled and seeded
1 garlic clove, coarsely chopped
3 scallions, including an inch of the greens, roughly chopped
¼ cup chopped cilantro
½ cup plus 2 Tbsp. olive oil or avocado oil

Put everything but the oil in a blender and puree. Gradually pour in the oil with the machine running.

This dressing will hold well, refrigerated, for several hours. Place plastic wrap directly on the surface to prevent browning.

Yield: 1 ½ cups

16. Asian Salad Dressing

This dressing is especially good on steamed broccoli and tofu.

½ cup canola oil
¼ cup rice vinegar (if you have a rice sensitivity, substitute apple cider vinegar or wine vinegar)
2 Tbsp. sesame oil
1½ Tbsp. peeled and minced fresh ginger
2 tsp. soy sauce (if you are sensitive to wheat, corn or rice, substitute barley miso)
Ground pepper

In a medium bowl whisk all of the ingredients together. Drizzle over mixed greens or steamed vegetables.

Yield: 8 (2 Tbsp.) servings

176

17. Japanese-Style Carrot Dressing

This bright orange dressing has great visual as well as taste appeal.

> 1 small carrot, shredded (about 1 cup)
> 2 Tbsp. wine (if you have a wheat, beef or poor sensitivity, substitute apple cider vinegar)
> 2 Tbsp. apple cider vinegar
> 1 Tbsp. barley miso
> OPTIONAL:
> ½ tsp. dark sesame oil
> 1 Tbsp. grated fresh ginger root
> ¼ cake silken tofu, about 3 ounces

Put all ingredients in a blender and whirl until smooth. Store chilled in a covered jar. Will keep about a week (less with tofu).

Yield: about 1 ½ cups

18. Nutritional Yeast as a Condiment

Nutritional yeast is rich in the B vitamins. Increasing intake of these vitamins can be an important part of healing from arthritis.

Nutritional yeast tastes good in many of the same dishes that cheese is traditionally used. This includes sprinkled on salads, stir-fried vegetables, lentils, rice and kasha. It is also good sprinkled on potatoes, popcorn and in vegetable broth.

Lentil Dishes

Lentils are high in protein, easy to digest and don't need to be soaked overnight like other beans, although they will be even easier to digest if you do. They are a satisfying and versatile food that lends itself to a variety of healthy recipes.

19. Dal—Version 1

In India the word "dal" refers to lentils and beans and also to a soup made from them. Masur dal is made from red lentils, and moong or mung dal from split mung beans. Chana and urad dal are made from still other varieties of lentils. All of these types can be found at Indian grocery stores and each is an excellent choice for this soup. Split peas also work well in this recipe.

Ghee is clarified butter. It can be purchased at Indian grocery stores or made by heating butter over low heat for an hour or two until the solids in the butter drop to the bottom of the pan. The clear liquid is the ghee. Alternatively, you can simply use unsalted butter or canola oil in place of ghee in this recipe.

Asafetida is a spice that can be purchased at Indian grocery stores. It has a distinctive taste and smell that some people love and other people strongly dislike. It is good for digestion. Unfortunately for those with a wheat intolerance, it is usually sold mixed with wheat flour. This recipe works just fine if you leave out the asafetida.

> 1 cup dal or split peas
> 8 cups water
> 1½ tsp. sea salt
> 2 bay leaves
> 1 cinnamon stick, 3 inches long, broken in half
> 1 tsp. turmeric
> 1 Tbsp. butter
> 10 oz. assorted vegetables, washed and cubed
> 2 Tbsp. ghee
> 1½ tsp. cumin seeds
> 2 dried chili peppers, crushed
> 2 tsp. grated ginger
> 1 tsp. chopped fresh cilantro leaves
> OPTIONAL:
> 1 tsp. asafetida, omit if sensitive to wheat
> 2 lemons, cut into 8 wedges each

Clean and wash the dal. Drain. Combine water, salt, bay leaves and pieces of cinnamon stick in a heavy saucepan or pot. Bring to a boil and add the dal.

When the water comes to a second boil, partially cover the pot, lower to medium heat, and cook for about 20 minutes, or until the dal grains are quite tender. Remove any froth that collects at the top. Then put in the turmeric and butter. Add vegetables, replace the lid, and continue cooking on the same heat until the vegetables are tender and the dal is completely broken up. Let the dal simmer while you prepare the seasonings.

Heat 2 Tbsp. ghee, unsalted butter or canola oil in a small frying pan and toss in the cumin seeds and crushed chili pepper. Stir once. When the cumin seeds darken, put in the grated ginger and asafetida, if using, and fry a few more seconds. Pour the seasonings into the dal, and simmer for 4 or 5 minutes. Serve with a steaming hot grain such as rice and, if desired, additional vegetables. See Chapter 10 for an extensive list of grains that you can substitute for rice.

Garnish with chopped cilantro and lemon wedges, if desired.

This dal should have a thin consistency. If it is too thick, add some hot water.

Yield: 8 servings

20. Dal—Version 2

This versions calls for whole black mustard seeds, which can be found at Indian grocery stores and international grocery stores that carry Indian spices. Using the whole white mustard seeds found in the spice section of most grocery stores also produces a tasty although slightly less authentic dish.

1 cup dal or split peas
4 cups water
1 tsp. turmeric
4 Tbsp. unsalted butter
½ tsp. whole black mustard seeds
½ onion, chopped
1 clove garlic, minced
1 tsp. grated ginger
¼ hot chili pepper
¼ tsp. ground cumin
¼ tsp. ground coriander
crushed seeds from one cardamom pod or ¼ tsp. ground cardamom
¾ tsp. sea salt

Carefully wash dal or split peas. Put in pot with water and turmeric. Bring to a boil, cover, and simmer for 1 hour or more, until the dal is tender. Add water as necessary.

In a small frying pan melt butter and begin cooking black mustard seeds until they begin to pop. Add onion and garlic and turn heat to low. Add ginger, chili pepper, cumin, coriander and cardamom. Simmer for about 5 minutes.

Add the spice mix and salt to the dal. Simmer 30 minutes and taste. Add more salt if needed. Serve as a thin gravy over a cooked grain such as rice.

Yield: about 4 servings

21. Lentils and Rice

This is another simple but satisfying lentil dish. The attended cooking time is short, so this is a good dish to make when you are tired. You can rest while it cooks. You can also substitute any grain you desire for the rice. Use rye berries for a pleasantly chewy alternative.

> 5 Tbsp. olive oil
> 1 large onion, chopped
> 1¼ cups green or brown lentils, sorted and rinsed
> ¾ cup brown rice
> Sea salt

Heat oil in a 2- or 3-quart sauce pan over medium heat. Add onion and cook until it turns translucent. Add lentils and rice. Stir until they are coated with the oil and onion liquid. Add water to cover; bring to a boil and then simmer on low heat for 30 to 45 minutes or until the water is absorbed and the grain and lentils done. Salt to taste. Serve alone or with a vegetable salad or cooked vegetable.

Yield: 4 servings

22. Lentil Salad

This salad is often just the right thing on a hot day. The lentils are earthy, the tofu absorbs the flavors of the marinade, and the green beans add a pleasant, fresh texture.

> 1½ cups dried lentils
> 1 bay leaf
> 1 lb. fresh green beans or pole beans
> 4 garlic cloves, minced
> 1/8 tsp. salt
> 3 Tbsp. apple cider vinegar
> ¼ cup olive oil
> 10 to 16 ounces firm tofu, cubed
> ½ cup fresh parsley
> 4 Tbsp. herbs such as fresh minced mint, lovage and/or sage

Rinse the lentils. Place them in a medium pot with a bay leaf and cover with an inch or two of water. Bring to a boil, turn down to a simmer and then cook covered with a lid for 20 to 30 minutes. The lentils should be cooked but still firm enough to hold their shape.

Wash and string beans. If you have a steamer, steam beans for about 20 minutes or until done. If you don't have a steamer, boil them, not quite covered with water, for about 20 minutes or until done.

Prepare the dressing. Place the garlic and salt in a small bowl. Using the back of a spoon or a pestle, press the garlic to a paste. Mix in the vinegar and olive oil.

When the lentils are cooked, drain and immediately toss in a large bowl with the dressing. Add the cooked beans. Gently mix in the cubed tofu. Set aside to marinate for 1 hour.

Before serving, toss in the parsley and herbs. Add a touch more vinegar if needed.

Yield: 4 servings

23. Baked Lentils with Cheese

This is a simple dish to make. I consider it a comfort food (hearty but easy to digest) with some of the same appeal as pizza since it also has tomatoes and melted cheese.

1¾ cups lentils, rinsed
2 cups water
1 whole bay leaf
1 tsp. sea salt
¼ tsp. black pepper
⅛ tsp. marjoram
⅛ tsp. sage
⅛ tsp. thyme
2 large onions, chopped
2 cloves garlic, chopped
2 cups canned tomatoes (if corn-sensitive buy a brand made with sea salt or no salt, or if necessary use a can of tomato paste which has no salt and mix with a little water to thin, or use fresh tomatoes)
2 large carrots, thinly sliced
½ cup celery, thinly sliced
3 cups grated white cheddar cheese (white cheddar made with sea salt is available in health food stores)
OPTIONAL:
1 green pepper, chopped
2 Tbsp. finely chopped parsley

Preheat oven to 375°F.

Combine the lentils, water, bay leaf, spices, onions, garlic and tomatoes in a shallow 9 x 13-inch or 2- to 3-quart baking dish, preferably one with a lid. Cover and bake for 30 minutes.

Uncover and stir in carrots and celery. Bake covered 40 minutes more until vegetables are tender.

Stir in optional green pepper and parsley. Sprinkle grated cheddar cheese on top. Bake uncovered 5 minutes, until cheese melts.

Yield: 6 servings

Chickpea Dishes

Chickpeas, also known as garbanzo beans, or in flour form as besan flour, are another high-protein, easy-to-digest food. They are popular in Indian and Middle Eastern cuisines. The recipes below represent just two of the many ways to fix chickpeas. See the chocolate cake in the dessert section for a surprising and delightful way to use chickpea flour.

24. Savory Bread

This bread from India is so colorful and delicious that you might forget how healthy it is. Because it is steamed instead of baked, it is a good bread to make in the summer when you don't want to heat up your kitchen.

For the batter:
1½ cups sifted chickpea flour (a.k.a. besan or garbanzo bean flour)
1½ Tbsp. peeled, minced fresh ginger root
¼ tsp. turmeric
½ tsp. sea salt
3 Tbsp. melted, unsalted butter, ghee or sesame oil, plus 1 tsp. for the pan
⅔ cup plain yogurt or buttermilk
½ tsp. grain-free baking powder
½ tsp. baking soda
3 Tbsp. warm water
OPTIONAL:
1 tsp. brown sugar
¼ tsp. cracked black pepper

For the garnish:
⅓ cup grated coconut

3 Tbsp. coarsely chopped fresh coriander leaves
¼ cup unsalted butter or ghee
½ Tbsp. black mustard seeds, sesame seed or black poppy seeds

Combine the flour, ginger, turmeric, salt and optional sugar and pepper in a medium mixing bowl and blend well. Stir in 3 Tbsp. of butter, ghee or oil and the yogurt or buttermilk and mix into a thick batter. Add warm water as needed to get to moist batter consistency. Cover and set aside at room temperature or in the refrigerator for 8 hours or overnight. Add more water if the batter gets too thick to stir.

Set up an arrangement for steaming. I use a 4-quart stockpot, an 8-inch spring-form pan and an empty tuna can with both the top and bottom removed. The tuna can sits in the bottom of the stockpot and holds the spring-form pan away from the bottom of the pot. I fill the stockpot with water to within ½ inch of the top of the tuna can. Have a clean dish towel ready to line the inside of the lid during steaming. Pour 1 tsp. melted butter or oil into the cake pan and tilt to spread it over the bottom and sides.

When you are ready to steam the bread, place the steaming pot over moderately high heat, covered to bring the water to a boil. (Because my particular steaming arrangement is so tight, to avoid being scalded when I lower my spring-form pan into the steaming pot, I do not heat the water to a full boil.) Sprinkle the baking powder and soda into the chickpea-yogurt batter and mix. Pour in the water and gently stir in one direction until the batter begins to froth. Immediately pour the batter into the prepared pan and set in the steaming pot.

A dish towel is used to keep the steam that condenses inside the pot from dripping on the batter. Stretch the towel across the top of the stockpot and then put the lid of the stockpot on to hold the towel in place. Alternatively, stretch the towel across the inside edge of the lid and put the lid on the pot. Place the edges of the towel on top of the lid to keep them away from the burner. Steam for about 15 minutes. Uncover and insert a toothpick into the bread. If it comes out clean, the bread is cooked. If not, steam a few more minutes. Remove the finished bread and set it aside, loosely covered, for 10 minutes.

On a cutting board, cut the bread into roughly 1 1/2 inch pieces. Sprinkle with grated coconut and chopped coriander leaves. Heat the unsalted butter or ghee or oil in a small pot over moderate heat. When it is hot, add the mustard seeds and fry until they sputter and pop. Pour over the bread. If you use sesame or poppy seeds, add the seeds to the pan and within 5 seconds, pour over the bread. Serve warm or at room temperature.

Yield: 24 pieces

25. Hummus

This is a good dip to take to parties. I also like to take it along, with vegetable dippers, as a snack on long car trips. Chickpeas and chickpeas are two names for the same thing.

> 1 cup dried chickpeas or 4 cups cooked chickpeas
> ½ cup water
> 3 Tbsp. tahini (sesame butter)
> 2 Tbsp. lemon or lime juice
> 1 or more cloves garlic
> OPTIONAL:
> 1 tsp. sesame oil
> 1 tsp. cumin
> salt and pepper to taste

If using dried chickpeas, soak overnight. Rinse several times and then cover with water. Bring to a boil and then for 20-30 minutes.

Then place all the ingredients in a food processor or blender. Blend until creamy. Chill before serving. Makes a great dip for pita bread and for vegetables such as broccoli, cauliflower and bell pepper cut into bite-sized pieces.

Yield: 4 1/2 cups

26. Falafel

Falafel is very popular in the Middle East. Instead of traditional deep-frying, this recipe calls for baking. It still has the same great taste, but is healthier and less of a hassle to make.

> 3 cups cooked chickpeas
> ¼ cup liquid from cooked beans
> ¼ cup wheat germ or cracker crumbs (if wheat- or corn-sensitive use crumbs left over from anything bready you have cooked from the breads recipe section)
> 1 small onion, finely chopped
> 2 garlic cloves, minced
> 4 Tbsp. chopped fresh parsley
> ¼ cup sesame seeds
> ¼ cup dried oregano
> 1 tsp. cumin
> 1 tsp. chili powder

¼ cup lemon juice
¾ cup wheat germ or cracker crumbs

Soak 1 cup chickpeas (garbanzo beans) 8 hours or overnight. Rinse thoroughly, cover with water and simmer for 45 minutes. This should yield about 3 cups cooked chickpeas, with perhaps a cup left over for other uses, including eating plain.

Preheat oven to 400°F. Blend chickpeas and ¼ cup liquid in blender. Place blended chickpeas in a large bowl and add other ingredients except for wheat germ or cracker crumbs. Mix well. Add just enough wheat germ or cracker crumbs so the mixture will hold together.

With hands roll mixture into balls 1 ½ inch in diameter. Arrange balls on a nonstick cookie sheet and bake for 20 to 30 minutes. Turn occasionally during baking to brown evenly.

Serve with tahini sauce (see tahini sauce recipe given below).

Yield: about 20 small patties

Sauces

Sauces can be used to dress up falafel, pasta, vegetables, meat and fish. Use your imagination.

27. Tahini Sauce

This sauce is especially good on falafel and spaghetti squash.

> 1 cup unsalted tahini (sesame seed paste, available in health food stores and Middle Eastern markets)
> ½ cup water
> OPTIONAL:
> 2 Tbsp. Fresh lemon juice
> 1/4 to ½ cup plain yogurt
> 3 cloves minced garlic

Place ingredients in blender. Blend until smooth.

Yield: 1 1/2 cups

28. Pesto

Pesto can be made with any leafy herbs, but it is usually made with basil leaves.

This recipe gives you an option of using basil, cilantro or parsley. Mixtures of any of these herbs also yield good pestos.

> 4 cups fresh basil leaves
> OR
> 4 cups fresh cilantro leaves
> OR
> 4 cups fresh parsley
> OR
> 4 cups of a mixture of basil, cilantro and parsley leaves
>
> ½ cup extra-virgin olive oil
> 6 cloves garlic
> ¼ cup walnuts, pecans or pine nuts
> ¼ tsp. sea salt

Wash herbs and remove stems. In a blender or food processor process herbs and olive oil into a fine puree. Add the rest of ingredients and process until smooth.

Freeze in small containers for future use or store in refrigerator for up to one week.

If you wish, you can blend the herbs and garlic with just enough olive oil to make processing efficient. Chopped nuts and salt can be added when serving.

Use about 2 Tbsp. per serving to flavor pasta, spaghetti squash, salmon, etc. or in place of tomato sauce on pizza.

Pesto also tastes great with a little Parmesan cheese.

Yield: about 1⅔ cups

Vegetable Dishes

Vegetables are an important part of any healthy diet. Especially if you have multiple food intolerances, you may have to rely heavily on vegetables as the mainstay of your diet. Find vegetable recipes that are hearty and satisfying and, most importantly, that you like. Recipes from countries like

India that have a strong vegetarian tradition are a good place to start, but keep your eye out for any recipes that work for you.

Here are a few of my favorites:

29. Scalloped Butternut Squash and Spinach

My 6-year-old-nephew loves spinach when served this way. The bright orange of the squash and the deep green of the spinach make this a festive Thanksgiving dish.

> 1 butternut squash (1 to 2 lbs.)
> 2 lbs. fresh spinach or 2 10-ounce packages of frozen chopped spinach
> 8 ounces white cheddar cheese (health food stores sell varieties made with sea salt)

Cut squash in half and remove seeds. Bake for 30 minutes at 400°F, with squash facing down in a baking pan filled with 1 inch of water. Let cool. Remove skin and mash or cut into small pieces.

If using fresh spinach, wash and chop. In a covered pan with ½ inch water in the bottom, heat spinach for about 10 minutes or until lightly cooked. Otherwise, thaw and drain.

Grate cheese.

Mix the three ingredients together in a baking pan. Just before serving, heat in 300°F oven for 15-20 minutes or until warm. Individual servings heat well in a microwave oven.

Yield: 10-12 servings

30. Spaghetti Squash

Spaghetti squash is great for those of us with grain allergies. It can be eaten any way that traditional spaghetti is eaten, including with tomato sauce or pesto. My personal favorite is spaghetti squash with a little tahini straight from the jar.

This type of squash keeps well at room temperature, so it is easy to keep a few on hand.

To cook:

Pierce skin in several places and microwave on high, about 6 minutes per pound. It is done when shell gives to the touch and feels soft. Cut open and scoop out seeds. Then scoop out "spaghetti" for use.

OR

Cut in half. Scoop out seeds. Bake face down in 1-inch of water at 350°F for one hour.

OR

Cut into pieces and boil for about 30 minutes or until done.

Yield: 6-8 servings

31. Carrot Cutlets

My friend Helen made these for me for my birthday. I loved them so much I just had to have the recipe. They were a perfect change of pace from the stir-fry and Indian food I usually ate.

2 cups cooked brown rice or millet
1 small onion, peeled and finely chopped
1 Tbsp. fresh parsley, finely chopped
1 cup carrots, cooked and mashed (about 3 raw carrots)
1 Tbsp. water or soy milk
2 Tbsp. arrowroot powder or other binder (see Chapter 10 for an extensive list of other binders)
¾ cup wheat germ (substitute more rice or millet if sensitive to wheat)
2 Tbsp. oil

Mix all the ingredients together in a bowl, except the oil. Form 12 small patties.

Heat the oil in a large frying pan over medium heat. Fry carrot cutlets for 5 minutes or until brown on one side. Flip over fry for another 5 minutes.

Serve cutlets warm, 2 per serving. They are good plain or with sautéed onions or mushrooms.

Yield: 6 servings

32. Cabbage and Carrot Sauté

This is a quick and tasty dish. The ginger powder and lemon juice really bring out the flavor.

½ medium cabbage, shredded
1 lb. carrots, peeled and grated

2 cloves garlic, peeled and minced
½ tsp. ginger powder
Salt and pepper to taste
2 tsp. oil
1 Tbsp. lemon juice.

Sauté all the ingredients, except the lemon juice, in a large frying pan over medium-high heat for 5 minutes. Add the lemon juice and continue to sauté for 2 more minutes. Serve warm.

Yield: 6 Servings

33. Saag with Tofu

This is a delicious Indian dish. Farmers markets often have fresh greens. Use whatever looks freshest. My favorite is beet greens. They are high in minerals, delicious and often available free for the asking at stands that sell beets.

2 lbs. fresh greens, such as spinach, mustard greens and/or beet greens
½ cup unsalted butter or vegetable oil
1½ tsp. whole cumin seed
1 small hot pepper, crushed
1 large clove garlic
1 tsp. turmeric
1 lb. firm tofu, drained and cut into 1-inch cubes
1½ tsp. ground cumin
2½ tsp. ground coriander
1 tsp. salt

Thoroughly wash the greens. Coarsely chop. If using a green such as mustard or turnip greens that tend to be bitter, add to boiling water, boil a few minutes and drain well. Boiling and draining minimizes bitterness.

Melt the butter or oil in a large frying pan. Add whole cumin seed, hot pepper, garlic and turmeric. When butter or oil is hot, add tofu cubes. Stir over high heat for a few minutes. Begin adding greens and continue frying until greens are wilted, or if pre-boiled, until hot. Add ground cumin, coriander and salt. Cover and simmer 10 minutes.

Yield: 4 servings

Breads

If you have problems with corn and/or wheat, or if you are gluten-intolerant, it will be difficult for you to find bread and other baked goods that are safe for you to eat.

Luckily there are many fine recipes that will allow you to make pancakes, muffins, wafers and bread that is safe. Below are a few to get you started.

34. Urad Flour Crepes, Blintzes or Tortillas

These crepes are very high in protein. The urad flour makes an almost creamy batter that is especially good as a thin batter for crepes.

You can also make a thicker batter and cook like a pancake, but the batter is so creamy that instead of cooking on the inside like a pancake, it will tend to remain soft and gooey, almost like a cream filling.

> 1 cup urad flour or other bean flour
> 1to 2 cups water (enough to make a thin batter)
> 3 tsp. ground cumin
> OPTIONAL:
> sugar or other sweetener to taste

Mix the ingredients above, until you have a smooth batter. Let batter rest 4 to 24 hours. As bean flours soak up water they become thick and creamy. Depending on how much water you added originally and how long you let the batter rest, you may need to add more water to get the batter thinned down to pancake or crepe batter consistency.

After letting batter rest 4-24 hours, add:
> 1 egg
> 1 tsp. grain-free baking powder

Cook as you would pancakes or crepes. Use a thinner batter for crepes. Serve with yogurt sauce, peanut butter, syrup or fruit. Can also be used for blintzes or as tortillas.

Yield: 10 crepes or blintzes or tortillas

35. Any Flour Pancakes and Waffles

Once you taste how good pancakes and waffles are with alternative flours, you may wonder why anyone would want any other kind.

> 1 cup oat flour or other flour
> 2 tsp. grain-free baking powder
> ⅛ tsp. sea salt
> 1 egg or egg substitute
> ½ to ¾ cup liquid, half soy milk or other milk substitute and half water
> 1 Tbsp. oil for pancakes, 2 Tbsp. oil for waffles
> OPTIONAL:
> 1 Tbsp. honey or other sweetener
> ½ cup frozen blueberries, thawed
> ½ cup chopped pecans or other nuts

Mix together dry ingredients. Make a well and add rest of ingredients. Mix well. Start with ½ cup liquid and add more if batter is too stiff. If blueberries are juicy, less liquid will be required. If egg or sweetener is omitted, more liquid may be needed.

For an egg substitute mix 1 Tbsp. psyllium seed husk in 3 Tbsp. of water. Let stand 2 minutes, then add to batter in place of egg. Alternatively, use any of the egg substitutes mentioned in Chapter 10.

Pour by spoonfuls onto a medium hot griddle, making small 4-inch pancakes. Cook well on one side, then turn to cook the other side.

For waffles add appropriate amount of batter to a hot waffle iron. Cook 5 minutes or until done.

Yield: 2 or 3 servings

36. Any Flour Muffins

Muffins are quick and easy. They can be made ahead of time for a quick breakfast or snack.

> 1½ cups any type of flour
> 2 Tbsp. arrowroot powder
> 2 tsp. grain-free baking powder
> 1 tsp. cinnamon
> ⅛ tsp. sea salt
> ½ to 1 cup chopped nuts

3 Tbsp. or more milk, soy milk, other milk substitute, fruit juice or water
1 Tbsp. oil

1 large ripe mashed banana
OR
½ to ¾ cup applesauce, pumpkin puree or shredded zucchini

OPTIONAL:
1 Tbsp. honey or other sweetener
1 egg

Preheat oven to 425°F. Grease a muffin tin with canola oil.

Combine dry ingredients. Make a well in dry ingredients and combine wet ingredients. Mix lightly. Add 3 Tbsp. liquid initially; add more in 2 Tbsp. increments if needed to moisten flour. Dough should be stiff.

Divide dough evenly among the 12 muffin cups. Bake about 12 minutes. Immediately after removing from oven, loosen muffins with a fork and turn them sideways in the cups to cool.

Yield: 12 muffins

37. Sunflower-Rye Muffins

These muffins are exquisite, especially on the day they are made. The sunflower seeds add the perfect touch of crunchiness.

1½ cups rye flour
⅓ cup sunflower seeds, coarsely ground
1½ tsp. cream of tartar
¾ tsp. baking soda
½ tsp. sea salt
½ tsp. cinnamon
6 Tbsp. nonfat dry milk powder
3 Tbsp. canola oil
3 Tbsp. Molasses
1 egg, lightly beaten
1 cup water

Preheat oven to 400°F. Combine dry ingredients. Make a well in the center and add liquid ingredients. Stir until moistened. Spoon into oiled muffin cups. Bake about 20 minutes.

Yield: 9-12 muffins

38. Oat Wafers

If you miss crackers, this is the recipe for you.

> 2½ cups rolled oats
> 2 tsp. dried dill
> 2 tsp. sesame or caraway seeds
> 1½ Tbsp. canola oil
> ½ cup water
> Coarsely ground sea salt

Preheat oven to 325°.

Grind 1 cup of oats into coarse powder in a blender. Transfer to bowl. Add other ingredients except salt. Stir until dough forms. Halve dough. Shape into smooth patties. Top with a bit of salt. Roll out until thin. Using 2-inch biscuit cutter, cut out rounds. Place on nonstick baking sheet.

Bake until pale gold (40-45 min). Cool on rack. Store in airtight container. Keeps well for 2 weeks. Crisp from oven but soften with storage. Good with soup or salad.

Yield: about 36 crackers

39. Sourdough Rye Bread

Rye bread is heavier than wheat bread, but if you like hearty bread, this is for you. The tricks are to make sure you start with an activated sourdough culture and that you allow enough rising time. Use these tricks and get good bread. Skip these tricks and get something resembling a rock.

> 8 cups freshly ground whole rye flour
> 3 cups warm water
> ½ cup sourdough culture, activated the day before*

Mix 7 cups of flour with water and sourdough culture. Cover and let stand in a warm place overnight, 12-18 hours. Add remaining flour and mix well. Place in pans greased with canola oil. Lightly oil the top of loaves with canola oil and cover with a damp towel. Let rise for approximately ½ to 3 hours, depending on how well the loaves are rising. Bake at 350°F, one hour or more if needed.

Always leave ½ cup of dough as a culture for the next baking. Keep the culture in a tight jar in your refrigerator. See the section on leavenings in Chapter 10 for instructions on how to make your own initial sourdough culture.

193

*If you haven't used your culture in a while, pour off any gray liquid smelling of alcohol and add a little sweetener, water and rye flour. Let the starter sit in a warm place for 12-24 hours before you need it, in order to reactivate it.

Yield: 2 loaves

Snacks

Use your imagination. There are many options for quick and easy snacks:

- Fresh fruit, such as bananas, cherries, apples, pears, grapes, watermelon, cantaloupe, honeydew melon, peaches, blueberries, raspberries, strawberries, etc.
- Dried fruit, such as pineapple, figs, raisins, dates, papaya, bananas, apples, etc. Try to find fruit that is unsulfured.
- Yogurt with fruit or nuts and sweetened with honey
- Unsalted nuts such as pecans, walnuts, hazelnuts, cashews, Brazil nuts, soy nuts, almonds or peanuts.
- Trail mix
- Granola
- Smoothies (recipes in the beverage section)
- Leftovers of anything you like

Desserts

What about those times when everyone else is having some sort of cookie, cake or pie?

Perhaps the recipes below will inspire you (or someone who would like to cook up a special treat for you!) to create desserts you can have.

Make sure that at least on occasion you get dessert, too!

40. In the Zone Almond Oatmeal Cookies

One popular theory in the diet world right now is that if you eat each meal or snack with the proper balance of protein, carbohydrate and fat, you will feel better. These cookies follow the proportions suggested in the book *In the Zone* and are tasty as well.

¼ cup almond butter or tahini or peanut butter
½ cup plus 1 Tbsp. brown sugar

2 egg whites
½ tsp. vanilla extract (if corn-sensitive find a brand without added corn syrup)
1 cup plus 2 Tbsp. soy powder or whey protein
½ tsp. baking soda
¼ tsp. ground nutmeg
½ tsp. ground cinnamon
¼ tsp. sea salt
1½ cups oatmeal
OPTIONAL:
½ tsp. almond extract
½ cup water

Preheat oven to 350°F.

In a large mixing bowl, mix almond butter and brown sugar until somewhat smooth with an electric mixer or food processor. Mix in egg whites, vanilla and optional almond extract.

In a second bowl mix soy powder, baking soda, nutmeg, cinnamon and salt. Add the water (if using). Add mixture to the almond butter/sugar mixture and stir well. Stir in the oatmeal.

Use nonstick cookie sheets. Divide batter into 24 cookies and place 9 to 12 cookies per sheet. Bake for 8 minutes, take off sheet and let cool.

The amount of water used determines the texture. No added water results in a very sticky batter and very dry, biscotti-like cookies. Adding water makes the cookies more cake-like and moist. Using soy powder instead of whey also contributes to a creamy, moist texture.

The taste will also vary depending on whether you use almond butter, tahini or peanut butter and whether you add almond extract.

Yield: 24 cookies

41. Oatmeal-Flaxseed Cookies

These are a favorite at my house, but my mother complains that though they are good, they are not really sweet enough to be called a cookie. To each their own. Add more sweetener if you like, or just think of them as a dessert biscuit.

½ cup canola oil
2 eggs
2 Tbsp. sorghum molasses

1 cup ground flaxseeds (grind in a hand mill shortly before using)
1 tsp. ground cinnamon
1 tsp. baking soda
½ tsp. salt
2 cups rolled oats
½ cup chopped nuts
1 cup unsulfured raisins
10 dates, chopped
several Tbsp. or enough quinoa or other flour to bind

Preheat oven to 400°F. Beat together oil, eggs and molasses. In a separate bowl mix together the ground flaxseeds, cinnamon, baking soda and salt. Add to the oil-egg-molasses mixture. Stir in the remaining ingredients. Use only enough flour to bind.

Drop by teaspoons onto an oiled or nonstick baking sheet. Bake for 8 to 10 minutes or until done. Cool on a wire rack.

Yield: 36 cookies

42. Moist Rye Gingerbread

Rye flour is the perfect flour for making gingerbread. Ginger is anti-inflammatory. The prune puree makes for a moist cake without much oil. Who said dessert couldn't be both tasty and healthy?

2½ cups rye flour
2 tsp. baking soda
1½ tsp. ginger
1 tsp. cinnamon
½ tsp. cloves
½ tsp. dry mustard
⅛ tsp. sea salt
½ cup packed brown sugar
⅓ cup prune puree (To make prune puree, soak a cup of chopped prunes with 1/3 cup hot water for about 20 minutes, then puree in a food processor or blender.)
2 Tbsp. canola oil
1 large egg white
1 cup dark molasses
2 tsp. vanilla (if corn-sensitive find brand without added corn syrup)
1 cup boiling water
Canola oil for greasing the pan

Preheat oven to 375°F. Lightly oil a 9 x 9-inch baking pan and dust with flour. In a medium bowl, sift together flour, baking soda, ginger, cinnamon, cloves, mustard and salt. Set aside.

In a large bowl, cream together brown sugar, prune puree and oil. Beat in egg white. Add molasses and vanilla and beat until smooth.

In 3 additions, alternately add dry ingredients and boiling water to the creamed mixture, beating well after each addition. Pour batter into prepared pan and bake for 30 to 35 minutes, or until a toothpick inserted in the center comes out clean.

Yield: 16 servings

43. Oma's Pecan Squares

My 95-year-old grandmother still makes these delicious squares as treats at Christmas time. I have converted her recipe from the German metric system of measure into the American system of measure.

> 4 ounces unsweetened chocolate
> ½ cup plus 1 Tbsp. butter
> ½ cup sugar
> 4 eggs, separated
> ½ cup pecan meal (or any type of ground nut)
> 1 Tbsp. flour (oat, rye, spelt, or whatever type of flour you can tolerate)
> 10 ounces apricot jelly

Preheat oven to 350°F.

Soften chocolate in a double boiler, cool until lukewarm.

Beat butter, sugar and egg yolks until foamy. Beat egg whites until they start to form peaks; set aside. Add the nuts to the butter, sugar and egg mixture, then the chocolate, then the flour and then the egg whites. Spread this on a cookie sheet and bake 20 minutes or until a toothpick inserted in the center comes out clean. Spread half of this with apricot jelly (or any other type of jelly that you can tolerate). Place the other half on top.

Cut into small pieces. Decorate with a pecan half or a piece of chocolate.

Yield: about 12 squares

44. Chocolate Chickpea Cake

I made this one Christmas and it was a great hit with my family. I didn't tell anyone what sort of chocolate cake it was until the praise started rolling in for its wonderful, rich, moist texture. My grandmother, who is an expert baker, didn't miss a beat. She told of how they ran out of flour when she was a girl in wartime Germany, but her uncle, the village baker, was still able to make a delicious pastry for her birthday using a paste made from cooked beans. She glowed as she told us how they cooked and mashed the beans. For her turning beans into pastries was part of the triumph of the human spirit.

⅔ cup dried chickpeas or 2 cups cooked chickpeas, drained
Canola oil for greasing the pan
⅓ cup orange juice
4 large eggs, room temperature
1 cup packed brown sugar
¼ cup cocoa
½ tsp. baking powder
¼ cup baking soda

Generously cover ⅔ cup dried chickpeas with water and soak overnight. Rinse well, cover again with water, and bring to a boil. Turn heat down and simmer for 30-40 minutes or until chickpeas are tender. Cool and drain.

Preheat oven to 350°F. Lightly oil an 8-inch round cake pan and line bottom with a circle of waxed or parchment paper.

In a food processor, process chickpeas and orange juice until very smooth. Add eggs, one at a time, pulsing after each addition.

In a medium bowl, whisk together sugar, cocoa, baking powder and baking soda. Add to processor and pulse until just blended.

Pour batter into prepared pan and bake for 50 minutes, or until a toothpick inserted in the center comes out clean. Remove cake from oven and let cool on a rack for 15 minutes before removing from pan. Serve warm or at room temperature.

Yield: 8 servings

45. Oil-Based Pie Crust

Pies are easy to make. This crust is especially simple.

Using oil for a crust makes a delicate, flaky crust. Vegetable oil also has the advantage of being much healthier than shortening. This crust can be baked and then filled or filled before baking. Use a pie filling of your choice.

> 1½ cups bean flour mix OR nongluten flour mix OR any gluten-containing flour
> 1 tsp. salt
> ½ cup vegetable oil
> 3 Tbsp. cold milk or nondairy liquid
> OPTIONAL:
> 1 tsp. baking powder
> 1 ½ teaspoons sugar

Bean flour mix is made by combining one part bean flour, one part arrowroot powder, and one part tapioca flour. For instance, use ½ cup each, which equals 1 ½ cups total.

Nongluten flour mix is made from rice or corn flour. Make up a mix with 6 parts nongluten flour, ⅔ parts potato starch flour and ⅓ part tapioca flour. For instance, use 1 cup rice flour, ⅓ cup potato starch flour and 1/6 cup (2 Tbsp. plus 2 tsp.) tapioca flour, which equals 1½ cups total.

Gluten-containing flour such as wheat, kamut, spelt, rye, barley or oat flour can be used as is.

Mix dry ingredients; set aside. Mix oil and milk, blending with a fork. Pour into dry ingredients and stir until the mixture is crumbly and almost sticks together.

Pat the mixture into a 9-inch or 10-inch oiled pie pan. Form a medium-thick crust.

If the pie is to be filled and baked, pour the filling in gently and bake according to the filling recipe.

If the crust is to be pre-baked, bake in a preheated 400°F oven for 13 to 15 minutes. Cool before filling.

Yield: one 9-inch or 10-inch pie crust

46. Oatmeal Pie Crust

This is a sweet crust with plenty of texture. It goes well with creamy, smooth fillings. Use the substitution suggestions in Chapter 10 to create safe versions of your favorite pie fillings.

1 cup oatmeal

⅔ cup chopped walnuts or pecans

2 Tbsp. brown sugar

1/3 cup melted, unsalted butter

Spread oats and nuts on a baking sheet. Bake in 350°F oven for 10 minutes or until light brown. Toss in brown sugar and butter. Press evenly on bottom and sides of a 9-inch pie plate. Refrigerate. When cool, fill with the filling of your choice.

Yield: one 9-inch or 10-inch pie crust

24 Other Recipes in Chapters 10 and 11

Chapter 10 and Chapter 11 also contain quick and easy recipes.

See Chapter 10 for:

1-2. 2 Corn Bread/Millet Bread Recipes

3-18. Chart of Water/Cooking Times for 16 Grains

See Chapter 11 for:

19-21. 3 Peanut Sauce Recipes

22. Parsley-Almond Sauce Recipe

23. Fresh Salsa Recipe

24. Kasha with Onions Recipe

Long-Term Benefits

The long-term benefits of tasty, healthy, healing food cannot be underestimated. Avoiding your problem foods stops the damage caused by food sensitivities. Getting healthy food gives your body what it needs to heal and paves the way for deep and successful healing. Along the way you get the comfort and joy of great-tasting food.

Resources

Marilyn Gioannini, *The Complete Food Allergy Cookbook* (Rocklin, CA: Prima Publishing, 1996).

Nicolette M. Dumke, *5 Years without Food: The Food Allergy Survival Guide* (Louisville, CO: Adapt Books, 1997).
Nicolette Dumke successfully healed from food sensitivities so extensive that the only way she could survive was on a very strict rotation diet that was based on many uncommon and exotic foods. Her book is a very practical guide that includes information on how to buy and cook these foods.

Bette Hagman, *The Gluten-free Gourmet Cooks Fast and Healthy* (New York: Henry Holt and Company, Inc., 1996).

Linda Edwards, *Baking for Health: Whole Food Baking for Better Health* (Garden City Park, NY: Avery Publishing Group Inc., 1988).
Linda Edwards explains in detail how to bake using minimally processed ingredients and still get good results.

Doris Janzen Longacre, *More-with-Less Cookbook* (Scottsdale, PA: Herald Press, 1976).
This cookbook is a collection of recipes from Mennonites who lived all over the world and learned to make good meals from simple, inexpensive, relatively unprocessed ingredients.

Debra Wasserman, *The Lowfat Jewish Vegetarian Cookbook* (Baltimore, MD: The Vegetarian Resource Group, 1994).
This gem of a book modifies Jewish recipes from all over the world. The results are some great low-fat versions of simple, tasty, traditional fare.

Yamuna Devi, *The Best of Lord Krishna's Cuisine: Favorite Recipes from the Art of Indian Vegetarian Cooking* (Poway, CA: Bala Books, Inc., 1991).

Chapter 13: Ridding Yourself of Current Food Intolerances And Avoiding New Ones—13 Strategies

Highlights:

❑ Thirteen methods for avoiding new food intolerances, for stopping an intolerance reaction once it has started, and for ridding yourself of current food intolerances.

Effort Involved:

❑ **The effort involved is variable.** Implementing ONE of the 13 strategies might be enough to cure you of your food sensitivities. Alternatively, you might have to use several strategies just to keep from developing new sensitivities and several more to see a reduction or elimination of your current food sensitivities.

❑ **Strategy 1**: Instituting a rotation diet involves considerable effort. You must learn about food families, keep track of what you have eaten in the last four days, and make sure that you don't eat foods that are in the same food families more often than once every four days.

❑ **Strategy 2:** Instituting an elimination diet can be simple or involved, depending on how many food sensitivities you have and what they are.

❑ **Strategy 3:** Correcting leaky gut syndrome can be easy or complicated, depending on your current food and drink habits and your medicine needs.

❑ **Strategy 4:** Alleviating symptoms caused by overwhelmed sulfoxidation and sulfation detoxification pathways can be easy or hard depending on your current food and drink habits, your medicine needs, your toxic chemical exposure, and your genetic makeup.

❑ **Strategy 5:** Improving detoxification by supporting the liver can be easy or involved, depending on your current food, drink and exercise habits. The liver can also be supported by supplements available through health food stores.

❑ **Strategy 6:** Avoiding damage from lectins involves avoiding eating certain foods based on your blood type and involves implementing Strategy 3, correcting leaky gut syndrome.

- ❏ **Strategy 7:** Improving thymus function includes taking a multiple vitamin and mineral pill and thymus extract pills that can be purchased in health food stores.
- ❏ **Strategy 8:** High-dose vitamin C is a quick and easy way to provide immediate relief from an intolerance reaction.
- ❏ **Strategies 9 and 10:** Provocation-Neutralization Treatments and Enzyme-Potentiated Desensitization (EPD) involve the effort and expense of repeated trips for months or years to a qualified doctor. EPD also involves staying on an ultraclean diet for a few weeks around treatment time.
- ❏ **Strategy 11:** Nambudripad Allergy Elimination Technique (NAET) involves acupressure and totally eliminating for 25 hours the problem foods being treated in a given session. It also involves the effort and expense of repeated trips (usually at least 10) to a qualified practitioner.
- ❏ **Strategy 12:** Machaelle Small Wright's Medical Assistance Program (MAP) is a comprehensive program involving a willingness to make a detailed inventory of symptoms, set priorities, and participate in 40-minute periods alone where you actively work with healing energies that are not generally included in standard medical models.
- ❏ **Strategy 13:** Meditation is easy to learn. See Chapter 15 for details.

Payoff:

- ❏ Short-term relief from food intolerances.
- ❏ In some cases, long-term, total elimination of food intolerances.

Introduction

This chapter will make the most sense if you already have at least a passing familiarity with the information in earlier chapters. Chapters 1 and 2 describe what food sensitivities are and how they arise. Chapters 3 and 4 describe how to test for them. Chapters 5-8 provide important information on how to tell from food labeling if a product contains problematic ingredients. Chapters 9-12 provide practical advice on how to get safe and tasty food once you have identified your food sensitivities.

13 Strategies for Minimizing and Eliminating Food Sensitivities

The following strategies will minimize symptoms of food sensitivities and in some cases even lead to their elimination. The high-dose vitamin C strategy will even stop an adverse reaction after it has been triggered.

Sometimes using just one of these strategies is enough to eliminate food sensitivities. Sometimes it takes several. Read through and determine which are most appropriate to your situation.

1. Rotation Diets

People with multiple food intolerances are prone to developing new food intolerances to any food that they eat too frequently. The worse your intolerances, the more likely you are to develop new ones. The best way to avoid this is by not eating any given food more often than once every four days. In EXTREME cases you may not be able to eat a given food AND any closely related foods more often than once every 10 days. Since people with multiple food intolerances seem to be most prone to developing new intolerances to grains, you should pay particular attention to using a rotation diet for grains such as wheat, corn, rye, oats, barley, millet, rice, wild rice and the heirloom varieties of wheat that some wheat-sensitive individuals can tolerate: kamut and spelt.

A full explanation of rotation diets and food families is beyond the scope of this book. I recommend reading one of the many good books on this subject. The books listed in the resource section at the end of the chapter are three that I found particularly helpful.

Rotation diets are appropriate in two cases. The first is for people with so many food sensitivities that they cannot eliminate all problem foods and still get a balanced diet. Rotation minimizes adverse reactions. The second is in conjunction with an elimination diet. In this case, totally eliminate everything to which you adversely react. Then use a four-day rotation schedule to minimize developing new sensitivities.

The good news about rotation diets, even without selective elimination, is that you may be able to use this type of diet to rid yourself of at least some of your food sensitivities. There is a tendency for adverse reactions to fade and sometimes even disappear on rotation diets.

Checklist: Starting a Rotation Diet

❑ Read one of the many good books available on rotation diets, such as those recommended in the resource section at the end of this chapter.
❑ Find and purchase some of the alternative foods recommended in these books to expand the number of allowable foods you have available. The following are good sources:
    ❑   Mail-order sources suggested in these books
    ❑   Health food stores
    ❑   Ethnic food markets

❑   Organic farmers (many organic farms have a subscription service where you are supplied each week for the entire growing season with a variety of fresh produce)
❑ Get a notebook for writing down everything you eat, especially if you deviate from your normal rotation diet plan, so you can adequately compensate on the following days.
❑ Buy several colors of tape to mark extra portions of food that you freeze, so you can quickly identify on which day of your rotation diet it can be eaten.

2. Elimination Diets

As the name suggests, elimination diets totally eliminate every trace of problem foods. This stops damage to the body by removing the triggering event. The body then has a chance to heal.

This type of diet is appropriate when you have only a relatively small number of foods to which you react poorly. For instance, using the information in Chapters 5-8 to ferret out all the hidden sources of problem foods, I was able to completely eliminate my problem foods from my diet. For me, this meant eliminating all sources of corn, rice, wheat, beef and food dyes. Although this meant the elimination of many types of food from my diet, I was still able to get enough to eat. If this is the case for you, be happy, because total elimination is one of the more reliable ways to heal.

As mentioned above for rotation diets, often the body is able to heal itself of a food sensitivity, if the problem food is eaten only on a rotation schedule for six months to two years. The same is true for total elimination, except that total elimination is even more likely to lead to healing. After this, a former problem food is often either no longer a problem or can be easily tolerated on a rotation diet.

If a food sensitivity doesn't disappear after two years on a total elimination diet, you will need some other help besides just elimination to overcome it.

One limitation of an elimination diet is that sometimes people react poorly to such a large number of foods (sometimes 20, 50 or more) that total elimination is impossible. In that case, pick the worst offenders for elimination, and eat everything else on a rotation schedule.

3. Correct Leaky Gut Syndrome

As explained in Chapter 2, one cause of food sensitivities is leaky gut syndrome. Correcting this syndrome often leads to spontaneous recovery from food sensitivities.

Leaky gut syndrome is characterized by considerable amounts of undigested or partially digested food leaking from the small intestines directly into the bloodstream. Risk factors are use of conventional NSAIDs, alcohol, anti-ulcer drugs such as Zantac and Tagamet, antacid tablets and/or antibiotics (including antibiotics taken years ago), diets high in simple carbohydrates, gulping food without chewing thoroughly, presence of parasites in the digestive tract, and a personal or family history of allergies or food sensitivities.

Symptoms can include any of the following: poor digestion, gas and bloating, food sensitivities, yeast infections, fatigue, joint pain, cloudy thinking, and difficulty maintaining weight.

A doctor can determine if leaky gut syndrome is present using a test described in Chapter 2 in the section called "Testing for Leaky Gut Syndrome." Since the corrective measures are largely healthy lifestyle changes, you may want to make these changes even without medical tests.

The way to correct leaky gut syndrome is to reduce intestinal permeability, improve digestion, and return intestinal flora to a healthy balance. To do this, take the following steps:

To Reduce Intestinal Permeability:
- Avoid foods to which you are intolerant. (See Chapters 3-8 for a detailed explanation of how to identify and avoid these foods.)
- Avoid coffee and other caffeinated products if you find that they tend to cause abdominal pain or discomfort.
- Avoid alcohol and conventional NSAIDs, both of which increase intestinal permeability.
- Be checked by a medical professional for parasites, yeast and pathogenic bacteria in your intestinal tract. Treat any problems that are found.

To Improve Digestion:
- Chew food until it has liquefied.
- Never eat when anxious or rushed.
- Eat in relaxed and pleasant surroundings.
- Take time to enjoy the taste and texture of food.
- Restore digestive power by taking supplements such as pancreatin, *Aspergillus orazeae* extracts, bromelain, papain and hydrochloric acid. (See Chapter 2 for a discussion of a test that is available to see if you need them. See the discussion below for instructions on how to use them.)

- Avoid antacid tablets and anti-ulcer drugs such as Tagamet (cimetidine) and Zantac (ranitidine) that inhibit the production of hydrochloric acid in the stomach.
- Avoid protease inhibitors. They impair protein digestion and are found in the raw and undercooked forms of the following foods: soybeans, peanuts, lentils, rice, corn and potatoes. Make sure that when you eat these foods they are thoroughly cooked

To Restore and Maintain Healthy Intestinal Flora:

- Avoid antibiotics whenever possible.
- Eat a diet low in animal protein and low in simple carbohydrates, such as those found in table sugar, milk and sweet fruits and fruit juices.
- Eat lots of legumes, whole grains and vegetables. Soak legumes and whole grain in water overnight before cooking to aid digestion and to discourage gas-producing intestinal flora that thrive on incompletely digested food.
- Eat foods such as yogurt, miso, tempeh and homemade sauerkraut that are a source of healthy intestinal bacteria and/or take commercial supplements containing healthy bacteria such as *Lactobacillus acidophilus* and *Bifidobacterium bifidum*. These supplements are known by the general name "probiotics" and are available in health food stores.
- See Chapter 14 for more complete details on the best type of healing diet for someone with arthritis.

How to Use Digestional Aids to Treat Leaky Gut Syndrome:

Digestive secretions such as gastric hydrochloric acid, pancreatic enzymes and bile inhibit the overgrowth of yeast and bacteria in the upper part of the small intestine. As mentioned in Chapter 2, overgrowth of microorganisms in this part of the intestine is a major cause of leaky gut syndrome. Restoration of normal digestive secretions is thus a key step in correcting this syndrome. Not surprisingly, restoration of normal digestive secretions also improves digestion. This means that less undigested food is present in the small intestines, where it can cause trouble by being absorbed into the bloodstream.

If you have undigested food in the stool, this indicates a deficiency in the secretion of hydrochloric acid by the stomach, of digestive enzymes by the pancreas, or both. The Comprehensive Digestive Stool Analysis (CDSA) discussed in Chapter 2 can help pinpoint the exact nature of the problem. Deficiencies can be corrected, at least in part, by the following supplements:

- Pancreatin, which is an extract from the pancreas of cows or pigs
- Extracts from the fungus *Aspergillus orazeae*

- Bromelain (from pineapple)
- Papain (from papaya)
- Hydrochloric acid

Each of these digestive aids is available through health food stores.

Hydrochloric acid supplementation should only be undertaken under the supervision of a health care practitioner. If not needed or taken in too large amounts it can cause ulceration of the stomach. Pancreatin and *Aspergillus orazeae* extracts provide broad-spectrum digestive aid and therefore are often very effective in improving digestion. Bromelain and papain aid only in protein digestion and do not improve fat and carbohydrate digestion. Because it is easy to develop new food sensitivities to digestional supplements, it is best to rotate their use, similar to how food is handled on the rotation diets described earlier in this chapter. In brief, use a different supplement each day and do not reuse a supplement more often than once every four days. You should also avoid antacid tablets and anti-ulcer drugs such as Tagamet (cimetidine) and Zantac (ranitidine), which inhibit the production of hydrochloric acid in the stomach.

4. Alleviate Symptoms Caused by Overwhelmed Sulfoxidation and Sulfation Detoxification Pathways

As explained in Chapter 2, overwhelming sulfoxidation and sulfation detoxification pathways can lead to a host of problems, including chemical sensitivities and arthritis. Your doctor can test how well these pathways are functioning using a test described in Appendix A.

If you suspect that you have suboptimal sulfoxidation and sulfation detoxification pathways, Dr. Stephen McFadden[35] recommends that you:

- Avoid the drugs D-penicillamine, sodium aurothiomalate (used in gold treatments) and acetaminophen (in Tylenol, etc.).
- Minimize exposure to toxic chemicals such as chlorine, natural gas, exhaust fumes, organic solvents and insecticides.
- Ask your health practitioner for advice about possible supplementation with magnesium sulfate, taurine and/or molybdenum.
- Avoid high-protein diets and avoid supplementation with cysteine, methionine and other thiol-containing nutrients, but make sure that you

---

[35] Stephen A. McFadden, "Phenotypic Variation in Xenobiotic Metabolism and Adverse Environmental Response: Focus on Sulfur-dependent Detoxification Pathways," *Toxicology* 111 (1996) 43-65.

are getting adequate amounts of nutritionally complete protein in your diet.

- ❑ Avoid glutamate (as in the flavor enhancer monosodium glutamate [MSG]).
- ❑ Avoid aspartate in free form (including supplements chelated with aspartate, since the aspartate is released in free form in the body).
- ❑ Go on a diet such as the Feingold diet[36] that eliminates all salicylates, food colorings and preservatives.
- ❑ If monoamine-containing foods, such as cheese (tyramine), chocolate (phenylethamine) and bananas, make you feel worse, avoid them.
- ❑ Avoid stimulants.
- ❑ Avoid exposure to anticholinesterase insecticides.
- ❑ Avoid oranges. (Some flavinoids, especially those in oranges, result in a temporary reduction in sulfation capacity.)
- ❑ Ask your doctor about dietary evaluation to determine if phenolic food constituents common to some food families should be avoided. Debra Lynn Dadd[37], a researcher who has done much to help individuals with multiple chemical sensitivities, has outlined one useful evaluation. A reference for her evaluation is in the resource section of this chapter.
- ❑ Consider treatment at a spa with water that has a high sulfate/sulfur ratio.
- ❑ Avoid phenolated allergy extracts and other phenolated medicinals. (Read labels and packaging carefully to find out if extracts or medicinals have any phenol added.)

5. Improve Detoxification by Supporting the Liver

According to Dr. Michael Murray, co-author of the Encyclopedia of Natural Medicine[38], a healthy liver is critical for detoxification of toxic chemicals. Sulfoxidation, and many other enzymatic detoxification reactions take place in the liver.

---

[36] Ben I. Feingold and Helen S. Feingold, *The Feingold Cookbook for Hyperactive Children and Others with Problems Associated with Food Additives and Salicylates* (New York: Random House, 1979).

[37] D.L. Dadd, R.C. Dadd, J.J. McGovern and R.W. Gardner, *Therapeutic Diets with Special Emphasis on the Rotary Diversified Diet (With Index of Phenylic Food Compounds)*, (San Francisco, CA: Nutritional Research Company, 1980).

[38] Michael Murray, N.D, and Joseph Pizzorno, N.D., *Encyclopedia of Natural Medicine* (Rocklin, CA.: Prima Publishing, 1998).

If the liver is even slightly damaged, immune function is compromised. Among other things, this can lead to overgrowths of intestinal flora. This is often enough to set into motion a whole series of events that ultimately results in arthritis. Improving liver function can be an important element in restoring health.

Dr. Murray suggests the following measures to support optimal liver function:
☐ Avoid alcohol.
☐ Exercise regularly.
☐ Eat a healthy diet. Avoid saturated fats and refined sugar. See Chapter 14 for more details on a healthy diet.
☐ Take lipotrophic agents like choline, betaine and methionine that promote the flow of fat and bile to and from the liver. Take a daily dose of 1,000 mg choline and 1,000 mg of methionine and/or cysteine. These agents increase levels of glutathione, one of the major detoxifying compounds in the liver. (Note that this suggestion conflicts with one of Dr. McFadden's suggestions for treating symptoms caused by overwhelmed sulfoxidation and sulfation pathways. Skip this suggestion if you suspect that your sulfoxidation and sulfation pathways may be overwhelmed.)
☐ Take silymarin, a special extract of milk thistle *(Silybum marianum)* that protects the liver and enhances detoxification by preventing the depletion of glutathione. Silymarin is available at health food stores. Standard dosage is 70 to 210 mg three times a day.
☐ Go on a three-day fast four times a year (each time the seasons change). Chapter 4 on explains how to do this. Fasting gives the liver a chance to process any backlog of substances to be detoxified.

If you suspect that you have suboptimal functioning of these detoxification pathways or the overwhelming of these pathways for any other reason, follow the steps given in Chapter 2 for coping with this problem.

6. Avoid Damage from Lectins

As explained in Chapter 2, a type of chemical called a lectin that is commonly found in food can cause arthritis. How you react to certain lectins depends on your blood type. Although people with any blood type can have problems, those of us with type A blood are particularly prone to arthritis induced by adverse reactions to certain lectins. Often, eliminating these problem lectins from your diet or healing your digestive tract so that they no longer pass undigested into your bloodstream will lead to improvement.

This is the strategy Gail Furman uses to eliminate her arthritis. She still occasionally eats "forbidden" foods, but knows she'll pay the price with pain later on. One interesting note is that Gail seems to crave the very foods that cause her arthritis to flare. Her story is told in Chapter 1.

To avoid damage from lectins:

❑ Use the lists from Dr. Peter J. D'Adamo's book, *Eat Right for Your Type*, to avoid foods that contain lectins that are bad for people with your blood type (A, B, AB or O).
❑ Soak beans and grains overnight before cooking.
❑ Cook all beans and grains thoroughly.
❑ Follow the steps listed in the section above called "Correcting Leaky Gut Syndrome."

7. Improve Thymus Function

Some themes recur throughout this book. One of these is the value of antioxidant vitamins and minerals, which aid healing in many ways. One way is improving thymus function. Taking thymus extracts also improves thymus function.

Thymus extracts (thymodulin) have been shown to normalize the ratio of T helper cells to suppressor cells, whether the ratio is low (as in AIDS or cancer) or high (as in allergies or rheumatoid arthritis).[39,40] A high helper-to-suppressor T-cell ratio is believed to be one of the causes of rheumatoid arthritis (RA) and other types of arthritis such as reactive arthritis. It is not surprising that since thymus extracts improve this ratio, they also improve the clinical symptoms of RA.

There are no industry standards for the production of thymus extracts, but products that are concentrated and standardized for polypeptide content are preferable to crude preparations. These products are available at health food stores. No side effects or adverse effects have been reported in the medical literature from the use of thymus preparations.[41] However, thymus

---

[39] Pietro Cazzola et al., "*In vivo* Modulating Effect of a Calf Thymus Acid Lysate on Human T Lymphocyte Subsets and CD4+/CD8+ Ratio in the Course of Different Diseases," *Curr Ther Res*, 42(6) (6 Dec. 1987):1011-1017.

[40] N.M. Kouttab et al., "Thymodulin: biological properties and clinical applications," *Med. Oncol & Tumor Pharmacother.*, 6(1) (1989):5-9.

[41] Michael T. Murray, N.D., *Chronic candidiasis–The Yeast Syndrome* (Rocklin, CA: Prima Publishing, 1997).

extracts are generally made from calf thymus, so if you have a beef sensitivity, you may want to avoid these extracts.

Dr. Michael Murray recommends taking the following daily dose of antioxidant nutrients to maximize thymus function:[42]

- ❑ Carotenes (found in especially high amounts in red and orange vegetables like beets, pumpkin and carrots)
- ❑ Vitamin C (1-3 g per day in divided doses)
- ❑ Vitamin E (400-800 IU per day)
- ❑ Zinc (15-45 mg per day; zinc bound to picolinate, acetate, citrate, glycerate or monomethionine are all excellent forms of zinc)
- ❑ Selenium (200 mcg per day)
- ❑ Vitamin B-6 (50 to 100 mg per day; do not take more than 50 mg at a time, and do not exceed recommended dosage since nerve toxicity results in some individuals at higher dosages)

Antioxidant supplements are available as multiple vitamin and mineral pills. Probably the easiest way to ensure that you get the daily amounts listed above is to take a high-level antioxidant supplement in addition to a lower level, more comprehensive vitamin and mineral supplement.

Dr. Murray suggests that a good daily dosage of thymus extract is 750 mg of crude polypeptide fractions. A study in the medical literature from Milan, Italy, used an alternative way of measuring dosage. This study obtained good results with rheumatoid arthritis using 2 mg thymomodulin per kilogram of body weight per day for three months.[43] Because thymus extracts labeled by thymomodulin content are harder to find than those marked by crude polypeptide fraction content, you will probably end up using the first guideline. Dr. Murray does not mention a time period, but if you are using a high-quality product and if this strategy is going to help you, you should see results within three months.

---

[42] Michael Murray, N.D., and Joseph Pizzorno, N.D., *Encyclopedia of Natural Medicine* (Prima Publishing, 1998. pp. 161, 745, and 788).

[43] Pietro Cazzola et al., "*In vivo* Modulating Effect of a Calf Thymus Acid Lysate on Human T Lymphocyte Subsets and CD4+/CD8+ Ratio in the Course of Different Diseases," *Curr Ther Res*, 42(6) (6 Dec. 1987):1011-1017.

8. High-Dose Vitamin C

Vitamin C is known to provide immediate, temporary relief of allergic reactions. The speed of treatment is the most important factor in stopping an allergic reaction. Some reactions, especially classical food allergies, cannot be reversed if treatment is not begun early enough. Although this remedy does not correct the underlying causes of food intolerance, it can provide temporary relief and also prevent some of the damage that occurs in the body as a consequence of a full-blown allergic reaction.

Buffered vitamin C is the most effective form of vitamin C for stopping reactions. The buffer (calcium carbonate, magnesium carbonate and potassium bicarbonate) works by reversing the body's tendency to become acidic during allergic reactions. The vitamin C itself (as opposed to the buffer) also aids in reversing or stopping allergic reactions, but by a different mechanism. It provides an antihistamine-like effect without the side effects of antihistamines.

Bicarbonate preparations such as Alka Seltzer Gold-TM (it contains corn products so it is not suitable for people with corn sensitivities), Vital Life Bi-Carb Formula-TM or Tri-Salts also work to reverse allergic reactions in the same way as the buffer in buffered vitamin C.

Some people become more alkaline when they have an allergic reaction. This can be determined with the use of nitrazine paper or litmus paper (available at most pharmacies). Both saliva and urine must be tested to determine the pH. These people will need to take the ascorbic acid form to stop their reaction.

It is best to take bicarbonate preparations or buffered vitamin C 20 minutes to one hour after a meal to which you react so that the buffer does not interfere with the stomach acid needed to digest that meal or your next meal.

According to Jacqueline A. Krohn, M.D., author of *The Whole Way to Allergy Relief and Prevention: A Doctor's Complete Guide to Treatment and Self-Care*, you should not exceed more than 5 teaspoons or 20 capsules daily (10 grams) of buffered vitamin C, because of the high levels of potassium, calcium and magnesium involved. If you need more vitamin C than this, use it in the ascorbic acid form.

Dr. Krohn also states that taking vitamin C at the level of bowel tolerance is the most effective dose. This means taking as much vitamin C orally as you can without inducing diarrhea. She recommends taking this as a daily supplement to allow the body time to heal, instead of just taking this at the beginning of an allergic reaction. She gives detailed instructions in her book on how much to take. In brief, start with 1 gram per day taken at mealtime and increase it gradually to just short of the point of inducing diarrhea. The doses should be spread out evenly over the day. If you take more than 20 to 30 grams per day, supplement with additional minerals to compensate for those lost through vitamin C, which acts as a diuretic at these extremely high doses.

Be careful of cutting back on high levels of vitamin C too quickly—a condition called rebound scurvy can result. Also be careful to rinse your teeth after each dose, since over time vitamin C powder can damage tooth enamel.

Vitamin C is available derived from many sources (beet, carrot, corn, tapioca and potato). You may want to rotate the source so you do not develop a new food intolerance from any one source of vitamin C.

9. Provocation-Neutralization Treatments

This treatment involves either subcutaneous (under the skin) injections or sublingual (under the tongue) drops that are carefully measured to contain the exact "neutralizing" dose of food extract needed to "turn off" food intolerance symptoms.

A neutralizing dose is determined by a series of intradermal injections of serial dilutions of a food extract. Intradermal injections place food extracts deeper in the skin than the skin-prick tests used to identify classical allergies. (See Chapter 2 for a discussion of the differences between classical allergies and food sensitivity reactions.) The highest dilution that does not produce a positive wheal is the neutralizing dose. (A wheal is a small, hard, raised spot on the skin.)

This testing is time-consuming and only a few substances can be tested during each session. Because neutralizing doses change, patients must be retested frequently to keep their neutralizing shots or drops current and working effectively. Although no one knows how these neutralizing doses are able to "turn off" food sensitivity reactions, this phenomenon has been repeatedly observed.

Once the neutralizing dose has been found, patients are taught to inject it into the skin of the upper arm, a process that is needed every two days at first, but only twice a week or even less frequently once the treatment has been under way for some months. The immune system eventually heals enough for some people to stop treatment altogether.

The neutralizing dose for sublingual therapy is determined in exactly the same manner as intradermal injection/wheal testing except that the neutralizing dose is supplied in the form of drops placed under the tongue. The drops provide neutralization of food sensitivities for only a few hours.

Studies of the effectiveness of provocation-neutralization therapy tend to show that with physicians who have had relatively little experience with this technique, it does not work well, but with physicians who have used this technique for years, it is more often successful.

Since the neutralizing doses of food extracts mentioned above turn off, at least for a short time, adverse reactions to given foods, they often allow people with numerous food sensitivities or allergies to have a more varied and healthy diet. Because the same technique also works for chemical sensitivities, it can also allow some people who would otherwise be confined to their homes to lead more normal lives.

10. Enzyme-Potentiated Desensitization (EPD)

This treatment is based on the ability of an enzyme, ß-glucuronidase, in the presence of food allergens, to regulate the immune system cells known as T-cells that would normally facilitate a food sensitivity reaction. By training T-cells not to react to food allergens, the body learns not to have adverse reactions to these allergens. EPD has been used in England for about 25 years and has recently become available in the United States. It works in about 85 percent of people and treats a wide range of allergens, including food, airborne and chemical allergens.

EPD treatment consists of food extract and the ß-glucuronidase enzyme being applied to a scratch in the skin or injected as a shot. A comprehensive mixture of food extracts is generally used and the same dose is used for all patients. Treatments are initially needed once every two to three months and eventually only once a year. Many patients can discontinue EPD and remain symptom-free after they have taken about 18 shots over a period of about seven years. For severely allergic persons it may take two to three years of treatment to achieve good results with all food allergens, but after that, most patients' diets are usually unrestricted except for around the time of their shots.

The advantage of EPD is that treatment tends to produce permanent improvements. The disadvantage is that right around treatment time, one must be hypervigilant about avoiding allergens, because one sometimes becomes hypersensitive and could even develop new allergies.

In 1999, when I was considering undergoing this treatment, there were clinical trials of EPD going on in the United States. These trials are now over. An application has been submitted for FDA approval. Although the FDA is expected to approve this application, in the interim EPD treatment is not available in the United States. However, the treatment is available in other parts of the world. For further information and the status of the FDA application call the American EPD Society at (505) 984-0004 or visit its web site at http://www.epdallergy.com

There are also other unofficial sources of EPD information sites on the Web. The best is a site created by Stan Rohrer. The address is http://www.dma.org/~rohrers/allergy/allergy.htm

11. Acupressure

Dr. Devi S. Nambudripad developed a technique called Nambudripad Allergy Elimination Technique (NAET) that relies on muscle testing and acupressure. Everything I have learned about this method is by word of mouth and from a single magazine article (Linda Weber, "The Man Who Couldn't Lift Peas," Natural Health, July-August 1998, pp. 106-111, 178-182). Unlike most techniques I mention in this book, I have neither tried this technique nor found support for it in medical journals. However, anecdotal accounts are promising. This technique was on my personal list of cures to try before my food sensitivities disappeared using other modalities.

The claim is an 80 to 90 percent success rate in clearing long-standing adverse food and chemical reactions using a series of treatments that involves the person being treated holding a problem substance in one hand while getting acupressure.

If you want to find out more about this form of treatment, one place to start is the Web site: http://www.naet.com. It has a directory that you can use to find a practitioner near you. I suggest you ask lots of questions and perhaps interview two or three people who have received these treatments. Make sure that anyone you see for treatment has a good track record, no matter what type of treatments you decide to receive. Be informed. Don't enter into this or any other treatment blindly. Make sure it is worth your time and effort.

12. Machaelle Small Wright and the Medical Assistance Program

Machaelle Small Wright's Medical Assistance Program (MAP) is unlike any other alternative health care modality that I have seen. It is based on something Wright calls co-creative science. As she describes it, it integrates the involuntary input of nature (order, organization and life vitality/action) with the evolutionary dynamic of man (direction and purpose). It requires that an individual become an equal partner in his or her health care and provides integrated treatment on the emotional, physical, mental and spiritual levels.

MAP costs nothing and is so simple that anyone can use it, but because it involves working directly with "spiritual energies" it will appeal to some people more than others. Wright uses words like nature spirits, devas, and conings to explain how the program works. I find it useful to think of it as a special kind of prayer or meditation that allows me to contact my higher self and special "energy healers" to assist me in the healing process. If this sort of thing appeals to you, then I recommend you read Wright's book (listed under references at the end of the chapter).

My experience was that my food intolerances vanished three weeks after starting the program. I have been able to eat absolutely anything I want since then, with absolutely no intolerance reaction.

At the time I started MAP I had been on an ultraclean diet for years. Most of my intolerances had greatly lessened or possibly even disappeared, except for my corn intolerance. I know this because one month before starting MAP I accidentally ate something containing wheat flour at my brother's wedding and suffered no ill effects.

In contrast, several months earlier at a meditation retreat I accidentally ate something containing corn allergens and became sick—I was achy all over, had trouble thinking clearly, and was continuously exhausted. Although I was thinking clearly enough to realize that most of the food served at the retreat was unsafe for me, I wasn't thinking clearly enough to figure out how to get enough safe food to meet my needs. By the time the retreat was over, my body chemistry was off from not having eaten a balanced diet. I had a metallic, copper-like taste in my mouth and was ravenously hungry.

Because I had trusted the retreat center to provide safe food, I had not brought along a large enough supply of my own. This led me to do a very stupid thing on the way home. I was so desperate that I snacked on airport and then airline food, even though I knew that what I chosen had corn products (table salt) and probably other problematic ingredients as well. My body must have gotten something of what it needed to rebalance from what I ate, because I was temporarily better, but within a few hours my food sensitivity reactions kicked in again. At home I spent several tired and achy days in bed. It took about two weeks on a clean diet for me to totally recover.

I had the idea from having gone through this food crisis during and immediately after a *vipassana* meditation retreat (when I was turned deeply inward and paying close attention to my body sensations) that a key to

217

losing my food intolerances would be to stop attacking my food. I had the idea at the time that my immune system was attacking out of fear. I would later learn through further meditation that I was attacking not only out of fear but also because of anger turned inward upon myself.

A large part of what had to happen for me to totally lose my food intolerances was for me to release some deep-seated fear and rage of which I was normally not aware but that was literally driving me to attack my food and my body at the level of my immune system. Because I had already contacted and released much of this fear and rage through the practice of *vipassana* meditation, it was relatively quick and easy to release the rest with the added support of MAP. I believe MAP accelerated the release process while also making it easier and smoother.

I think MAP is wonderful. It has been useful for every physical, mental, emotional and/or spiritual issue to which I have applied it. I am impressed with how quickly and easily it allows me to move through even long-standing problems.

13. Meditation

Meditation has been a powerful tool for me. It has helped me deal with chronic pain and been a major factor in healing from my food sensitivities. See Chapter 15 for an overview of meditation and simple instructions for the two types I have personally found to be most useful.

Summary

Drugs may cover up the symptoms of arthritis, but currently they offer no cure. Only removing the underlying problems (in many cases, food intolerance reactions) will allow the body to fully recover. Rotation diets and elimination diets are two tools that alone will sometimes allow full recovery. Sometimes further strategies must also be implemented.

These further strategies that you can largely implement on your own include correcting leaky gut syndrome, alleviating symptoms caused by overwhelmed sulfoxidation and sulfation detoxification pathways, improving detoxification by improving liver function, avoiding damage from lectins, and improving thymus function. There is also high-dose Vitamin C, which if taken soon enough can provide immediate relief from an intolerance reaction once it has started, and which taken on an ongoing basis can promote healing.

Further strategies that involve treatments from a skilled practitioner include desensitization procedures such as provocation-neutralization treatment, enzyme potentiated desensitization (EPD) and acupressure. These three strategies are capable of offering at least some people long-term relief from food sensitivities.

Machealle Small Wright's Medical Assistance Program (MAP) is quite different from standard medical models and other alternative treatments, but in my case MAP, plus meditation (see Chapter 15) contributed to total eradication of all of my intolerance reactions.

Long-Term Benefits

For people like Gail Furman and Shirley and Angela Crenshaw, profiled in Chapter 1, removing the foods to which they are sensitive has meant the difference between crippling illness and a healthy, high-energy lifestyle. The strategies in this chapter take these benefits one step further. Instead of avoiding illness by avoiding certain foods, implementing the strategies in this chapter leads to even deeper healing. Previous problem foods once again become safe to eat.

Resources

Rotation Diets

Marilyn Gioannini, *The Complete Food Allergy Cookbook: the Foods You've Always Loved Without the Ingredients You Can't Have* (Rocklin, CA: Prima Publishing, 1997).
This book has a particularly good section on rotating grains and on using alternatives such as teff, amaranth, buckwheat, quinoa and bean flours.

John Postley with Janet M. Barton, *The Allergy Discovery Diet: A Rotation Diet for Discovering Your Allergies to Food* (New York: Doubleday, 1990).
This book explains the use of a rotation diet for food intolerance testing.

Nicolette M. Dumke, *5 Years Without Food: The Food Allergy Survival Guide* (Louisville, CO Adapt Books, 1997).
This book has an excellent rotation diet plan complete with recipes and sources for a large variety of unusual foods to expand otherwise restricted diets. In addition to the usual assortment of alternative products available at health food stores, this book gives sources for items such as game meats, chestnut flour, milo, tuber flours (white sweet potato, cassava, malanga, true yam, water chestnut, etc.), noncorn sources of vitamin C and alternative sweeteners.

Elimination Diets
See Chapters 1-12.

Leaky Gut
Jonathan Brostoff and Linda Gamlin, *The Complete Guide to Food Allergy and Intolerance* (New York: Crown Publishers, Inc., 1992).

Lectins
Peter J. D'Adamo with Catherine Whitney, *Eat Right for Your Type: The Individualized Diet Solution to Staying Healthy, Living Longer & Achieving Your Ideal Weight* (New York: G. P. Putnam's Sons, 1996).

Sulfoxidation and Sulfation Detoxification Pathways
Stephen A. McFadden, "Phenotypic Variation in Xenobiotic Metabolism and Adverse Environmental Response: Focus on Sulfur-dependent detoxification Pathways," 111 Toxicology (1996)43-65.

Ben I. Feingold and Helen S. Feingold, *The Feingold Cookbook for Hyperactive Children and Others with Problems Associated with Food Additives and Salicylates* (New York: Random House, 1979).

D.L. Dadd, R.C. Dadd, J.J. McGovern and R.W. Gardner, *Therapeutic Diets with Special Emphasis on the Rotary Diversified Diet (With Index of Phenylic Food Compounds)* (San Francisco, CA: Nutritional Research Company, 1980).

Thymus Function
Michael Murray, N.D., and Joseph Pizzorno, N.D., *Encyclopedia of Natural Medicine—Revised 2nd Edition* (Rocklin, CA: Prima Publishing, 1988, pp. 161, 745, and 788).

Vitamin C Therapy
Jacqueline Krohn, Francis A. Taylor and Erla Mae Larson, *The Whole Way to Allergy Relief and Prevention: A Doctor's Guide to Treatment and Self-Care* (Point Roberts, WA: Hartley and Marks, Inc., 1991).

Allergy Research Group
PO Box 489
400 Preda Street
San Leandro, CA 94577-0489
800-782-4274
A source of buffered and unbuffered vitamin C from beets.

Provocation-Neutralization Treatments
Joseph B. Miller, "Chapter 54: Intradermal Provocative-Neutralizing Food Testing and Subcutaneous Food Extract Injection Therapy," in *Food Allergy and Intolerance,* edited by Jonathan Brostoff and Stephen J. Challacombe (Philadelphia: Bailliere Tindall, 1987).

Doris J. Rapp, "Chapter 56: Sublingual Testing and Treatment," in *Food Allergy and Intolerance*, edited by Jonathan Brostoff and Stephen J. Challacombe (Philadelphia: Bailliere Tindall, 1987).

William P. King et al., "Provocation-Neutralization: A Two-Part Study Part I. The Intracutaneous Provocative Food Test: a Multicenter Comparison Study," *Otolaryngology—Head and Neck Surgery* 99(3) (Sept 1988):263-271.

William P. King et. al., "Provocation-Neutralization: A Two-Part Study Part II. Subcutaneous Neutralization Therapy: a Multicenter Comparison Study," *Otolaryngology—Head and Neck Surgery* 99(3) (Sept. 1988):272-277.

Jack L. Pulec, M.D., "Enzyme-Potentiated Desensitization: A Major Breakthrough," *Ear Nose Throat J*, 17(Oct. 1996):642.

American EPD Society, 505-984-0004, http://www.epdallergy.com

Unofficial source of EPD information provided by Stan Rohrer, http://www.dma.org/~rohrers/allergy/allergy.htm

Acupressure

Linda Weber, "The Man Who Couldn't Lift Peas," *Natural Health*, (July-August 1998):106-111, 178-182.

Dr. Devi S. Nambudripad's Web site: http://www.naet.com

MAP

Machaelle Small Wright, *MAP: The Co-Creative White Brotherhood Medical Assistance Program* (Warrenton, VA: Perelandra, Ltd., 1990).
http://www.perelandra-ltd.com
800-960-8806 United States and Canada
1-540-937-2153 Overseas and Mexico

Meditation
See Chapter 15.

Chapter 14: Superior Nutritional Support—How to Eat to Maximize Healing

Highlights:

- ❑ The basic healing diet.
- ❑ Thirteen good effects of this healing diet.
- ❑ Eight types of foods and supplements that further promote healing.

Effort Involved:

- ❑ Change your eating habits to improve your diet, if necessary.
- ❑ You may need to shop at a health food store for some of the food and supplements.

Payoff:

- ❑ Less joint pain.
- ❑ Less morning stiffness.
- ❑ Less disability.
- ❑ Better digestion.
- ❑ More energy.
- ❑ Repair of some or all of damage to joints.

Good Food

My grandfather, who survived two world wars, told me, "Never go without good food or good shoes. Even if you don't have money for anything else, make sure you have good food and good shoes."

Wartime and its aftermath made the evils of malnutrition very obvious. Losing most of his material possessions made it obvious how little is actually essential.

As he saw it, good food and good shoes were essential foundations. Good health requires good food. Moving about, at least in a cold climate, requires good shoes. With those two things, one could still carry on.

This chapter is not about good shoes. It is about how to heal through the power of good nutrition. If this is what you want to learn about, you are in the right place. Read on.

Bad Foods vs. Good Foods

Some foods trigger autoimmune responses that lead to arthritis. These foods, no matter how "healthy" they are, must be eliminated from your diet. As long as you eat these personal problem foods, your body will be busy destroying itself. Chapters 3-12 explain how to identify these foods, eliminate them from your diet, and still eat well. Despite what some books will try to tell you, there is no single list of "no-no" foods for people with arthritis. The list varies from one person to the next.

Some foods actively promote healing from arthritis. They give your body what it needs to recover. As long as these foods do not appear on your personal "no-no" list, including them in your diet will speed your recovery.

Many books have been written on what to eat to heal from arthritis. Some of these books are excellent. Some aren't so great. Most fail to point out that the groups of foods, which are good to eat BECAUSE they promote healing, may also include foods, which YOU PERSONALLY MUST ELIMINATE because they trigger autoimmune responses in you.

Remember, even the "healthiest" food in the world, even the ones included in this chapter, will not be healthy for you if you REACT adversely to it.

The Basic Healing Diet

The basic healing diet is high in fresh, preferably organically grown, fruits and vegetables and minimally processed foods. The most extreme diet of this type is an uncooked vegan (no animal products) diet sometimes called a "living foods diet." Studies have shown that this type of diet leads to improvements in both rheumatoid arthritis[44] and in fibromyalgia[45].

---

[44] O. Hanninen, K. Kaartinen, A. L. Rauma, M. Nenonen, R. Torronen, A. S. Hakkinen, H. Adlersceutz and J. Laakso, "Antioxidants in Vegan Diet and Rheumatic Disorders," *Toxicology* 155(1-3) (2000):45-53.

[45] K. Kaartinen, K. Lammi, M. Hypen, M. Nenonen, O. Hanninen and A. L. Raumal, "Vegan Diet Alleviates Fibromyalgia Symptoms," *Scand J. Rheumatol* 29(5) (2000):308-13.

For most people a strict, uncooked vegan diet is safe and beneficial but too extreme to be practical. Some meat and dairy products are generally OK, but to promote healing, the bulk of your diet should be whole grains and minimally processed nuts, seeds, beans, fruits and vegetables. Say good-bye to junk foods like soft drinks, white bread, donuts, Chee-tos®, highly processed lunchmeats and most fast food. Check out health food stores and see Chapters 10-12 for healthy alternatives.

The basic healing diet also includes the eight types of specific foods and supplements listed. These eight give your body what it needs to maximize healing from arthritis.

13 Advantages of a Diet High in Fresh Fruits and Vegetables and Minimally Processed Foods

This type of diet provides many healing benefits that our ancestors enjoyed automatically. Before the advent of the modern food-processing industry, a more natural diet was the only type available.

A diet high in fresh fruits and vegetables and minimally processed foods has 13 advantages. This type of diet:

1. Calms inflammation
2. Regulates blood sugar
3. Promotes healing
4. Enhances elimination of wastes
5. Improves blood cholesterol levels
6. Lowers cancer risk
7. Lowers heart disease risk
8. Lowers risk of obesity
9. Prevents free-radical damage
10. Supplies vitamins
11. Supplies minerals
12. Contains fewer toxic additives and contaminants
13. Contains fewer hidden allergens

1. The Magic of Omega-3 Oils—Calming Inflammation

The ratio of omega-3 to omega-6 oils in your body determines how easily inflammation is triggered in your body. Omega-3 calms inflammation. Omega-6 turns it on.

Getting enough omega-3 oil (also called omega-3 fatty acids) plus enough antioxidant vitamins and minerals (discussed below) is now recognized in the medical literature as an effective treatment for both rheumatoid and osteoarthritis.[46]

Most unprocessed food has a good omega-3 to omega-6 ratio. Unfortunately, food processing leaves omega-6 oils but removes virtually all omega-3 oil. This is because while omega-6 oils are relatively stable, omega-3 oils are relatively fragile and not suitable in products that are designed to have a long shelf life. The result is that most of us don't get enough omega-3 oils and get much too much omega-6.

Your omega-3 to omega-6 ratio automatically improves if you eat fresh fruits and vegetables and minimally processed foods.

To further ensure this good ratio, make sure you avoid omega-6 oils. Omega-6 oils are prevalent in all refined oil except canola oil, and they are at especially high levels in corn oil, safflower oil and sunflower oil. Avoid these oils. Also avoid products that contain these oils, such as baked goods, salad dressings and sauces. If you wish to cook with or otherwise add oil to your food, use canola oil or extra-virgin olive oil. Instead of being high in omega-6, they are high in omega-9 oil, another type of healthy oil, which is neutral as far as inflammation is concerned. Flaxseed oil is high in omega-3 oils and makes an excellent oil for salad dressings. As suggested later in this chapter, cod liver oil is also high in omega-3 oils and can be taken as a daily supplement.

2-8. The Multiple Good Effects of a Low Glycemic Index—Better Blood Sugar Regulation, Promotion of Healing, Enhanced Elimination of Wastes, Improved Cholesterol Levels, and Reduced Risk of Cancer, Heart Disease and Obesity

Having a low glycemic index means that when a food is eaten, glucose enters the bloodstream relatively slowly. Fresh fruit and vegetables and minimally processed food have lower—sometimes dramatically lower—glycemic indexes than their more processed counterparts.

Low glycemic index foods have many healing actions at once. They work their magic through the soluble and insoluble fiber that has not been removed by processing.

---

[46] L.G. Darlington and T. W. Stone, "Antioxidants and Fatty Acids in the Amelioration of Rheumatoid Arthritis and Related Disorders," *Br J Nutr* 85(3) (2001):251-69.

Because these foods foster a slower, more even absorption of glucose into the bloodstream, they:

1. Lower high blood glucose levels that impair healing.
2. Prevent uneven energy and hypoglycemic slumps. Hypoglycemia is a risk factor for trigger points. As explained in Chapter 17, trigger points in muscles set up a cycle of perpetual pain.
3. Reduce the glucagon/stress response. This allows the body to stay in healing mode instead of going into fight-or-flight mode.

These high-fiber foods also:

1. Improve elimination. This is important because constipation is a risk factor for arthritis.
2. Improve blood cholesterol levels.
3. Lower cancer risk.
4. Lower heart disease risk.
5. Lower obesity risk

Some of these good benefits arise from the fact that low glycemic index foods increase levels of HDL (so-called good cholesterol) and reduce levels of LDL (so-called bad cholesterol) in the bloodstream. Another benefit is that low glycemic index foods reduce insulin resistance.

Insulin resistance increases the amount of insulin the body must have to use blood sugar properly. This results in high levels of insulin circulating in the bloodstream. A high level of insulin can trigger an unwanted cell proliferation and is a risk factor for cancers such as colon cancer. A high level of insulin has also long been associated with a condition known as Syndrome X, a constellation of abnormalities that include high blood pressure and increased heart attack risk. Too much insulin is also a factor in other health problems, such as polycystic ovarian syndrome. Finally, a high level of insulin makes it difficult for the body to utilize reserves of fat. In other words, it makes it difficult to lose weight. It is easy to see why the ability of low glycemic index foods to reduce insulin resistance is so important.

Low glycemic index foods also tend to be low in calories. That means you can eat larger portions without gaining weight.

If you want to gain weight on this type of diet, be sure to get enough calories by including healthy oils, such as olive oil and flaxseed oil, in your food.

9. Antioxidants—Prevention of Free-Radical Damage

A diet high in fresh, preferably organically grown fruits and vegetables and minimally processed foods contains a rich and complex array of antioxidants. Anyone who has followed the nutritional headlines in the last decade probably knows by now that antioxidants are the good guys who fight off free-radical damage in the body. Antioxidants keep the order in Dodge City. When the bad guys ride in, the antioxidants shut them down before they can shoot up the town.

Highly processed food has much of its antioxidant capacity removed. These antioxidants include vitamins, pigments, and a host of other substances that are still being discovered. What is added back to highly processed food in the form of vitamin supplementation is only a fraction of the rich and complex array of protective substances that had been there originally. The antioxidants in fresh, organically grown food are like a highly dispersed, highly trained anti-terrorist team that eliminates trouble before it gets started. What is added back to processed food amounts to just a few SWAT team members who are run ragged without the resources to do the job completely.

10-11. Better Supply of Vitamins and Minerals

Many of the methods used to process food have a detrimental effect on nutritional quality[47,48]. Blanching vegetables and refining carbohydrates, for example, both result in loss of vitamins and minerals. Milling and extrusion can cause the physical removal of minerals.

Eating fresh, minimally processed food is the best way to prevent such losses. Here are a few ways to do that:

□ Eat fresh, raw vegetables instead of cooked vegetables.
□ Eat whole grains such as cooked wheat grains instead of products made from wheat flour.
□ Eat products made from whole-grain flour instead of white flour.

---

[47] M. B. Reddy and M. Love, "The Impact of Food Processing on the Nutritional Quality of Vitamins and Minerals," *Adv Exp Med Biol* 459 (1999):99-106.

[48] N. J. Temple, "Refined Carbohydrates-A Cause of Suboptimal Nutrient Intake," *Med Hypotheses* 10(4) (1983):411-24.

12. Fewer Toxic Additives and Contaminants

Highly processed food, especially food produced by current agribusiness practices, contains many additives and contaminants. These include food preservatives and pesticide residues. Even when these are within "safe" limits, they represent stresses to the body.

For instance, the body uses up vitamins E and vitamin C when it detoxifies nitrite, a commonly used preservative.[49] The detoxification of other preservatives and pesticide residues also requires that the body use up some of its supply of vitamins. The more preservatives and pesticides the body must detoxify, the greater the stress on its detoxification pathways and the greater the vitamin depletion.

How can you avoid this depletion? Once again, the answer is eating fresh organically grown fruits and vegetables and other minimally processed foods. Fresh avoids problems with preservatives. Organic avoids problems with pesticide residues.

13. Fewer Hidden Allergens

Modern food processing adds many substances to food. Since not all of these are indicated on product labeling, these additives can become problematic sources of hidden allergens.

For instance, if you have a corn allergy and you don't know that most baking powder is half cornstarch, it may take you a long time to figure out why eating baked goods leavened with baking powder makes you sick. Even more problematic, if you have a corn allergy and don't know that the dextrose that is added to table salt is commercially derived from corn and therefore contaminated with corn allergens, you may not realize why you get sick every time you eat something that contains table salt. Since table salt is such a prevalent food additive, you may stay at least mildly sick most of the time and have problems pinpointing the problem. This happened to me.

Chapters 6-8 have extensive lists of hidden allergens commonly found in processed food. If you have food sensitivities, it may be necessary to rely almost totally on fresh, preferably organically grown fruits and vegetables and minimally processed foods, in order to avoid having your sensitivities triggered by these hidden allergens.

---

[49] E. Quattrucci and V. Masci, "Nutritional Aspects of Food Preservatives," *Food Addit Contam* 9(5) (1992):515-25.

8 Types of Foods and Supplements to Maximize Healing from Arthritis Specifically

1. Omega-3 oils
2. Vitamins and minerals
3. Digestive tract healers
4. Digestive aids
5. Indian spices
6. Alfalfa
7. General health tonics
8. Glucosamine and chondroitin

1. Omega-3 oils

Improving your omega-3 to omega-6 oil ratio calms inflammation. To improve this ratio, it helps not only to eat minimally processed food but also to supplement your diet with a good source of omega-3 oil, such as flaxseed oil, flaxseeds, cod liver oil, and fresh or frozen mackerel, trout, herring, tuna or salmon. Don't count on canned fish for omega-3 oils. The heat involved in the canning process destroys these oils.

Avoid farm-raised fish because their diet of processed fish food causes them to have a much poorer omega-3 to omega-6 ratio than their wild counterparts. Usually the only way to know if you are getting farm-raised fish or wild fish is if you know the fisherman or if it is revealed on the packaging.

To make sure you get enough omega-3, get a daily dose of one of the following: 1 to 2 tsp. cod liver oil, 1 to 2 tsp. flaxseed oil, OR 3 ½ ounces of one of the fish mentioned above.

Increasing the ratio of omega-3 to omega-6 oil in your diet is often enough to relieve arthritis. Because the turnover of oils in the body is slow, it generally takes one to two months on a diet high in omega-3 and low omega-6 oil to see a change.

2. Vitamins and Minerals

Healthy joints require adequate levels of vitamins and minerals such as vitamin B-1 (thiamine), B-5 (pantothenic acid), B-6 (pyridoxine), B-12 (cyanocobalamin), C (ascorbic acid), D and E (tocopherol) and folic acid, beta-carotene, calcium, potassium, iron and several trace minerals including selenium. Elimination of pain caused by myofascial trigger points also requires adequate levels of these vitamins and minerals. Myofascial trigger points, which are discussed in Chapter 17, are tight spots in muscles, which often produce symptoms that mimic the pain and restricted range of motion of arthritis.

Damage done by free radicals in the body contributes significantly to the development of both osteoarthritis and autoimmune types of arthritis such as rheumatoid arthritis. Adequate levels of antioxidant vitamins and antioxidant minerals, including vitamin C, vitamin E and selenium, help stop the damage and promote healing. Others like vitamin D and calcium are needed to build and maintain healthy bones. The rest are essential in various ways for proper metabolism.

Levels of these vitamins and minerals tend to be low in people with arthritis.[50, 51, 52, 53, 54] Raising these levels leads to measurable improvements. Several studies have shown improvements in arthritis using a cocktail of antioxidant vitamins and minerals.[55, 56, 57]

---

[50] J. Stone, A. Doube, D. Dudson and J. Wallace, "Inadequate Calcium, Folic Acid, Vitamin E, Zinc, and Selenium Intake in Rheumatoid Arthritis Patients: Results of a Dietary Survey," *Semin Arthritis Rheum* 27(3) (1997):180-5.

[51] G. W. Comstock, A. E. Burke, S. C. Hoffman, K. J. Helzlsouer, A. Bendich, A. T. Masi, E. P. Norkus, R. L. Malament and M. E. Gershwin, "Serum Concentrations of Alpha Tocopherol, Beta Carotene, and Retinol Preceding the Diagnosis of Rheumatoid Arthritis and Systemic Lupus Erythematosus," *Ann Rheum Dis* 56(5) (1997):323-5.

[52] M. Sklodowska, J. Gromadzinska, M. Biernacka, W. Wasowicz, P. Wolkanin, A. Marszalek, H. Brozik and K. Pokuszynska, "Vitamin E, Thiobarbituric Acid Reactive Substance Concentrations and Superoxide Dismutase Activity in the Blood of Children with Juvenile Rheumatoid Arthritis," *Clin Exp Rheumatol* 14(4) (1996):43309.

[53] M. Heliovaara, P. Knekt, K. Aho, R. K. Aaran, G. Alfthan and A. Aromaa, "Serum Antioxidants and Risk of Rheumatoid Arthritis," *Ann Rheum Dis* 53(1) (1994):51-3.

[54] E. D. Rosenstein and J. R. Caldwell, "Trace Elements in the Treatment of Rheumatic Conditions," *Rheum Dis Clin North Am* 25(4) (1999):929-35,viii.

[55] T. E. McAlindon, P. Jacques, Y. Zhang, M. T. Hannan, P. Aliabadi, B. Weissman, D. Rush, D. Levy and D. T. Felson, "Do Antioxidant

A few studies have also shown improvements using elevated levels of a single vitamin such as vitamin E, pantothenic acid (B-5), or vitamin C.

One placebo-controlled, double-blind trial has shown that 600 mg vitamin E given twice a day for 12 weeks to rheumatoid arthritis patients, in addition to their other drugs, lowered pain levels.[58] In another study, vitamin E was shown to increase the effectiveness of aspirin in inhibiting inflammation.[59]

Ninety-four patients participated in a double-blind study of a placebo versus oral, high-dosage calcium pantothenate.[60] The dose of calcium pantothenate started at 500 mg a day and gradually increased to 2000 mg a day, given in four equal dosages during the day. Calcium pantothenate was shown to have highly significant effects in reducing the duration of morning stiffness, the degree of disability and the severity of pain in those patients with rheumatoid arthritis.

Micronutrients Protect Against the Development and Progression of Knee Osteoarthritis?" *Arthritis Rheum* 39(4) (1996):648-56.

[56] G. Wilhelmi, "Potential Influence of Nutrition with Supplements on Healthy and Arthritic Joints. II. Nutritional Quantity, Supplements, Contamination," *Z Rheumatol* 52(4) (1993):191-200.

[57] J. Aaseth, M. Haugen and O. Forre, "Rheumatoid Arthritis and Metal Compounds—Perspective on the Role of Oxygen Radical Detoxification," *Analyst* 123(1) (1998):3-6.

[58] S. E. Edmonds, P. G. Winyard, R. Guo, B. Kidd, P. Merry, A. Langrish-Smith, C. Hansen, S. Ramm and D. R. Blake, "Putative Analgesic Activity of Repeated Oral Doses of Vitamin E in the Treatment of Rheumatoid Arthritis. Results of a Prospective Placebo Controlled Double Blind Trial," *Ann Rheum Dis* 56(11) (1997):649-55.

[59] A. Abate, G. Yang, P.A. Dennery, S. Oberle and H. Schroder, "Synergistic Inhibition of Cyclooxygenease-2 Expression by Vitamin E and Aspirin," *Free Radic Biol Med* 29(11) (2000):1135-42.

[60] "Calcium Pantothenate in Arthritis Conditions. A Report from the General Practitioner Research Group," *Practitioner* 224 (1980):208-211.

Vitamin C is involved in a remarkable number of essential body functions, including collagen synthesis, degradation of amino acids, and the synthesis of two neurotransmitters.[61] Collagen (and thus vitamin C) is essential to the formation of connective tissue and the cartilage in joints. Collagen (and thus vitamin C) is also essential for the deposit of calcium phosphate crystals to form bone. Because of this, it is easy to see why sufficient vitamin C is essential for healthy joints.

The importance of vitamin C for arthritis is supported by a study that shows that it reduces the risk of cartilage loss and disease progression in people with osteoarthritis.[62] Its importance is further supported by a study that shows that vitamin C reduces inflammation in the joints of rats used as an animal model for autoimmune types of arthritis such as rheumatoid arthritis.[63]

In addition, high doses of vitamin C, as detailed in Chapter 14, have been found to be useful in treating leaky gut syndrome and food sensitivities.

Dr. Janet G Travell, M.D., recommends up to 500 mg of vitamin C per day to bring the level of vitamin C in the body up to optimum levels for eliminating trigger points.[64]

Because the vitamins and minerals mentioned above work synergistically, it is generally more effective to take a balanced multiple vitamin and mineral supplement than to supplement with high levels of only one or a few of these vitamins and minerals.

---

[61] Janet G. Travell, M.D., and David G. Simons, M.D., *Myofascial Pain and Dysfunction: the Trigger Point Manual, Vol. 1*, (Baltimore, MD: Williams & Wilkins, 1983, 137-138).

[62] T. E. McAlindon, P. Jacques, Y. Zhang, M. T. Hannan, P. Aliabadi, B. Weissman, D. Rush, D. Levy and D. T. Felson, "Do Antioxidant Micronutrients Protect Against the Development and Progression of Knee Osteoarthritis?" *Arthritis Rheum* 39(4) (1996):648-56.

[63] A. Sakai, T. Hirano, R. Okazaki, N. Okimoto, K. Tanaka and T. Nakamura, "Large-dose Ascorbic Acid Administration Suppresses the Development of Arthritis in Adjuvant-Infected Rats," *Arch Orthop Trauma Surg* 119(3-4) (1999):121-6.

[64] Janet G. Travell, M.D., and David G. Simons, M.D., *Myofascial Pain and Dysfunction: the Trigger Point Manual, Vol. 1* (Baltimore, MD: Williams & Wilkins, 1983, 141).

3. Digestive Tract Healers

As explained in Chapter 2, one of the underlying causes of arthritis is leaky gut syndrome. Foods that help heal the digestive tract help heal what is often a major contributing factor to arthritis at its very source.

Cabbage juice, fiber, yogurt, miso, sauerkraut, vitamin C and colostrum are some of the many foods that help heal the digestive tract.

Cabbage and cabbage juice have been known for centuries as stomach healers. Modern science now knows that cabbage is high in proteins called mucins that form a protective coating in the stomach. This coating protects the stomach from stomach acids and mechanical stresses, giving it a chance to heal. Freshly made cabbage juice, in particular, is a potent healer. Because of its strong taste, you might want to mix it with carrot juice to make it more appealing.

Adequate fiber in your diet promotes healthy intestinal flora and timely elimination. Both of these are important for a healthy digestive tract.

Yogurt, miso and sauerkraut are good sources of the healthy flora you want living in your intestines. Yogurt is fermented milk. Miso is a traditional Japanese fermented soybean paste that sometimes also contains a grain such as rice or barley. Sauerkraut is fermented cabbage. Because of the health-promoting bacteria that cause the fermentation, each of these products is a good source of healthy varieties of bacteria. These products are good to eat on a regular basis, but are especially important after a round of antibiotics. Use them to reseed your gut with healthy intestinal flora.

Vitamin C, perhaps because it is so good at reducing inflammation, helps the gut. See Chapter 14 for details.

Bovine colostrum comes from cows in the first few days after they give birth. It is marketed in health food stores as a health food supplement. Perhaps because it is a rich source of growth factors, it has been shown to help heal the damage to the gut caused by nonsteroidal anti-inflammatory drugs (NSAIDs).[65]

---

[65] R. J. Playford, D. N. Floyd, C. E. Macdonald, D. P. Calnan, R. O. Adenekan, W. Johnson, R. A. Goodlad and T. Marchbank, "Bovine Colostrum is a Health Food Supplement Which Prevents NSAID Induced Gut Damage," *Gut* 44(5) (1999):653-8.

4. Digestive Aids

The type of imbalances in intestinal flora that lead to arthritis can be caused by not digesting your food well. See Chapter 2 for a full discussion of this issue. It explains how to determine if you need digestive aids and which you might want to use. In short, aids like hydrochloric acid, digestive enzymes, pineapple and papaya, all available in health food stores, can lead to dramatic improvements in your condition.

5. Indian Spices

Several Indian spices have been shown to improve arthritis. These spices work their magic in at least two ways.

First, they stimulate digestive enzymes. In this sense, Indian spices could also be considered with the other digestive aids mentioned in the section above. Spicing with turmeric (or with just the active principle, curcumin), hot pepper (or with just the active principle, capsaicin), black pepper (or with just the active principle, piperine), ginger, fenugreek, cumin and/or asafetida has been scientifically shown to make food easier to digest.[66]

Second, Indian foods improve arthritic conditions through an anti-inflammatory effect. Turmeric has been reported to reduce inflammation and disability in double-blind clinical trials on patients with rheumatoid arthritis.[67] Studies show that powdered ginger provides varying degrees of relief from pain and swelling from rheumatoid and osteoarthritis.[68] Ginger also provides pain relief for patients with muscular discomfort. Unlike conventional anti-inflammatory medicines, no adverse effects have been reported for ginger. Fresh ginger used in cooking also has excellent anti-inflammatory effects. Jean Carper, author of the book *Food—Your Miracle Medicine*, quotes Dr. K. C. Srivastava of Odensee University in Denmark, who recommends about 1/3 teaspoon fresh ginger three times a day for his patients with arthritis.

---

[66] K. Platel and K. Srivivasan, "Influence of Dietary Spices and Their Active Principles on Pancreatic Digestive Enzymes in Albino Rats," *Nahrung* 44(1) (2000):42-6.

[67] R. Lodha and A. Bagga, "Traditional Indian Systems of Medicine," *Ann Acad Med Singapore* 29(1) (2000):37-41.

[68] K. C. Srivastava and T. Mustafa, "Ginger (*Zingiber officinale*) in Rheumatism and Musculoskeletal Disorders," *Med Hypotheses* 39(4) (1992):342-8.

6. Alfalfa

Alfalfa is a folk remedy for arthritis and one that helped me get well. The dried leaves can be made into tea, taken in capsules, or taken as an extract. It is believed to help correct arthritis by adjusting the pH of the body to a range more conducive to healing. Arthritis is thought to be a disease of acidity. Alfalfa is a corrective because it is a great alkalizer.

7. General Health Tonics

Some foods and extracts have a centuries-long history as general health tonics. They help heal because anything that builds your general health and vitality will make it easier for you to heal from whatever ails you, including arthritis. To identify some of these foods, just think of the old sayings such as "An apple a day keeps the doctor away," and Popeye's boast "I'm strong to the finish, 'cause I eat my spinach."

Garlic, onions, ginger, and ginseng are also some of the many foods and herbs that have been used since antiquity to maintain and restore health.

Modern research is now documenting some of these good effects. Raw garlic has been shown to have potent anti-inflammatory properties.[69] A study from Russia found a garlic preparation called alisate to be at least as effective a treatment for rheumatoid arthritis as conventional therapy.[70] We now know that the ancient cure-all, onion, is chock full of antioxidants and anticancer agents. Onions are also anti-inflammatory, antibiotic, antiviral, and good for your cholesterol levels. Ginger, mentioned above as an Indian spice, has more than one hundred good health effects and is also a health tonic. It fights nausea, helps stomachs heal and acts as an anti-inflammatory. Ginseng, which has long been popular in Asia, is a tonic herb that functions as an adaptogen. An adaptogen helps the body perform optimally and cope better with stress.

Andrew Weil, M.D., in his book *Eight Weeks to Optimum Health*, mentions other general health tonics. His list includes ashwagandha, a herbal remedy from the Ayurvedic tradition of India; astragalus, made from the roots of a Chinese species *A. membranaceus;* cordyceps, made from a fungus that grows in the bodies of certain moth larvae; dong quai, made from the root

---

[69] M. Ali, "Mechanism by which Garlic (*Allium sativum*) Inhibits Cyclooxygenase Activity. Effect of Raw versus Boiled Garlic Extract on the Synthesis of Prostanoids," *Prostaglandins Leukot Essent Fatty Acids* 53 (1995):397-400.

[70] L. N. Denisov, I. V. Andrianova and S. S. Timofeeva, "Garlic Effectiveness in Rheumatoid Arthritis," *Ter Arkh* 71(8) (1999):55-8.

of *Angelica sinensis*; maitake, the Japanese name for the mushroom *Grifola frondosa*, known in America as "hen of the woods"; milk thistle, made from the seed of *Silybum marianum*; reishi, made from the mushroom *Ganoderma lucidum*, and Siberian ginseng, made from the root of a large shrub called *Eleutherococcus senticosus*. Ashwagandha and reishi are general tonics, astragalus and maitake improve immune system function, cordyceps functions as an adaptogen, dong quai helps circulation, and milk thistle protects the liver.

The point in mentioning all these tonics is not to overwhelm you with information. You don't need to know about or take all of them. Just picking one or two is enough. Regularly taking one or more health tonics will promote your overall health and your ability to heal.

8. Glucosamine and Chondroitin

Glucosamine and chondroitin are two substances with a good track record for helping people heal from arthritis. They have been used in Europe for years for this purpose. In the last few years, they have also become popular in the United States. They are usually taken together.

The body makes both glucosamine and chondroitin, although in lesser amounts as we age and not always in great enough quantities to rebuild damaged cartilage and heal intestinal problems without oral supplementation.

Glucosamine inhibits free-radical production and inflammation. It also speeds wound-healing and reduces scarring.[71] It does this both when placed directly on a wound and when taken orally. It speeds the healing of surgical wounds, traumas such as cuts and bruises, injury to the gastrointestinal tract, and arthritic joints.

The two modes by which glucosamine heals arthritis are healing at the site of the arthritic joints and healing of the gastrointestinal tract.[72] This second mode of action will be of no surprise to you if you have already read Chapter 2, which provides a detailed explanation of the link between gastrointestinal problems and arthritis.

---

[71] M. F. McCarty, "Glucosamine for Wound Healing," *Med Hypothesis* 47(4) (1996):273-5.

[72] A. L. Russell, "Glucosamine in Osteoarthritis and Gastrointestinal Disorders: An Exemplar of the Need for a Paradigm Shift," *Med Hypotheses* 51(4) (1988:347-9.

Glucosamine promotes gastrointestinal healing by increasing the number of cells making protective mucins and by upping the amount of mucins that each of these cells makes.

Several types of gastrointestinal disturbances disrupt the protective mucin layer. For example, *Helicobacter pylori*, an infection associated with ulcers, reduces these mucins.[73] Abnormalities in colonic mucin synthesis have also been implicated in ulcerative colitis and Crohn's disease.[74] Because glucosamine synthesis is the bottleneck step in the biosynthesis of mucins, it is easy to see why oral supplementation with glucosamine can speed healing from these conditions. Supplementation simply bypasses the bottleneck, allowing cells to make more protective mucins.

In a review of 16 trials of glucosamine alone for treating osteoarthritis, it was found that glucosamine is a safe and effective treatment that works as well as or better than conventional NSAIDs.[75] In addition, unlike NSAIDs, glucosamine seems to have no toxic side effects.

Chondroitin sulfates stimulate the production of cartilage and stop the action of enzymes that break down cartilage. They also speed the healing of bones and skin wounds.

A different review of 17 studies, this time of glucosamine and chondroitin, found that the combination of both helps heal osteoarthritis.[76] Presumably because chondroitin helps rebuild damaged cartilage and thus corrects the underlying problem, instead of only reducing inflammation and thus merely

---

[73] J.C. Byrd, C. K. Yunker, Q. S. Xu, L. R. Sternberg and R. S. Bresalier, "Inhibition of Gastric Mucin synthesis by Helicobacter pylori," *Gastroenterology* 118(6) (2000):1072-9.

[74] M. C. Winslet, V. Poxon, A. Allan and M. R. Keighley, "Mucosal Glucosamine Synthetase Activity in Inflammatory Bowel Disease," *Dig Dis Sci* 39(3) (1994):540-4.

[75] T. E. Towheed, T. P. Anastassiades, B. Shea, J. Houpt, V. Welch and M. C. Hochberg, "Glucosamine Therapy for Treating Osteoarthritis (Cochrane Review)," *Cochrane Database Syst. Rev* 1 (2001):CD002946.

[76] T. F. McAlindon, M. P. LaValley, J. P. Gulin and D. T. Felon, "Glucosamine and Chondroitin were Found to Improve Outcomes in Patients with Osteoarthritis," *J Bone Joint Surg* 82 (2000):1323.

treating the symptom, one study using treatment with only chondroitin showed that improvements continued for a month post-treatment.[77] One can speculate that if the study had gone on longer, it may well have found that the improvements continued to last for much longer than only a month.

Although there are no published clinical trials that show that glucosamine and chondroitin have a favorable impact on rheumatoid arthritis and other autoimmune types of arthritis, this is probably only a matter of time. The preliminary results from animal studies and tissue culture studies indicate that these agents can help heal all sorts of arthritis.[78]

Luke Bucci, Ph.D.[79], suggests a daily dose for people with arthritis of 1,500 mg glucosamine salts (preferably glucosamine hydrochloride) and 1,500 mg chondroitin sulfates (find a purified source; avoid cartilage powder, trachea powder and mussels). These supplements are sold at health food stores and drugstores, often combined as 500 mg each per pill. If this is the case, take one pill morning, noon, and evening.

Long-Term Benefits

Your body is amazing. Given the right nutrients, it has a tremendous ability to heal itself. The healing foods and supplements in this chapter maximize your ability to heal from arthritis by giving your body exactly what it needs to heal.

Some of these foods and supplements have many good effects throughout the entire body, some provide a natural way to reduce inflammation, some improve digestion, and some give the body what it needs to heal arthritic joints. Taken as a whole, this type of diet has the power to unleash previously dormant healing.

---

[77] B. Mazieres, B. Combe, Van A. Phan, J. Tondut and M. Grynfeltt, "Chondroitin Sulfate in Osteoarthritis of the Knee: A Prospective, Double Blind, Placebo Controlled Multicenter Clinical Study," *J Rheumatol* 28(1) (2001):173-81.

[78] J. Beren, S. L. Hill, M. Diener-West and N. R. Rose, "Effect of Pre-Loading Oral Glucosamine HCl/Chondroitin Sulfate/Manganese Ascorbate Combination on Experimental Arthritis in Rats," *Exp Biol Med* 226(2)(2001)144-51.

[79] Luke Bucci, Pain Free: The Definitive Guide to Healing Arthritis, Low-Back Pain, and Sports Injuries through Nutrition and Supplements (Fort Worth, TX: The Summit Group, 1995).

If you switch to the nutritional program outlined in this chapter, you are likely to begin noticing less joint pain, less morning stiffness, less disability, better digestion, more energy, and eventually repair of some or all of the damage to your joints.

Resources

Jean Carper, *Food—Your Miracle Medicine* (New York: HarperCollins Publishers, Inc., 1993).

Andrew Weil, M.D., *Eight Weeks to Optimum Health* (New York: Alfred A. Knopf, Inc., 1997).

Luke Bucci, *Pain Free: The Definitive Guide to Healing Arthritis, Low-Back Pain, and Sports Injuries through Nutrition and Supplements* (Fort Worth, TX: The Summit Group, 1995).

Chapter 15: Transforming Your Relationship to Pain—How to Use Meditation as a Powerful Aid in Healing

Highlights:

❑ Directions for two simple meditations.

Effort Involved:

❑ Only a few minutes of effort are involved in initially trying the two meditation techniques described. However, the more you use these tools, the more you will benefit.

Payoff:

❑ Radical reduction in suffering.

Not Just for Mystics Anymore — What Meditation is and Why it is so Useful for Dealing with Chronic Pain

What is Meditation?

Meditation is a SPECIAL WAY of focusing attention. There are many kinds of meditation and without asking it is almost impossible to know what someone using the term meditation might actually mean. Some people mean creative visualization, targeted thinking, systematic relaxation of muscles, sitting still without talking, or any number of other activities. For our purposes here, NONE of these activities qualifies as meditation. What does qualify is A SPECIAL KIND OF ATTENTION that makes it possible to radically retrain your relationship to pain.

Why is Meditation so Useful?

Meditation is USEFUL in treating chronic pain because it is an EXCELLENT TOOL for retraining your response to pain. Even if your pain never goes away, you can learn to experience it not as a problem, but as something that just is. In some cases you may even find that what you formerly experienced as hard, solidified pain becomes a pleasant, empowering flow of energy that makes your life easier and more joyful. That may sound like science fiction, but it is not.

In 1993 the Bill Moyers TV special called "Healing and the Mind" introduced millions of Americans to Dr. Jon Kabat-Zinn and the program of the Stress Reduction Clinic at the University of Massachusetts Medical Center. This program, run by Dr. Kabat-Zinn and offered in a hospital setting, has had great success teaching the use of mindfulness meditation for dealing better with chronic pain. These good results are all the more impressive because most of the participants in this Stress Reduction Clinic are very ill, and modern medicine has otherwise reached the end of what it has to offer them in terms of improvement.

Meditation is a good tool for dealing with stress and pain. Because these are major issues for people with rheumatoid arthritis and other autoimmune types of arthritis, meditation works particularly well for these types of arthritis. Preliminary research published in medical journals supports this. One paper concludes that people with rheumatoid arthritis who use meditation in combination with traditional medications appear to live better lives and may have better long-term outcomes.[80] Another suggests that meditation-based stress reduction is effective for people with fibromyalgia.[81]

My Experience with Tonglen and Vipassana Meditation

The two examples of meditation I will be discussing come from the vast array of Buddhist meditative practices.

The first example is *tonglen* meditation. It comes from the Tibetan tradition. I first read about it in a book called *The Tibetan Book of Living*

---

[80] D.E. Yocum, W.L. Castro, and M. Cornett, "Exercise, Education, and Behavioral Modifications as Alternative Therapy for Pain and Stress in Rheumatic Disease," *Rheum Dis Clin North Am* 2000 Feb; 26(1):145-59, x-xi.

[81] K. H. Kaplan, D. L. Goldenberg, and M. Galvin-Nadeau, "The Impact of a Meditation-Based Stress Reduction Program on Fibromyalgia," *Gen Hosp Psychiatry* 1993 Sep;15(5):284-9.

and Dying by Sogyal Rinpoche. It was the first type of meditation that ever gave me pain relief. When I was lying in bed at night in too much pain to sleep and sometimes almost out of my mind in pain, I would do the *tonglen* practice. For as long as I could do it, the results were magical. At first this relief was for only a moment or two. Later I could hold it for five minutes at a time and eventually much longer. It became fascinating to me that one minute I could be out of my mind in pain and the next I could be having a profound break from the otherwise unremitting pain. Training my attention, moment by moment, was the key.

The second example is *vipassana* meditation. It comes from the Therevadan school of Buddhism. In the West this type of meditation is often called insight meditation or mindfulness meditation. It has come to America from Southeast Asia. My first introduction to this practice came from a set of tapes called "Break Through Pain" by Shinzen Young. On one of these tapes Shinzen stated that if you could stay conscious through fainting intensities of pain, your life would never be the same again. Upon hearing these words I finally understood what had been spontaneously happening to me during the worst of my arthritis pain.

More Reasons to Use Meditation to Deal with Chronic Pain

1. It provides a way to understand experiences that you may already have been having but have been reluctant to talk about.
2. It provides a systematic way to cultivate certain highly desirable states of consciousness that you might otherwise seldom or never stumble upon.

Before listening to Shinzen's "Break Through Pain" tapes, I didn't have the words or the concepts to even begin to formulate why the pain I experienced during the first years of my arthritis seemed like one of the greatest gifts of my life. I never talked about this to anyone, because I didn't want people to think I was crazy.

Shinzen's clear explanations helped me to realize what had happened when I was in intense pain. Pain naturally tends to put a person into a special state of high concentration that Buddhist teachings refer to as *samadhi*. This state of high concentration or focus can occur not only spontaneously in moments of intense pain but can also be cultivated through meditation. Instead of passing out from the intense pain, what would sometimes happen was that through the grace of spontaneous moments of *samadhi* I would enter a state of great peacefulness.

Given my levels of pain, it is not surprising that I don't remember these years of my life very well. The great gift from this period was the conviction that no matter what happened, I would be OK. When the pain was more than I could bear, I would rest in a place of great love that was beyond any sense of having a body or rational thought. Even just the memory of a moment in this timeless place was enough to make all the confusion, pain and loss that I was experiencing seem bearable.

Systematically Cultivating Special States of Consciousness

Shinzen's "Break Through Pain" tapes gave me a clear, systematic way to cultivate special and highly desirable states of consciousness. Even though fainting intensities of pain are now rare for me, I still have plenty of sensations with which to work. It turns out that it is possible to use any body sensation, whether it be pleasant, unpleasant or neutral, as a training ground. The sensations can be almost undetectably faint, almost unbearably extreme, or anywhere in between.

In the seven years since I was introduced to *vipassana* meditation, I have found—again and again—that it is often only the quality of my attention that means the difference between experiencing a sensation as pain or pleasure. I experience this rather dramatically on long bike rides. If I can meditatively focus on a cramp, even one severe enough to make me get off my bike, the cramp will often open up into a pleasant flow of energy. Not only that, but the energy that had been trapped in the cramp then becomes available to power the ride. Suddenly I find myself riding almost effortlessly and much more quickly and joyfully than normal. Meditation is what makes the difference.

As stated earlier, meditation is useful in treating chronic pain because you can use it to retrain yourself to experience it not as pain but as a pleasant, empowering flow of energy that makes your life easier and more joyful.

Deep Healing

Unlocking the energy trapped in pain can also lead to deep healing. For 10 years I had extensive food sensitivities. My corn allergy, in particular, was so severe that the conventional medical opinion was that I would never be cured of it. Conventional medical opinion was wrong.

On August 2, 1999, over the course of one hour, my physiology changed dramatically. I was completely cured of all my food sensitivities. This happened as the culmination of many meditative releases of fear and anger.

On a *vipassana* meditation retreat in January 1999, I worked at a deep level with fear of food. Even at that time I had a sense that releasing fear was a key to releasing my food sensitivities.

On a *vipassana* meditation retreat in June 1999, I found that I had a lot of anger and learned to work with anger meditatively. I found myself working this way with anger all summer. On August 2, at the end of a meditation which was the culmination of a week of dramatic meditative releases of anger, I suddenly knew something had radically changed. I knew that I no longer had any of my food sensitivities. Meditative releases of my fear and anger had resulted in deep healing.

After a day of anguish and trepidation, I rather rashly tested myself on August 3, 1999, with a celebratory pizza. Although I knew on a deep level that this would be OK, it was still hard to voluntarily eat the very substances that had made me so very sick for years. To my utter joy, I suffered no ill effects—absolutely no joint pain, fatigue, or foggy mind. After years of getting very ill from even the smallest trace of many foods, most of which were a part of that pizza, I had absolutely no problem with food sensitivities. I have been completely free of food sensitivities ever since.

The Paradox

One of the paradoxes of meditation is that although the desire to change yourself is a good reason to meditate, you are unlikely to experience any of the benefits of meditation if you fall into the trap of expecting certain changes or trying to make certain changes happen.

On the contrary, what meditation requires is staying in the present moment and just noticing what is, without a particular agenda for what should happen. You must suspend any desire for your pain to go away and any desire to be healed in any way. The key to this type of meditation is becoming fascinated with exactly what is and accepting it exactly the way it is, whatever that may be.

If you would like to read more about how to let go of your expectations and agendas, I recommend Shinzen Young's article titled "Equanimity." It is available on the Internet at:
http://www.shinzen.org/shinsub3/theoryEquanimity.htm

Different Meditative Traditions

I have used examples of meditation that come from the Buddhist tradition because that is what appealed to me, but these basic types of meditation have been discovered and rediscovered by individuals and cultures all over the globe and throughout history. These meditation techniques have been most extensively developed and preserved within Buddhism, but they found in all of the major religions of the world including Christianity, Judaism, Islam and Hinduism, and are also practiced by tribal peoples.

No particular set of religious beliefs is required to make effective use of the two types of meditation described below.

The Mechanics — Step by Step Guide to 2 Simple and Powerful Meditation Techniques

Tonglen Meditation— Soygal Rinpoche

Tonglen meditation is known as the practice of giving and receiving. It has many forms. The form I use is very simple. It is related to breathing in and out. On my in-breath I imagine breathing in the pain of everyone in the whole world who is experiencing, at that exact moment, exactly the same kind of pain as mine. As I breathe in, I focus on exactly where in my body I am feeling pain. Sometimes I even imagine breathing directly into the pain and letting it expand however much it needs to. On the out-breath I imagine breathing out to each of those people, including myself, exactly what each of us needs to be free of our suffering.

Although this practice may seem too simplistic to be of help, I heartily recommend trying it. I find it to be profoundly powerful. If breathing in that much suffering seems too intimidating, start with just your own pain or some small subset of your pain. Start with a short meditation period, perhaps just one minute if your pain is great. Lengthen the meditation period as you are able.

If you want to learn more about *tonglen* meditation, I recommend reading the chapter on compassion in *The Tibetan Book of Living and Dying* by Sogyal Rinpoche. This chapter has full descriptions of many different variations of *tonglen* meditation.

Pain Meditation— Shinzen Young

Shinzen Young teaches a form of meditation called *vipassana* meditation, also known as mindfulness or insight meditation.

This type of meditation cultivates two qualities: mindfulness and equanimity.

245

The basic technique is to sit or lie quietly while bringing these qualities to your experience of pain.

Mindfulness, when dealing with pain, means being aware of the exact location, shape and intensity of the pain, how the pain's location, shape and intensity vary with time, and also the exact "flavor" of the pain. A few of the possible "flavors" include burning, itching, stabbing, and crushing.

Equanimity means not interfering with the flow of sensation. Equanimity means letting the pain expand or contract as much as it wants, and in any direction that it wants. It means letting it get as intense or as faint as it wants. It means letting it last as long or as short as it wants. Giving pain such radical permission to move can be scary, especially at first, and sometimes it might even seem to make the pain seem worse. However, if you can maintain equanimity, what generally happens is that the pain will eventually start to break up.

If you are interested in this type of meditation I recommend listening to the "Break Through Pain" available through Sounds True catalog, 800-333-9185. The first tape clearly explains how this type of meditation works and the second and third tapes take you through guided meditations that facilitate learning how to fully use the techniques.

How to Get the Most Out of Meditation — 2 Hints

1. Find a qualified teacher. Although it is useful to learn about meditation by reading about it, nothing beats learning directly from a qualified teacher. The one-on-one feedback and the personal example are invaluable. Going on meditation retreats is an excellent way to meet teachers and receive personal guidance. At the end of this chapter, contact information is given for several organizations that sponsor *vipassana* retreats.

2. Practice on a regular basis. Daily practice is best. Meditation is a only a tool. A tool is only useful to the degree that you use it and use it well.

Long-Term Benefits

Meditation will not magically remove all the problems and obstacles in your life. What it will do is give you a tool that with practice can make pain more bearable. As you train yourself to experience pain with mindfulness and equanimity, you will find that pain that used to cause you great suffering is not as much of a problem. You may even find that, as your skills in meditation grow, what used to be hard, solidified pain melts into a pleasant flow of sensation. Some people, and I am one of them, have even found that over time, meditation has led to dramatic healing of physical conditions.

As you train yourself in meditation, you will also likely notice yourself feeling more alive. Your experience of the taste and texture of food may become more rich and varied. Your experience of not just pain but all body sensations may become more complex and satisfying. Your experience of sight and sound may become more vivid. In short, even without your external circumstances changing, you are likely to find your life more satisfying and intense.

Resources

Books and Tapes
The Tibetan Book of Living and Dying by Sogyal Rinpoche, 1992, HarperSanFancisco.

"Break Through Pain," tapes by Shinzen Young, Sounds True catalog, 800-333-9185.

www.shinzen.org This Web site is a place to learn about meditation and its application to pain management. Shinzen has many good articles on meditation on his Web site. He also posts answers to questions posed by readers.

Full Catastrophe Living by Jon Kabat-Zinn, 1990, Dell Publishing.
In 1993 the Bill Moyers TV special called "Healing and the Mind" introduced millions of Americans to Jon Kabat-Zinn and the program he founded at the Stress Reduction Clinic at the University of Massachusetts Medical Center. This program, offered in a hospital setting, teaches the use of mindfulness meditation for dealing with chronic pain. The book describes this program and serves as an excellent guide for anyone who wants to use meditation as a tool to work with stress, pain or illness.

Retreats
My primary meditation teacher has been Shinzen Young. What I have to say about meditation has been greatly influenced by what I have learned from him and the aspects of meditation that he emphasizes. However, there are many other aspects of meditation that can be emphasized and many other models that can be used to describe it. Even within the *vipassana*

247

tradition, different teachers teach differently both in emphasis and in the models they use.

People like Shinzen Young and Jon Kabat-Zinn have a very clear sense of how to use pain as an opportunity for personal and spiritual transformation. In more traditional Buddhist training situations, such as those at the Insight Meditation Center in Barre, MA and Spirit Rock Center in Woodacre, CA, you may find the emphasis is not so much on with working with the pain as a vehicle but more on generic standard techniques such as working with breath, achieving spaciousness, and so forth. These procedures, if mastered, bring a state of liberation from suffering and therefore represent the ultimate pain management tool. If you go to a retreat with an IMS or Spirit Rock teacher, you should be prepared to work within their framework.

With that in mind, I recommend the following organizations, all of which are providers of quality retreats.

Vipassana Support Institute
3330 Hannibal Road
Burlington, Ontario
Canada L7M 1R7
Toll-free Phone: 866-666-0VSI (0874)
Fax: 905-336-2616
E-mail: vsi@shinzen.org
This organization, founded by Shirley Fenton and Shinzen Young, offers retreats and other activities that teach and support the practice of *vipassana* meditation.

Spirit Rock Center
PO Box 169
Woodacre, CA 94973
Info line: 415-488-0164
http://www.spiritrock.org
This organization, founded by Jack Kornfield, offers retreats and other activities that teach and support the practice of *vipassana* meditation.

Insight Meditation Center (IMS)
1230 Pleasant St.
Barre, MA 01005
978-355-4378
http://www.dharma.org/IMS/IMSschedule.htm

This organization, founded by Sharon Salzberg and Joseph Goldstein, offers retreats and other activities that teach and support the practice of *vipassana* meditation.

Mid America Dharma
PO Box 414411
Kansas City, MO 64141-4411
http://www.midamericadharma.org/
This umbrella group sponsors retreats in the Midwest. It can also put you in touch with local sitting groups throughout the Midwest. Sitting groups are groups of people who help support each other's practice by gathering to sit in meditation together.

Inquiring Mind
PO Box 9999
Berkeley, CA 94709
This publication comes out twice a year. It contains articles related to *vipassana* meditation, and more importantly an extensive list of sitting groups and upcoming meditation retreats in the United States and elsewhere. There is no set cost to receive the publication; it relies on donations.

Chapter 16: Partaking of the Elixir of Youth—How to Gain Maximum Benefits from Exercise Even if You are Still Quite Ill

Highlights:

❑ Four keys to getting the greatest benefits from exercise.
❑ The seven types of exercise that are best for arthritis.

Effort Involved:

❑ Ideally, a few minutes a day for range of motion exercises.
❑ 30 minutes a day, several times a week, for the strengthening and conditioning program of your choice.

Payoff:

❑ Greater strength, endurance, flexibility and resilience.
❑ Better mood and attitude.
❑ Healthier everything, including muscles, bones, joints, circulation and immune system. Even the very frail and the very ill can often benefit from exercise.

Why Exercise?—Inactivity Alone Can Cause Pathological Changes

It has long been known that prolonged bed rest can cause degenerative joint disease, even in healthy volunteers who had nothing wrong with them at the beginning of the test period.[82] Immobilization, for instance in a cast, of an otherwise healthy joint can cause degenerative joint disease. Both prolonged bed rest and immobilization cause the cartilage matrix

---

[82] D. K. Dittmer and R. Teasell, "Complications of Immobilization and Bed Rest. Part 1: Musculoskeletal and Cardiovascular Complications," *Can Fam Physician* 39 (1993): 1428-32, 1435-7.

composition to change quantitatively and qualitatively.[83] This means less cartilage overall and destructive changes within the cartilage that is still there.

The amazing fact is that inactivity alone can cause pathological changes that are indistinguishable from rheumatoid arthritis.

Inactivity can also cause many other complications, including loss of muscle strength and endurance, disuse osteoporosis, and cardiovascular complications. These cardiovascular complications come in several forms, including a marked decrease in the capacity of the cardiovascular system to control pulse and blood pressure, and an unhealthy constellation of blood abnormalities that increases the risk of heart attack and stroke. Inactivity can also cause diabetes.[84],[85]

Dramatic changes in muscle mass occur within four to six weeks of the beginning of bed rest, accompanied by a decrease of 6 to 40 percent in muscle strength. Luckily, the effect on muscle is reversible. However, the detrimental effects immobilization has on bone, are much more difficult to reverse.

As explained later in the chapter, it takes special measures such as weight lifting, to rebuild bone density. The regular exercise of day-to-day living, which is enough to rebuild muscle strength, is not enough to rebuild bone density.

The sobering fact is that bone mineral density in able-bodied men after bed rest is not fully recovered after six months of normal weight-bearing activity.[86] This is compounded by the frightening fact that bone loss due to osteoporosis from bed rest or immobilization is five to 20 times greater than with other causes of bone loss.[87] This makes this type of inactivity

---

[83] P. Diekstall, W. Schulze and W. Noack, "Immobilization Damage Sportverletz," *Sportsschaden* 9(2) (1995):35-43.

[84] H. Blotner, "Effect of Prolonged Physical Inactivity on Tolerance of Sugar," *Arch Intern Med* 75 (1945):39.

[85] P. Myllynen, V. A. Koivisto and A. Nikkila, "Glucose Intolerance and Insulin Resistance Accompany Immobilization," *Acta Med Scand* 222(1) (1987):75-81.

[86] S. A. Bloomfield, "Changes in Musculoskeletal Structure and Function with Prolonged Bed Rest," *Med Sci Sports Exerc* 29(2) (1997):197-206.

particularly dangerous for anyone with arthritis, and it also makes the bone-building weight-lifting exercises described later in this chapter particularly important.

So, how can all of these problems be avoided in the first place? The answer is exercise.

Because the changes in bone and joints are difficult to reverse, an ounce of prevention is worth much more than a pound of cure. Exercise is the only known prevention for these changes. Exercise is also the only known cure, short of joint replacement surgery, for those unhealthy changes in joints, bone and muscle that are able to be reversed.

Documented Benefits of Exercise for People with Arthritis

Exercise is good medicine, especially for someone with arthritis.

Patients with rheumatoid arthritis and osteoarthritis benefit from treadmill exercise programs.[88]

Several studies document physiological improvements in patients with RA who participated in a stationary cycling exercise program.[89] One found that a bicycling program did not exacerbate joint symptoms in patients with rheumatoid arthritis and osteoarthritis. The program improved functional capacity, muscle strength, and aerobic capacity.[90]

Exercise in a heated swimming pool has also been proven to be of benefit to people with RA. One study showed significant increases in strength and

---

[87] P. Diekstall, W. Schulze and W. Noack, "Immobilization Damage," *Sportverletz Sportsschaden* 9(2) (1995):35-43.

[88] T. M. Harkom, R. M. Lampman, B. F. Banwell, et al., "Therapeutic Value of Graded Aerobic Exercise Training in Rheumatoid Arthritis," *Arthritis Rheum* 28 (1985):32.

[89] A. Nath, R. R. Webel, D. Kay, et al., "Training Effect of Aerobic Exercise in Arthritis Patients," *Clin Res* 35 (1987):566A.

[90] C. A. Beals, R. M. Lampman, B. F. Banwell, et al., "Measurement of Exercise Tolerance in Patients with Rheumatoid and Osteoarthritis," *J Rheumatol* 12 (1985):458-461.

aerobic capacity.[91] Another showed improvements in joint tenderness and knee range of motion.[92]

Yet another study concluded that high-intensity strength training is feasible and safe in selected patients with well-controlled RA and leads to significant improvements in strength, pain and fatigue without exacerbating disease activity or joint pain.[93]

Some studies involved more than one type of exercise. In one, 18 patients with rheumatoid arthritis engaged in a graded-progressive exercise program that used both aerobic and strength-training components.[94] The number of swollen joints decreased by 35 percent and the patients' hemoglobin levels, strength and aerobic capacity increased. The authors concluded that patients with active rheumatoid arthritis, even with chronically swollen joints, receive substantial benefits from a physical training program.

Yet another study involved 64 patients who were admitted to a hospital because of active RA. They were randomly assigned to an intensive exercise program or to a conservative exercise program. The average age of these patients was 60, and the average disease duration was eight years. The intensive program consisted of knee and shoulder strengthening exercises against resistance five times a week and conditioning bicycle training three times a week. It was also supplemented with the conservative exercise program, which consisted of only range-of-motion and isometric

[91] B. Bannekiold-Samsoe, K. Lyngberg, T. Risum and M. Telling, "The Effect of Water Exercise Therapy Given to Patients With Rheumatoid Arthritis," *Scand J Rehabil Med* 19(1) (1987):31-5.

[92] J. Hall, S. M. Skevington, P. J. Maddison, and K. Chapman, "A Randomized and Controlled Trial of Hydrotherapy in Rheumatoid Arthritis," *Arthritis Care Res* 9(3) (1996):206-15.

[93] L. C. Rall, S. N. Meydani, J. J. Kehayias, B. Dawson-Hughes and R. Roubenoff, "The Effect of Progressive Resistance Training in Rheumatoid Arthritis. Increased Strength Without Changes in Energy Balance or Body Composition," *Arthritis Rheum* 39(3) (1996):415-26.

[94] K. Lyngberg, B. Danneskiold-Samse and O. Halskov, "The Effects of Physical Training on Patients with Rheumatoid Arthritis: Changes in Disease Activity, Muscle Strength and Aerobic Capacity. A Clinically Controlled Minimized Crossover Study," *Clin Exp Rheumatol* 6 (1988):253-260.

exercises. The short-term intensive exercise program was found to be more effective in improving muscle strength than the conservative exercise program. The disease did not get worse as a results of the intensive program, even in these patients with active RA.[95]

Other more meditative forms of exercise, such as yoga and tai chi, can also help restore health to people with arthritis. Traditional medical texts describe the benefits of yoga for many types of arthritis. Personal testimonies abound for the effectiveness of yoga and tai chi in improving arthritic conditions. Preliminary scientific studies looking at the use of yoga and tai chi to treat arthritis also show promising outcomes.[96]

The 4 Keys For Exercising For Anyone With Arthritis

1. Respect Your Limits

To maximize benefits, exercise must be done properly. As anyone who has experienced a major arthritis flare-up knows, exercise at the wrong time can cause more harm than good. You want to avoid exercising until you are over a flare-up. You also want to avoid exercise that is strenuous enough to cause a flare-up.

I found that paying careful attention to my body was the key to being able to exercise without causing a flare-up. I have the kind of personality that likes to push my limits. I always want to go faster and farther than the previous time. I finally realized that with arthritis my limits were constantly and dramatically fluctuating depending on stress, weather, and a host of other factors that were difficult to figure out. My limits fluctuated from day to day, and often from minute to minute.

If I tried to base my performance on what I did yesterday, or even five minutes before, I was likely to hurt myself. If I performed based on exactly where I was moment by moment, I didn't get hurt and ultimately was able to do much more.

---

[95] C. H. vanden Ende, F. C. Breedveld, S. le Cessie, B. A. Dijkmans, A.W. de Mug and J. M. Hazes, "Effect of Intensive Exercise on Patients with Active Rheumatoid Arthritis: A Randomized Clinical Trial," *Ann Rheum Dis* 59(8) (2000):615-21.

[96] M. Garfinkel and H. R. Schumacher, "Yoga," *Rheum Dis Clin North Am* 26(1) (2000):125-32.

I finally realized that if I rested at the first signs of a flare-up, I recovered more quickly. If I ignored the first signs for as little as 30 minutes, I might have had to spend several days in bed recovering. If I ignored the first signs for five or 10 minutes, I might have had to spend one day in bed recovering. However, if I rested immediately upon the first signs of inflammation, I often needed only about five minutes of rest or meditation to completely avoid a flare-up.

Not a bad trade-off.

Five minutes of rest at the right time could save me hours or days of misery and incapacitation. After such a brief rest I could often continue the exact activity that I had been doing when I noticed the warning signs.

At my worst, even when I wasn't having a flare-up, I was too weak to walk farther than from one room to the next or to sit upright for more than 30 minutes at a time. Monitoring my moment-to-moment limits was necessary for almost all activities. What was strenuous exercise for me looked like next to nothing to a healthy person. Standing long enough to brush my teeth was a major physical challenge. My roommates from this period in my life will tell you that for that very reason they often found me sitting on the vanity!

The point is that I was working on such a small margin of tolerance that even while brushing my teeth I had to be conscious of whether or not I was about to go into a flare-up. If I could stand, I would. It was good for my muscle strength. However, if it was more than I could tolerate at the time, I would sit. A few minutes of rest at critical moments helped me to remain more active.

2. Pay Close Attention to What Your Body is Telling You

The more in tune you are with your body, the easier it is to use key No. 1—respect your limits. How else are you even going to know what your moment-to-moment limits are?

By paying close attention to what my body was telling me, I eventually got to where I could recognize the first signs of a flare-up before there was any pain. By carefully observing the early stages of what it felt like to go into a flare-up and constantly trying to detect the beginning signal at earlier and earlier points, I could actually identify it when it was still just a slight twinge or "funny feeling."

Once upon a time, I would have thought resting, because of such a minor sensation, was a sign of weakness. Eventually I realized that not resting

255

when I felt such a minor sensation actually *caused* weakness. Failing to notice or even purposefully ignoring those first pain precursors led to a dramatic escalation of inflammation that was difficult to control once it got started. The inflammation left me weak and in pain. Catching and reversing this tendency toward inflammation before it got started, when it was still easy to reverse, kept me from experiencing the weakness and pain.

Instead of being mad at the pain, even the first sensations, I came to see it as my ally. Just like the oil light in your car warns you when to add oil in order to avoid major damage to your engine, pain warns you when to back off in order to avoid major damage to your body. Just like the dipstick allows you to know when you have added enough oil, the reversal of the pain lets you know when it is OK to exert yourself again.

In our society people often brag about having a high threshold for pain. Being able to withstand high levels of pain can be useful, but if it means being insensitive to all but the highest levels of pain, then this "talent" is actually a liability. Without sensitivity to the early warning signs from pain, such a person lacks the ability to recognize their own feedback mechanisms, and hence the ability to manage their body well. Without the equivalent of a good dipstick, it is hard for them to monitor when it is OK to continue and when they need to rest.

Proper reaction to the first signs of pain paves the way for miraculous recoveries. Further damage to the body can be avoided before it even starts, freeing up great resources for self-healing.

The more you are in tune with your body sensations, the better. If you "listen," your body will inform you, moment by moment, how to function at your best. It will let you know when it is safe to push yourself. It will let you know when you need to rest. If you pay attention, you will learn which sensations indicate an impending flare-up and which indicate a pain that will actually diminish if you continue your exercise for a while.

By listening to my body, I was eventually able to orchestrate an amazing recovery. I now participate in 30- to 50-mile bike rides. I take martial arts classes. I lift weights. I walk for miles at a time. However, my strategy for exercising has never changed. This strategy works at any level of health or conditioning. In a nutshell this strategy is: HONOR WHAT YOUR BODY IS TELLING YOU. Your body knows its own limits. It will teach you when to back off and rest. It will also teach you when it is OK or even desirable to exercise harder, faster or longer.

Don't buy into the myth, "no pain, no gain." Don't automatically "just push through the pain". The wrong kind of pain means you are destroying your body. This kind of pain definitely means no gain. To improve your strength and conditioning you will need to push yourself, but only with discretion. It is much better to find the "sweet spot" where you are working hard and feeling good while you are exercising, and feeling even better when you are done.

3. Accepting Yourself from Moment to Moment

This third key is critical to getting the most out of exercise. In this context, accepting yourself means a *deep body-level acceptance*. It's permission not only to feel whatever sensations you happen to be feeling, but also permission to let those sensations spread freely through the body. This key has the power to turn what you may have just been experiencing as a hard or sharp pain into an empowering flow of pleasure. It is one of the keys to finding the "sweet spot" I mention above.

Most people tend to tighten up around pain in an effort to keep it from spreading. This tightening actually creates a pain cycle. The more it hurts, the more you tighten. The more you tighten, the more it hurts. The original pain may be long gone, but unless you can break this cycle, the pain kept alive by tensing lingers on and on.

The way to break up this pain cycle is a deep body-level acceptance that lets pain and other sensations spread through you like the ripples in a pond. At first this may seem scary. Who wants to let pain spread through their body? Nobody, until you realize that once you let a wave of pain go, it is gone. This may sound ludicrous unless you have experienced it yourself, but when you get good at this body-level acceptance, what used to be experienced as hard, lasting pain often becomes brief, pleasant ripples of energy.

So what, you might be asking yourself, does this approach look like when exercising?

This time I'll use a bicycling example. What I love about bicycling is all the body sensations. I like the heavy breathing. I like feeling my leg muscles. I like the wind on my skin. I like how my body feels as the scenery rushes by. And the more I pay attention to all these body sensations, the better it gets. Once I exceed a certain threshold amount of attention, I can even tap into an energy source that almost effortlessly powers the ride.

Tapping into this energy source may sound miraculous or like science fiction, but it is really quite simple. I have found that if I *pay close attention to my body sensations*, including all their little shifts and changes, *if I totally accept each discomfort as it arises* (that means not trying to avoid it or make it go away, but rather letting it spread however it wants to through my body), and *if I don't push beyond my moment to moment physical limitations* (that may mean slowing down or even stopping for a while), then the discomfort tends to break up into pleasant sensations that fuel the ride. Many athletes call this energy a *second wind* or *being in the zone.*

For me, the amazing thing is how quickly a major discomfort can turn into a second wind. For example, last summer I was riding along and suddenly got a sharp pain in my side. It was so strong that I couldn't even pedal. I dismounted, but stayed in very close contact with all those physical sensations. After about a minute, all those unpleasant cramping sensations started breaking up into waves of sensation. I ended up speeding away on very strong, very pleasant surges of energy that lasted the rest of the ride. For a couple of days afterward friends even commented on how radiant I looked. This was none other than a second wind or being in the zone.

If you use my keys for exercising, it is simple to train yourself to know how to enter the zone and to be in the zone more frequently and for longer periods of time. In fact, theoretically it is possible to live your whole life in the zone. Any activity can be a great excuse to enter the zone.

You will find that after you have had a few of these zone experiences, it will be much easier to accept your limitations. You will know from your own repeated experience that if you can just pay enough attention and have enough body-level acceptance, those limits are likely to dissolve at any second into waves of pure energy. You will begin to look at each and every limitation that arises as a storehouse of energy just waiting to be tapped. And as more of your limitations dissolve, your ordinary, everyday levels of energy and joy will also increase dramatically.

Not a bad payoff.

4. Have Fun!

You might have figured out by now that these keys are not just for anyone with arthritis. They are for everyone.

In order to get the most out of exercise it should be enjoyable. At least one study suggests that if you force yourself to do exercises you hate, you may not gain many overall health benefits.[97] This is because the chronic stress

---

[97] A. Moraska, T. Deak, R.L Spenser, D. Roth and M. Fleshner, "Treadmill Running Produces Both Positive and Negative Physiological Adaptations in

responses triggered by aversive reactions negate many of the otherwise healthy side effects of exercising.

For example, the stress from forced exercise has adverse effects on neuroendocrine tissues and immune responses. On the other hand, the same exercise, when not forced, improves overall health, including improving the functioning of the immune system and protecting the body from stress.

So enjoy your exercise time. Put on music that you enjoy and that makes you want to move. Find workout partners you enjoy. Find places that lift your spirits. Find ways to make your workout a game. Do whatever you can to make your exercise periods a treat. Attitude is important.

In the words of Mary Poppins, "In every job that must by done there is an element of fun. Find the fun, and snap, the job's a game."

If you aren't having fun, something is wrong. Figure out what it is, and fix it pronto. It may be something as easy as reminding yourself this isn't meant to be torture or an endurance contest. Then find the joy, no matter how slight. See if you can locate exactly where in your body you feel joy. Is it in your face? Your arms? Your hips? Your feet? If you let it, does the joy want to spread to other parts of your body? Changing your focus to the joy can quickly shift the quality of the whole exercise session.

If you aren't enjoying yourself because you are pushing yourself too hard or are in pain, then reread the sections immediately above on working within your limits, listening to what your body is telling you, and accepting yourself moment by moment.

By having fun and working within your limits, you will get the quickest, greatest and longest-term benefits. In addition, you will receive all these benefits by expending the least possible amount of effort.

The 7 Types of Exercise that are Best for Arthritis

1. Range of motion (ROM) exercises
2. Hatha yoga
3. Tai chi
4. Walking

Sprague-Dawley Rats," *Am J Physiol Regul Integr Comp Physiol* 279(4) (2000):R1321-9.

5. Swimming
6. Cycling
7. Strength training

I compiled this list from recommendations from several sources: the Arthritis Foundation, the medical literature, and a book called *Arthritis: What Exercises Work*. An expanded list would include dancing, gardening and any other activities that give you great joy, get you moving and are easy on your joints.

ROM exercises are important for maintaining the integrity of affected joints.

Yoga, tai chi, and other exercise systems that have a strong meditative component tend to foster not only strength and flexibility, but also to train practitioners in the very useful skills of releasing stress and pain and relaxing at will.

Walking, swimming and cycling are relatively low-impact, joint-friendly activities that foster cardiovascular conditioning and endurance.

Strength training improves muscle strength, balance and bone health.

1. Range of Motion (ROM) Exercises – The Joint Savers

Inactivity and immobilization cause degenerative joint disease.[98] If you hurt, there is a tendency not to want to move the parts that hurt. This sets up a vicious cycle, whereby the very thing that you are doing to protect the joint (keeping it still) causes further degeneration. For this reason, it is important for anyone with arthritis to do range of motion exercises, preferably each day. This is a high-stakes game of "use it or lose it."

If you are very sick, have someone gently move your joints through their range of motion for you. If you can take your joints through their range of motion yourself, so much the better. However, either way, it is of critical importance that you gently move your joints through their full range of motion at least several times a week.

Remember as you move your joints *to respect your limits*. We are talking about *your* full range of motion moment by moment, not some idealized

---

[98] D.K. Dittmer and R. Teasell, "Complications of Immobilization and Bed Rest. Part 1: Musculoskeletal and Cardiovascular Complications," *Can Fam Physician* 39 (1993):1428-32, 1435-7.

range of motion or the range of motion you had 10 years ago, yesterday, or even five minutes ago.

To learn more about range of motion exercise, contact the Arthritis Foundation. Information is at the end of this chapter in the resource section.

2. Regaining Strength and Flexibility—The Benefits of Hatha Yoga

The Ability to Exercise with Minimum Motion

When I first started exercising, almost any motion, especially repetitive motion, would send me into a flare-up. The only way I knew to avoid pain and inflammation was to stay very still most of the time. As a consequence I became very weak. I finally got so weak that it was difficult for me to even sit up for more than 30 minutes at a time. Because of pain in my right hip, standing up for more than two minutes at a time would cause pain of near-fainting intensity. My dilemma was how to exercise with minimal motion and without needing to stand. The answer was yoga *asanas*.

Asanas

Yoga *asanas* are postures that help develop strength, flexibility and balance. I was particularly interested in developing strength. At the point in my life when I discovered yoga, the jarring motion of riding in a car was enough to send me into a flare-up, so traveling to a yoga class was out of the question. I did what most yoga instructors say you should never do. I learned from a book. One of my roommates was kind enough to check out a yoga book from the library for me, *The Complete Illustrated Book of Yoga* by Swami Vishnu-devananda.

My back was particularly weak, so my initial strategy was to pick out several back-strengthening *asanas* from this book. I tried to do one posture each day for a week. That took all the strength and energy I could muster.

Once a day, I would hold this single posture for a long as I could. Then I would rest. While I was resting I followed the relaxation instructions from the book. What happened next amazed me. If I could relax deeply enough, I could actually "untie" the pattern of sensation I associated with going into a flare-up. My goal became to not move from the relaxation posture until all signs of a flare-up were gone. With practice, this would only a take a few moments.

As I got physically stronger and better at "untying" flare-ups, I gradually added more *asanas*. Between each I would rest in the relaxation posture until all signs of a flare-up were gone. In this way I gradually became able to move more without going into a flare-up. The skill I gained at reversing flare-ups became invaluable in my eventual recovery.

Eventually I became strong enough and well enough to attend yoga classes, which is how I recommend learning yoga, if you have the choice. Books are good, but a good instructor is even better.

Breathing

Hatha yoga has many breathing exercises. These exercises are sometimes called *pranayama*. They are beneficial for at least three reasons:

1. Breath awareness makes it easier to recognize and release tensions, including the kind that can cause flare-ups.
2. These special breathing exercises are something you can do almost anytime, almost anywhere. They require no special equipment. They require no special strength or flexibility. No matter how sick you are, if you can still breathe, these exercises are something you can actively do to calm, strengthen and heal yourself.
3. Despite being so simple, these exercises offer big payoffs in terms of increased health and well-being.

How to Learn Yoga

Ideally, I recommend learning from a qualified instructor. See the resource section at the end of this chapter for contact information for the Yoga Alliance, an organization that offers a registry of Yoga schools and teachers.

If you learn well from books, they can get you started if your health makes getting to a yoga class too difficult. To learn the important awarenesses and intentions that are held during the practice of yoga as well as the mechanics of practicing yoga, I recommend the book, *Yoga: The Spirit and Practice of Moving Into Stillness* by Erich Schiffmann.

3. Tai Chi – An Ancient Martial Art Form as Therapy

Tai chi is an ancient form of exercise used widely in China. It is a graceful self-defense and fitness system that helps promote the flow of vital energy (chi) by using gentle motion, meditation, guided imagery and relaxation.

Studies have shown that alternative therapies such as tai chi and meditation are beneficial for people with arthritis.[99] The Arthritis Foundation has even joined with a nonprofit group called the ROM Dance Institute to promote an exercise program called ROM Dance. It makes use of the slow, gentle movements from tai chi to help people with arthritis get the widest motion from their joints. The ROM Dance program can be used separately or incorporated into the Arthritis Foundation's PACE (People with Arthritis Can Exercise) classes which promote fitness and strength.

One researcher who has moderately severe ankylosing spondylitis, a type of arthritis of the spine, has published his personal experience with tai chi[100] in a medical journal. At the time of publication he had practiced tai chi daily for 2½ years and felt stronger and healthier than before. However, he found that pain, weakness and general malaise returned if he neglected to practice for as little as one week. He listed improved skeletal muscle strength, limb co-ordination, balance, chest movement and ability to relax as further benefits of his tai chi practice.

Because tai chi is done from a standing position and I had difficulty standing when I still had arthritis, I chose to learn hatha yoga instead of tai chi. However, both of these systems provide many of the same benefits.

4. Walking – The Exercise for a Lifetime

When everything goes right, walking is truly the exercise for a lifetime. It is the quintessential form of human locomotion. It requires no special equipment and no fancy gym. For most of us, walking is a birthright.

Emotionally, walking is deeply tied to the transition from being a dependent infant to an intrepid toddler who suddenly has whole new worlds open to his or her eager grasp. Losing the ability to stand and to walk is difficult, especially for an adult, because it returns us to a dependent state. Regaining the ability to stand and walk returns new vistas, new avenues of exploration, and a renewed sense of independence.

Standing and walking touch the human psyche deeply. Anyone who has ever had to spend much time in a wheelchair or an electric cart, as I did for five years, knows just how rare it can be to be treated as a fully functioning

---

[99] D.E. Yocum, W.L. Castro and M. Cornett, "Exercise, Education, and Behavioral Modification as Alternative Therapy for Pain and Stress in Rheumatic Disease," *Rheum Dis Clin North Am* 26(1) (2000):145-59, x-xi.

[100] T.C. Koh, "Tai Chi and Ankylosing Spondylitis—A Personal Experience," *Am J Chin Med* 10(1-4) (1982):59-60.

adult. Because your eye level is at that of a child's, other adults often overlook you. When they do see you, you are often unconsciously treated as a child.

If you are physically capable of doing it, the advantages of walking for exercise are many. It is easy to do, easy to arrange, and inexpensive. It requires minimal equipment, can be done alone or in groups, uses large muscles (and thus makes it easy to get a good cardiovascular conditioning effect), and is a wonderful way to experience the world.

If you are not physically capable of walking, regaining your ability to walk has tremendous physical and psychological benefits. A strength-training program designed by a physical therapist is one excellent way to regain the muscle strength and joint stability needed to walk. Yoga postures are another possibility. Exercising in water and bicycling are also two good ways to stay in shape and rehabilitate the muscles and joints needed for walking.

5. Aquatic Exercise – Whole-Body Benefits Plus A Reprieve from Gravity

Exercising in water, including swimming, has the advantage that much of your weight is supported by buoyancy. Jumping, running in place, stretching, and range of motion exercises are often much easier when water is supporting your weight. On the other hand, the force needed to move in water provides resistance that can be used to build strength and cardiovascular conditioning.

The Arthritis Foundation offers special aquatic exercise programs for people with arthritis. Generally these are offered in community pools that are kept warmer than the average pool to make the water more comfortable for tender joints. Contact the Arthritis Foundation, www.arthritis.org, 800-283-7800, for information on classes in your area.

6. Bicycling – For the Pure Joy of It

For anyone with arthritis, bicycling has many advantages.

Cycling is nearly four times more mechanically efficient than walking or running. It allows people of modest physical prowess to travel faster and farther than the finest runners.[101] There are various types of bicycles (and tricycles) with many types of modifications available that can restore

---

[101] T.C. Namey, "Adaptive Bicycling," *Rheum Dis Clin North Am* 16(4) (1990): 871-886.

mobility to people with a wide variety of different physical limitations. A physical therapist or occupational therapist can help you find special equipment suited to your needs.

Bicycling is easier on the joints than walking or running. It is excellent for the rehabilitation of people with various knee problems, including problems from rheumatoid arthritis. A physical therapist can help you design a recovery program. Be aware that in order to avoid worsening knee problems, it is particularly important to make sure that your bicycle is properly fitted to you and that you ride in low gears.

Another advantage of cycling is that power output is continuously spread throughout much muscle mass, making the perception of exertion relatively low and reaching an aerobic heart rate more easily accomplished.

Bicycling is a recreational sport open to people of all ages. Serious cyclists often report that their performance improves well into their 50s, 60s and beyond. It can be an individual or group activity. It can be done indoors and outdoors. Perhaps best of all, *bicycling is fun.*

7. Weight Lifting – Great for Bones, Great for Reduction of Pain and Fatigue, and Great for Strength and Balance

Who would have predicted that lifting weights could be good for arthritis recovery? A study has found that even people with rheumatoid arthritis who found walking and other weight-bearing exercise painful were able to engage in strength training. In addition, this training decreased their pain and fatigue, increased their strength and did not exacerbate disease activity or increase the number of painful joints. These folks also improved their balance and their ability to walk.[102]

Weight lifting is also excellent for building and maintaining strong, healthy bones. As described earlier in this chapter, immobilization and bed rest cause rapid and extensive bone loss. Strength training is one very good way for people with arthritis to prevent this loss. Bone growth is maximally stimulated by extremely short exposures to dynamic loading. Static and repetitive loading such as found in standing and walking have a

---

[102] L. C. Rall, S. N. Meydani, J. J. Kehayias, B. Dawson-Hughes and R. Roubenoff, "The Effect of Progressive Resistance Training in Rheumatoid Arthritis. Increased Strength without Changes in Energy Balance or Body Composition," *Arthritis Rheum* 39(3) (1996):415-26.

minimal influence on bone structure. In contrast, vigorous and diverse stresses, such as found in a good weight-lifting routine, build bone.[103]

To learn more about weight lifting, I recommend the book *Strong Women Stay Young* by Miriam E. Nelson, Ph.D., with Sarah Wernick, Ph.D. Although the title of the book might imply that this program is only for women, it was developed using both genders and also works very well for men.

This book provides excellent, easy to follow, clearly written instructions that will teach you how to do a weight-lifting program adapted for home use. This program was originally tested in nursing homes on the oldest of the old. Previously frail seniors regained strength and balance. Some who were initially too weak to stand up regained the ability to stand and walk.

The progressive use of heavier weights as strength is gained makes this a fun, challenging and rewarding workout. Even in my presently healthy state, I continue to feel better as I gain strength and balance. This easy-to-use program is excellent in that it is easily adaptable to your current level of fitness, from very frail to very robust.

If you have had joint replacement surgery or your illness has caused joint damage, it is especially important to consult with your physician and physical therapist before undertaking any weight lifting. They can help you modify the lifting exercises to accommodate your altered muscular and/or altered joint structure.

Remember, with all of these exercises: *respect your limits*. If one pound is your limit, get stronger by lifting one pound. No matter what your limit is, don't exceed it. You will just hurt yourself. This is about getting stronger, healthier and having fun. It is not about getting hurt.

Long-Term Benefits

Long-term benefits of exercise include greater strength, endurance, flexibility and resilience, better mood and attitude, and healthier everything, including muscles, bones, joints, circulation and immune system. Even the very frail and the very ill can often benefit from exercise.

---

[103] *The Textbook of Rheumatology, Fifth Edition,* Edited by William N. Kelley, M.D., Shaun Ruddy, M.D., Edward D. Harris, M.D., and Clement B. Sledge, M.D., (Philadelphia, PA: W.B. Waunder Company, 1997, 71).

Additional Resources

"In the Zone" Training

"In the Zone," a 2 tape set by Shinzen Young, Sounds True catalog, 800-333-9185.

The first tape gives an overview of what entering the zone means and how to do it. The second tape is designed to be used while you exercise. It helps you train yourself in the techniques used for entering the zone.

Range of Motion Exercises

To learn more about range of motion exercise, contact the Arthritis Foundation at www.arthritis.org or 800-283-7800. The foundation offers ROM videos, books and classes for people with arthritis.

Hatha Yoga

Ideally, I recommend learning from a qualified instructor. The Yoga Alliance offers a registry of schools and teachers. It is available on the organization's Web site, www.yogaalliance.org, or by calling 877-964-2255 (877-YOGAALL) or by writing to the Yoga Alliance, 120 South Third Ave., West Reading PA 19611.

Books can be a useful way to further your understanding of yoga. My favorite yoga book is: *Yoga: The Spirit and Practice of Moving Into Stillness* by Erich Schiffmann, (New York: Simon & Schuster, Inc., 1996).

Information about yoga for specific medical conditions is available from the American Yoga Association. Send a self-addressed, business-sized envelope, stamped with 57 cents postage, to American Yoga Association, P.O. Box 19986, Sarasota, FL 34276. Information is also available on the association's Web site: www.americanyogaassociation.org

Tai Chi

A special program called "Tai Chi for Arthritis" was created by Dr. Paul Lam and his team of Tai Chi and medical experts. Information on this program is available at: www.taichiforarthritis.com

The organization's contact information in the United States is: PO Box 752, Butler, NJ 07405, fax 800-889-2082; 973-283-9698, e-mail: taichiproductions.us@worldnet.att.net

The organization's contact information in Australia is: 4 Fisher Place, Narwee NSW 2209, tel. 61 2 9533 6511; 9540 5048, fax. 61 2 9534 4311, e-mail: service@taichiforarthritis.com

Walking

If you are looking for a level, indoor place to walk, consider walking inside a mall in the morning before the stores open. Many malls have mall walking clubs.

If you are looking for group walking activities outside, contact your local YMCA, YWCA, or the American Volkssport Association. The address for the latter is 1001 Pat Booker Road, Suite 101, Universal City, TX 78148, tel. 210-659-2112, fax 210-659-1212, info line 800-830-WALK.

The Web site for the American Volksport Association, AVAHQ@aol.com, http://www.ava.org/, lists walking events and walking clubs throughout the USA.

Aquatic Exercise

Contact the Arthritis Foundation, www.arthritis.org, 800-283-7800, for information on classes and heated pools in your area.

Bicycling

Contact local bicycle shops to find out about group rides and good places to ride in your area. Contact local health clubs for group workouts and classes on stationary bicycles. These stationary bicycle workouts are quite popular and are often referred to as "spinning."

Weight Lifting

I recommend the book *Strong Women Stay Young* by Miriam E. Nelson, Ph.D., with Sarah Wernick, Ph.D. (New York: Bantam Books, 1997).

A General Guide for Exercises for Arthritis Recovery

I recommend the book *Arthritis: What Exercises Work* by Dava Sobel and Arthur C. Klein (New York: St. Martins Press, 1993).
The exercises in this book were chosen based on a survey of arthritis sufferers who revealed what actually works. This book explains how to get started, how to tailor an exercise program to your exact needs, and what exactly to do once you are exercising.

Chapter 17: Clearing Up Residual Pain and Stiffness—How to Erase Pesky Myofascial Trigger Points (TPs)

Highlights:

- Description of myofascial trigger points (TPs).
- Causes and perpetuating factors.
- Three methods for releasing TPs.

Effort Involved:

- Find a qualified therapist or learn to do releases yourself.
- Relatively new TPs can be released in a matter of minutes.
- Long-established TPs usually require release over a period of days.
- Sometimes perpetuating factors need to be corrected before lasting results are seen.

Payoff:

- Release of long-standing pain, including pain that mimics arthritis.
- Greater ease of motion.
- Renewed muscle strength.
- More restful sleep.
- Relief from headaches, sinus conditions, menstrual pain and balance problems.
- A tremendous sense of well being.

The Real Cause of Much Pain and Stiffness— How Tight Spots in Muscles Mimic Joint Pain and Limit Range of Motion

Learning about myofascial trigger points was a revelation to me. In fact, it was yet another magical answer in my quest to recover from arthritis. Like each of the other methods I describe in my book, the simple act of erasing these TPs took me to a whole new level of wellness.

Shortly before I discovered myofascial TPs, I was discouraged. The strategies in Chapters 1-16 had led to vast improvements in my condition, but as I became acclimatized, I found that I was hungry for even more improvement. The problem was that although the inflammation had left my body, I still had unexplainable aches and pains. I felt much better than I had for years, but I still didn't feel totally well. I started to wonder if perhaps I had found only a partial cure for my condition or if I had permanent joint damage.

In particular, my hands hurt. It wasn't the extreme pain and aversion to pressure or cold that I had when my arthritis was active, but a dull ache, especially after exercises that used my arms. I was worried that structural damage from arthritis might have rendered my hands unable to support much weight.

It was at this time that I took a fateful trip to my local library. On the give-away table was a book called *Pain Erasure* by physical therapist Bonnie Prudden. This book changed my life. From it, I learned that tight, irritable points in muscle can cause pain at other locations in the body and that these pains can mimic the pain and stiffness associated with arthritis. Better yet, I found that it is a relatively simple process to erase these TPs. Using the charts in Ms. Prudden's book, I learned I could do this process myself without ever leaving home. I could also train my friends to erase spots that were harder to reach. The book even provides exercises for strengthening and stretching muscles. These exercises help prevent relapses.

I never would have guessed this before trying out the instructions in Bonnie Prudden's book, but the dull ache in my hands was quickly and easily eliminated by releasing TPs in the back of my arms. Releasing TPs has now become a favorite way of releasing pain and stiffness. For me, it works on persistent but otherwise unexplainable aches, including headaches, stiff neck, sore back, and sore spots in arms, legs, knees or feet. Releasing TPs has also helped reduce the severity of my menstrual cramps.

Because Bonnie Prudden credited Dr. Janet Travell so highly in her books and because I noticed that Dr. Travell's books on TPs were used as textbooks in some massage schools, I made the effort to find a copy of Dr. Travell's books[104] at a local medical school library. What I found astounded me. With painstaking (no pun intended) care, Dr. Travell and her co-author Dr. David Simons spent more than 30 years mapping out the referred pain patterns for TPs in each muscle of the body. They then paired this with very clear drawings that laid out, step by step, exactly how to remedy the problem. Although the language is highly technical, these books comprise a magnum opus of supreme usefulness. You may never choose to own or study these medical textbooks, but rest assured that the existence and treatment of myofascial TPs are very well researched and documented. Even if you never read the text, the pictures in these books make it a wonderful learning tool.

Before going any further, a few simple definitions are in order. The "myo" in myofascial means muscle. The "fascial" in myofascial means the covering that surrounds a muscle and attaches it to tendons. Referred pain means that there is pain at some other location than the spot causing the pain. For instance, TPs in the upper arm can refer pain to the hand.

Because Dr. Travell was willing to believe that her patients hurt as much and in the way they said they did, she was able to discover and map pain patterns that at the time were unexplainable. She deserves a great deal of credit, especially in light of the long history of practitioners who have declared that a patient's pain is not "real" or is "all in the head" when confronted with pain that did not make logical sense to them. Due in large part to Dr. Travell's diligent and pioneering work, we now know that the central nervous system powerfully modulates pain input from the muscles in ways that can explain the characteristics of pain referral patterns caused by myofascial TPs. Better yet, because of her work we also know how to erase these pesky sources of pain.

As an interesting side note, perhaps the most famous beneficiary of Dr. Travell's work was John F. Kennedy. She was his personal physician. It was her successful treatment of his chronic back pain from his war injuries that enabled him to subsequently run for the presidency.

---

[104] Janet G. Travell, M.D., and David G. Simons, M.D., *Volume 1, Myofascial Pain and Dysfunction: The Trigger Point Manual, The Upper Extremities* (Baltimore, MD: Williams & Wilkins, 1983).

Janet G. Travell, M.D., and David G. Simons, M.D., *Volume 2, Myofascial Pain and Dysfunction: The Trigger Point Manual, The Lower Extremities* (Baltimore, MD: Williams & Wilkins, 1992).

How to Determine if You have Myofascial Trigger Points

The **easiest way** to determine if you have myofascial trigger points is to consult with a health care practitioner trained in the art of TP release. (See the resource section at the end of this chapter for information on finding a practitioner.)

The **second easiest way** is to flip through Dr. Travell's Trigger Point Manuals. (See the resource section at the end of the chapter for the complete citations for these manuals.) Look for pictures with pain marked in the same area that you experience pain or stiffness. When you find one, notice the location of trigger points (marked with an "X" in these figures) that can cause this pain. Press firmly at each of these locations. If pressing causes your pain or stiffness, you have just located a trigger point.

The **third easiest way** is to flip to the back of Bonnie Prudden's book *Pain Erasure*. (See the resource section at the end of the chapter for the complete citation for this book.) Find the charts of common TPs. Press on your own body at each point that is indicated. If you experience pain or stiffness somewhere in your body when you press at any of these locations, you have just located a trigger point.

How Myofascial Trigger Points are Caused and Perpetuated—Many Factors Contribute

Causes

Many factors can cause myofascial TPs. Direct causes include overloading a muscle, working it to fatigue, holding it in a shortened position for a long time, chilling it, or subjecting it to severe injury. Indirect causes include activation of other TPs, emotional distress and physical pain. This includes pain caused by arthritis. Almost everyone suffering from chronic pain will have TPs. Unless released, TPs can persist for years. They can last long after their initial cause is gone.

Proper exercise, including stretching and strengthening exercises, is one way to make your muscles much less susceptible to TP formation. Stronger muscles are less prone to overload and fatigue. Routine stretching prevents a muscle from being held in a shortened position for a long period. It also releases newly formed TPs before they become set and more difficult to release. See Chapter 16 for information on exercises that provide stretching and strengthening.

Minimize problems like chilling, trauma, emotional distress and physical pain, but recognize that they are sometimes unavoidable. The good news is that TPs caused by these and other factors can be released, preventing the ongoing accumulation of TP-induced aches and stiffness that is sometimes mistakenly considered the inevitable result of growing older.

Perpetuating Factors

Many factors can perpetuate TPs. These include mechanical stresses, nutritional deficiencies, metabolic and endocrine problems, psychological factors, chronic infection and other factors.

For TP release to have long-lasting effects, you must eliminate the factors causing and perpetuating your TPs. Perpetuating factors are considered in detail below.

Mechanical stresses include stresses on muscles caused by poor posture, poorly fitting furniture, or prolonged immobility. If you have poor posture you may need to work with a physical therapist to improve your posture and to strengthen supporting muscles that may have gotten too weak. This is especially true if you are weak because of prolonged immobility. If habit rather than weakness is the problem, you may want to have a few sessions with someone who teaches the Alexander Technique. These lessons focus on helping you improve your posture as you sit, stand, bend and walk. If your furniture does not fit you, you may wish to consult with someone specializing in ergonomics. A specialist can help you recognize poorly fitting furniture, help you modify this furniture, and/or help you acquire more appropriate furniture. If you flip through Dr. Travell's textbooks, you will also find several illustrations that can guide you in this matter.

Nutritional problems include vitamin and mineral inadequacies. Suboptimal or low "normal" levels of vitamins B-1, B-6, B-12 and or folic acid are often responsible when only transitory relief is obtained from myofascial TP release. Vitamin C deficiency causes post-exercise stiffness and is usually low in smokers. Adequate calcium, potassium, iron and several trace minerals are also necessary for normal muscle function and recovery from TPs. In short, taking a good multiple vitamin and mineral pill every day may be an important part of your recovery.

Metabolic and endocrine factors include suboptimal thyroid function, anemia, hypoglycemia and hypoxia (poor oxygen intake). Any condition that impairs muscle metabolism perpetuates TPs. If you suspect any of these conditions, work with a medical professional to screen for and correct them.

Psychological factors include hopelessness, depression, tension caused by anxiety, the "good sport" syndrome, and secondary gain.

Hopelessness often sets in when someone believes that their pain is due to untreatable physical factors such as degenerative joint disease. If you think there is no hope and live in dread of all painful movements, you will also avoid those movements that stretch the muscles and help them recover function. Even though I was doing the best I knew how at the time, I know now that my chronic pain led to years of excessively restricted motion which in turn aggravated and perpetuated my TPs.

Depression is a tricky subject. Treating an underlying clinical depression can definitely help a person have the energy and outlook to take better care of him or herself and to engage in exercises and activities that support recovery. However, some responses often viewed as signs of depression can just be a natural response to chronic pain. They do not necessarily indicate that someone is chemically unbalanced or clinically depressed. Chronic pain makes it hard to sleep well, and drains energy even when people are awake. Many so-called depressive symptoms in people with chronic pain are actually just fatigue.

In my case, my doctor misread my fatigue and eventually refused to continue to treat me unless I went on antidepressants. Given that ultimatum, I did. According to the doctor, the antidepressants were supposed to help me sleep better and function better by raising my threshold of pain. Unfortunately, since I did not need antidepressants, what actually happened was that they messed up my body chemistry. They did nothing to alleviate my fatigue and instead caused a whole new set of classic overdose symptoms that my doctor did not recognize. I would suddenly get very shaky and literally collapse in sudden and unpredictable exhaustion, sometimes while attempting to walk or drive. These dangerous situations occurred only while I was on Prozac, and this despite the fact that I was never on more than half the lowest recommended therapeutic dose.

Anxiety is often expressed as muscle tension. This tension overloads muscles and perpetuates TPs. Exercises that help one recognize and release unnecessary tension can be very useful in correcting this tendency. See Chapter 16 for a discussion of yoga and tai chi, two forms of exercise that help release muscle tension. Meditation is another useful practice for recognizing excess muscle tension and learning to let it go. See Chapter 15 for more details.

A good sport doesn't let pain get in the way. This type of person believes that pain is a sign of weakness and pushes on to demonstrate his or her mastery of it. Because good sports tend to abuse their muscles, they tend to aggravate existing TPs and create new ones. If this describes you, see the four keys to exercising in Chapter 16. These keys will give you a new way of doing things. They will minimize pain and maximize your ability to get things done.

Secondary gain means getting something out of being sick, incapacitated or in pain. Some people enjoy the perks of being sick. That might mean extra attention, avoiding certain unpleasant interactions, or being exempt from normal chores or duties. Often this gratification is unconscious. If some part of you would rather stay sick, it is very easy to find small, seemingly insignificant, often unconscious ways to sabotage your recovery.

If you suspect you might be enjoying some secondary gains and that this might be interfering, even at an unconscious level, with your desire to become completely well, you might try making a list of every benefit you get from being sick. Then make another list detailing how each of those needs could be equally well or even better met if you were totally well. The idea is to bring any hidden motivations you have to the surface, where you can deal with them in the open. You want to make sure you have healthy means to get your needs met, so that there is no need to depend on the secondary gains.

Chronic infections and infestations can also perpetuate TPs. TPs tend to become more active during any systemic viral disease. Viral infections that aggravate TPs include influenza and herpes simplex virus type 1, the type of herpes that causes cold sores and canker sores. TPs are also exacerbated by chronic bacterial infection. This includes infections found in abscessed or impacted teeth, sinus infections and urinary tract infections. Infestations that perpetuate pain from TPs include fish tapeworms, giardiasis and amebiasis. Have any infections or infestations treated by a health professional.

The final factors that perpetuate TPs are hay fever and dust-type allergies, impaired sleep and chronic pain. Do what you can to control or eliminate these conditions.

The Cure—How to Erase Trigger Points

There are many ways to release TPs. These methods include the stretch and spray method, local injection and ischemic compression.

Stretch and Spray

Dr. Travell's books rely heavily on a method called stretch and spray. She found this to generally release myofascial TPs more quickly, and with less patient discomfort, than local injection or ischemic compression. This is especially true when there are large numbers of TPs, and TPs in multiple muscles that can all be stretched at the same time.

In the stretch and spray method, the muscle or muscles with TPs to be released are stretched just short of causing pain. The skin over the entire length of the muscle(s) plus the referred pain areas is then sprayed two or three times with a vapocoolant spray, using a quick sweeping motion. A quick sweeping motion is important because the goal is to maximize the distraction value of the cold, while minimizing any cooling of the skin or muscle. Hot packs can be used before, between and after treatments to warm the skin. This method works best if the person being treated is comfortably warm and relaxed.

In the stretch and spray method, the stretch is the action. The spray is a distraction. The brief but extreme cold distracts the central nervous system long enough for the stretch to release the TPs. Since the vapocoolant spray that Dr. Travell relied on was eventually found to harm the ozone layer of the upper atmosphere, she later recommended two alternative distractions. The first is sweeping a piece of ice on a wooden stick along the skin in the same pattern and at the same quick speed as used with the vapocoolant spray. Keeping the ice very cold so that it does not leave water on the skin aids in the effectiveness of this method. The second distraction, for patients using this method on themselves at home, is hot running water, especially a hot shower. Sitting instead of standing in the shower generally aids in obtaining the relaxation needed for this method to work. Just let the hot water run over you, while you stretch.

Injection and Stretch

The second method that Dr. Travell developed is injection and stretch. Injection is used for those muscles that are impossible to stretch, such as the sternalis muscle, which is found under the collar bone. It is also used when a few TPs remain that are unresponsive to stretch and spray. The injection consists of a 0.5 percent procaine solution. Procaine is a local anesthetic that disrupts the feedback mechanism between the TP and the central nervous system long enough for the TP to release. Because the injections require a detailed knowledge of anatomy to be done safely, only highly trained professionals are qualified to offer this service. Immediately after injection, when possible, the muscle is additionally subjected to the stretch and spray method.

Ischemic Compression

The third method for releasing myofascial TPs is ischemic compression. It is the method championed by Bonnie Prudden in *Pain Erasure*. Ischemia means a lack of blood flow to a body part due to constriction or blocking of a blood vessel. Ischemic compression applies pressure to a TP so it is denied its normal flow of blood. Without the oxygen supplied by the blood, the TP does not have enough energy to maintain its tenseness. It then has no choice but to relax.

Ischemic compression can be applied using two approaches. The first approach is to completely inactivate the TPs in one treatment. In the case of recent, moderately active TPs, this is often successful. The second approach is to progressively eliminate the TP activity in a succession of small steps that may take days. This is often necessary for long-term, highly irritable TPs.

To apply ischemic compression, the relaxed muscle is stretched to the verge of discomfort. A finger, thumb or elbow, or mechanical aid such as a tennis ball or dowel, is pressed directly on the TP to create a tolerably painful, sustained pressure. As the discomfort lessens, pressure is gradually increased. Sometimes only light pressure and a period of time as short as five seconds are needed for a release. Other times pressures of 20 to 30 lbs. and longer times of up to one minute or more are needed for a release.

Sensitivity to the release process is important. Pressing too hard, too soon, only makes TPs worse. Pressing too hard before the TP has had a chance to begin relaxing causes involuntary tensing of the muscle. Tensing the muscle prevents release, because tensing protects TPs from the pressure. It also irritates existing TPs and may even create more TPs, since they form in response to pain.

The application of pressure should be gradual and sustained long enough for a release. Initially apply light pressure. Gradually increase the pressure as the TP releases. Do not release until the trigger point has completed released. A subtle flush of heat from the area followed immediately by a disappearance of pain will often signal the end of a release.

If you are like me, you will only be able to apply this method to yourself effectively when you are relatively well-rested and resilient. At those times I have enough sensitivity to detect the gradual releasing of a TP and to gradually adjust the amount of pressure I am applying to help the process along. When I am too tired, I usually end up just making myself more sore.

Although it requires a certain amount of sensitivity to apply correctly, and it takes longer than the stretch and spray method, once you learn the ischemic compression method you can use it on yourself anytime you have enough focus. Many fancy and useful tools are on the market that make it easier to reach and apply pressure to TPs. Tennis balls, doorknobs, doorframes and any number of other common objects can also be used to reach and apply pressure to TPs. In its simplest form it takes no tools other than your finger, thumb or elbow.

To my mind, Yamuna Zake has raised release through ischemic compression to an art form. She describes her methods in the book *Body Rolling*. In brief, she has found that muscles connect to each other in functional groups. What affects one muscle in a group affects the other muscles in the group. For instance, a knee problem will affect the muscles in the foot, the hip, and all the muscles in between. Releasing only the tension that refers pain to the knee will provide relief, but can leave problems elsewhere in the muscle group that can later reactivate the initial problem. Systematically releasing tension, including TPs, along the entire length of the muscle group can provide deeper and longer-lasting relief.

Zake's method is based on using a person's own body weight against a 6- to 10-inch ball to supply compression, using body positioning to supply a stretch, and using breath work and visualizations to aid the release process. Her book was written to guide body workers such as massage therapists and yoga teachers in learning more about the subtleties of muscle and tendon release. As such, the descriptions of the release routines assume a high degree of familiarity with anatomical terms. If you don't have this type of background but you are interested in learning the release routines, don't be needlessly discouraged. Purchasing a set of flash cards illustrating the muscles of the human body and using them as you read through the step-by-step instructions will make it possible to follow the Zake's methods.

Post-Traumatic Hyperirritability Syndrome— Even This Can be Treated

When I read what Dr. Travell wrote about post-traumatic hyperirritability syndrome, I felt like she was describing exactly what I experienced for years. She writes that the symptoms include "constant pain, which may be exacerbated by the vibration of a moving vehicle, by the slamming of a door, by a loud noise (a firecracker at close range), by jarring (bumping into something or being jostled), by mild thumps (a pat on the back), by prolonged physical activity, and by emotional stress (such as anger). Even with mild experiences of this type, it can take many minutes or hours to return to baseline pain levels. Stronger encounters with these stimuli can cause severe exacerbation of pain that can require days, weeks or longer for recovery." She went on to say that these patients almost always have a history of having coped well in life prior to their injury, having paid no more attention to pain than their friends or family. However, from the onset of the initial trauma, pain suddenly became the focus of life.

The sad fact is, people with this syndrome and other variations of chronic myofascial pain are often treated very poorly by the medical community. Because the causes and treatments for these conditions are not widely understood, instead of receiving quick and appropriate treatment, we are frequently treated as slackers, fibbers or mentally ill. I certainly had this problem when dealing with my doctors.

The good news is that although recovery from these chronic conditions is more difficult and time-consuming than garden-variety TP problems, it is possible to recover. I am living proof.

Enlisting the Help of a Massage Therapist, Physical Therapist or Other Healing Professional—Finding Someone with the Right Training

See the resource section at the end of this chapter to find:

1. A therapist with special certification in Janet Travell's myofascial TP release.
2. A therapist with special certification in Bonnie Prudden's myotherapy techniques.
3. A certified Alexander Technique teacher.
4. Help with ergonomics.

If you have no luck finding a certified therapist in your area, don't despair. Good help may still be available. Some massage schools use Janet Travell's Trigger Point Manuals as textbooks. Some physical therapy programs may as well. Ask around your area for a good massage or physical therapist, especially someone who is known to have a good track record treating chronic pain.

Once you have some likely candidates, call and interview them. Ask if they are familiar with myofascial release work or with Janet Travell's work on TPs. One word of caution. Many therapists will say yes at this point, even if they are not familiar with myofascial TPs. This is because they hear the words "trigger points" and think you mean acupressure points. Make sure you clarify with them what they mean. Trigger points and acupressure points are two very different sets of points and are part of two very different systems of treatment.

How to Benefit the Most

First, take care of any digestive system problems that may be contributing to your arthritis (see Chapters 1-13). Next, follow the guidelines in Chapter 14 on superior nutrition. TPs release is more effective when you have a diet high in vitamins and minerals. Then follow the guidelines in Chapter 16 on exercise. Proper exercise helps remove existing trigger points and makes you less likely to develop new ones. Finally, developing skill in meditation (see Chapter 15) will aid in noticing and skillfully releasing even minor TPs.

Long-Term Benefits

Sometimes arthritis can be long gone, but pain and stiffness that mimic arthritis are still all too present. Pain patterns triggered by tight spots in muscles can persist for decades without some kind of release. Myofascial TP release provides a quick and easy way to get rid of this pain and stiffness. In some cases, releasing myofascial TPs can also relieve muscle weakness, poor sleep, headaches, sinus conditions, menstrual pain and balance problems. The result is often a tremendous sense of lasting well-being.

Resources

Books

Bonnie Prudden, *Pain Erasure: The Bonnie Prudden Way* (New York: Ballantine Books, 1980).
This book changed my life by introducing me to the concept of myofascial trigger points.

Janet G. Travell, M.D., and David G. Simons, M.D., *Volume 1, Myofascial Pain and Dysfunction: The Trigger Point Manual, The Upper Extremities* (Baltimore, MD: Williams & Wilkins, 1983).

Janet G. Travell, M.D., and David G. Simons, M.D., *Volume 2, Myofascial Pain and Dysfunction: The Trigger Point Manual, The Lower Extremities* (Baltimore, MD: Williams & Wilkins, 1992).
These two volumes by Travell and Simon are broad in scope and rich in detail. They represent a stellar achievement. The authors not only report

on a colossal amount of highly detailed, primary research, they also present this research in a highly integrated, comprehensive, highly useful form. The clear, beautifully done illustrations are a particular joy.

Yamuna Zake and Stephanie Golden, *Body Rolling: An Experimental Approach to Complete Muscle Release* (Rochester, VT: Healing Arts Press, 1997).
I love this book. Zake's routines take muscle release to a whole new level. However, because the text assumes familiarity with anatomical terms, for many of us it is not easy to read without a little help. Having a set of muscle flash cards, and pulling out the cards for each muscle in a given routine, is an excellent aid in understanding exactly what Zake is talking about, even if you haven't studied anatomy.

Other Aids

Muscle Flash Cards
I have a set of cards that I like called *Flash Anatomy Flash Cards: The Muscles* by Bryan Edward Publications, 1284 E. Katella, Anaheim, CA 92805. Flash cards of this type can be purchased at bookstores serving universities that have medical schools, physical therapy programs and occupational therapy programs. They can also be purchased through stores associated with massage schools.

Foam Roller
A foam roller is my all-time favorite device for releasing trigger points. It allows me to totally relax while using my own body weight to apply pressure to many hard-to-reach spots. The roller is a cylinder of Ethafoam, 6 inches in diameter and 3 feet. Ethafoam cylinders are often stocked by packaging businesses. Just ask for a 3-foot section. You can also purchase one from The Massage Store, Ltd., P.O. Box 2247, Boulder, CO 80306; 800-728-2426.

Thera Cane
The Thera Cane is another one of my favorite tools for reaching trigger points in parts of the body like the back and shoulders that are hard to reach with fingers and elbows. It is shaped somewhat like a shepherd's crook with handles and knobs. You can order one through Stretching, Inc., P.O. Box 767, Palmer Lake, CO 80133, 800-333-1307, or The Massage Store, Ltd., P.Pl Box 2247, Boulder, CO 80306, 800-728-2426.

Certified Therapists and Instructors

The Academy For Myofascial Trigger Point Therapy
1312 East Carson Street
Pittsburgh, PA 15203

412-481-2553 tel
412-481-3279 fax
www.npimall.com/amtpt/links.html
This academy has a full course of study that teaches TP Therapy. It also has shorter continuing-education seminars for medical professions based on Janet Travell's work. The Web site offers a listing, by state, of therapists that the academy has certified to do this type of work.

Bonnie Prudden Pain Erasure, Inc.
P.O. Box 65240
Tucson, AZ 85728-5240
800-221-5634
520-529-3979
520-529-6679 fax
E-mail: info@bonnieprudden.com
http://www.bonnieprudden.com/
This organization offers a two-year training program that teaches Bonnie Prudden's methods for TP release. Fifteen-hour weekend workshops on the same topic are also taught. The Web site lists Bonnie-Prudden-certified myotherapists by state.

American Society for the Alexander Technique
http://www.alexandertech.com/rightside.html
An Australian stage actor developed the Alexander Technique last century. It is usually taught one-on-one and is excellent for improving posture and ease of motion. Improving posture helps prevent trigger points from reforming. The organization listed above has a list, by state, of certified Alexander Technique teachers. It also has links to sites with information on ergonomics and the Feldenkrais Method, another system that uses gentle motion to improve posture and release restrictions from the body.

Conclusion—How to Get the Most Bang for Your Buck, Plus 5 Bonus Secrets

As I mentioned in the introduction, all of the nine secrets in this book work together synergistically. That means the whole is greater than the sum of the parts. Every time you correct an underlying cause of your arthritis, you become healthier and more able to heal. Every time you take a step that increases your overall health, whether it specifically addresses an underlying cause of arthritis or not, you also become healthier and more able to heal.

The goal is to increase your healing capacity enough to start getting well again. At that point, the synergy really starts to kick in. Instead of creating a "vicious cycle" you create what might be called a "virtuous cycle." As you keep removing the underlying causes of the illness and you keep making changes that improve your overall health, you will eventually reach a point where positive changes start to snowball. Soon it becomes easy to feel good again.

The Best Order for Implementing the 9 Secrets

Because of the synergy, you can benefit from implementing many of the secrets in any order. However, common sense dictates that implementing the strategies in the following order is most likely to bring about the quickest results. This order was already mentioned in the introduction, but it is important enough to be repeated. This order is:

1. Learn about how food allergies, sensitivities and intolerances may be the cause of your arthritis. (Chapters 1-2)
2. Check for food allergies, sensitivities and intolerances. (Chapters 3-4)
3. Activate your healing potential by therapeutically fasting. (Chapter 4)
4. If you have food allergies, sensitivities or intolerances avoid your problem foods. (Chapters 5-8) and procure safe food. (Chapters 9-12)
5. If you have food allergies, sensitivities or intolerances, take steps to eliminate the underlying causes. (Chapter 13)
6. Take supplements and eat foods that specifically promote the healing of arthritis. (Chapter 14)

7. Learn how to break the vicious stress-tension-pain cycle and replace it with the virtuous pleasure-relaxation-pain-reduction cycle using meditation. (Chapter 15)
8. Learn strategies that will allow you to get the most out of exercise even if you are very weak or very sick. (Chapter 16)
9. Clear up residual pain and stiffness by erasing pesky myofascial trigger points. (Chapter 17)

By following this order you **first eliminate** any food allergies, sensitivities or intolerances. A problem handling specific foods is one of the major underlying causes of arthritis. **Next** you give your body the nutritional support it needs to heal. **Then** you give yourself a meditation practice that allows you to retrain your response to pain; a gentle exercise program that allows your body to regain strength and flexibility; and massage work that allows your muscles to release the restrictive pain patterns that they have been holding, often below the level of conscious awareness. If you need or want to do still more, implement the five Bonus Secrets.

How many of the secrets you need to implement in order to heal depends on how sick you are and your unique blend of underlying causes. If you are very sick, you may need to implement all the secrets. If you are only a little sick, implementing only one or two secrets may be enough.

6 Examples of How the Healing Strategies Work Together Synergistically

Each of the nine secrets provides a powerful means of getting better. Each of these nine secrets also becomes more powerful when they are used in conjunction with one or more of the other secrets.

1. Once you realize that food allergies, food sensitivities and food intolerances can cause arthritis (Secret 1) you have powerful motivation to test for problem foods (Secret 2), eliminate problem foods from your diet (Secret 4) and heal your body of the tendency to react adversely to your problem foods (Secret 5). As you may already know, identifying your problem foods aids in eliminating them from your diet. Eliminating them from your diet aids in healing your body. With enough healing you may even be able to eat former problem foods again without trouble.

2. Therapeutic fasting (Secret 3) can be naturally coordinated with the other secrets to greatly increase the effectiveness of each method. Not only does therapeutic fasting activate the healing potential of the body, it also helps uncover hidden food sensitivities (Secret 2), and can work as a back-up pain-fighting mechanism when meditation (Secret 7) isn't enough.

Therapeutic fasting can also make it easier to reach healing states of consciousness when meditating.

3. Before I started therapeutically fasting (Secret 3), I had too much inflammation in my body to move much at all. Movement tended to cause my inflammation to flair. As a consequence, I became very weak from lack of exercise. My first fast gave me profound relief from pain and inflammation and thus made it possible to exercise (Secret 8) without making my condition worse. In turn, as I regained strength and endurance through exercise, I had more energy with which to implement the other secrets.

4. Eating healing foods (Secret 5) is good anytime, but it is especially important after therapeutic fasting (Secret 3), since the body is then primed to heal and needs high-quality nutrients to do this. In addition, identifying your problem foods (Secret 2) and learning all the tricks necessary to totally eliminate them from your diet (Secret 4), allows you to screen out foods that are generally considered healing but that in your particular case are actually an underlying cause of your arthritis.

5. Exercise (Secret 8) is usually always beneficial, but during and after therapeutic fasting (Secret 3), exercise is especially important because it supports and accelerates the healing changes brought about by fasting.

6. Once underlying causes are identified and corrected by the first six secrets, trigger point therapy (Secret 9) can then erase underlying myofascial tightness, a final step in eliminating residual arthritis pain and in regaining range of motion. Meditation (Secret 7) and exercise (Secret 8) aid in releasing TPs. In turn, erasing TPs makes meditation and exercise more pleasant.

Taken together, these nine secrets are a powerful healing system.

The last four secrets are particularly powerful for increasing health even after your arthritis is gone. I found that once I identified and rid myself of food sensitivities (Secrets 1-5), that these last four secrets (eating healthy, healing foods; meditation; exercise; and myofascial trigger point release work) have continued to contribute to ever-increasing levels of wellness.

I am one of the few people I know who continues to feel better with each passing year. I credit this to continuing to use Secrets 6-9 which continues to lead to healing at deeper and deeper levels.

5 Bonus Healing Secrets—How To Find and Implement the Perfect Mix of Healing Strategies for Your Unique Situation

"You don't have to go very far off the interpreted path to find yourself in very difficult situations. The courage to face the trials and bring a whole new body of possibilities into the field of interpreted experience for other people to experience—that is the hero's deed."—Joseph Campbell

"This time, like all times, is a very good one, if we but know what to do with it."—Ralph Waldo Emerson

There are many more healing modalities available than I have mentioned in this book. The nine healing secrets that I used to heal my arthritis and that I concentrate on in this book are certainly not the only ones that can benefit someone seeking to heal their own arthritis or food allergies—they are just the ones that were most powerful for me. Your situation may be different. The perfect healing strategy for you may be something I never even mentioned. Perhaps it is something I have never even heard of. You are unique and it stands to reason that what you need to heal might be unique as well. How can you best find your unique answers to what will best help you heal?

To supplement the nine healing secrets in this book, I recommend five bonus healing secrets:
1. Ask empowering questions.
2. Set positive, attainable goals.
3. Make use of your resources.
4. Don't squander your most important resource.
5. Take an active role.

1. Ask Empowering Questions

"If you think you can succeed, you are right; if you think you will fail you are also right" –Henry Ford

"Every adversity, every failure, carries with it the seed of an equivalent or greater benefit."—Napoleon Hill

So much of how we experience the world depends on our attitudes. Thinking of ourselves as a success breeds success. Thinking of ourselves as a failure breeds failure. What we focus on tends to be what we get. One of the best ways to leave behind the failure track and start living on the success track is to upgrade the quality of questions we ask ourselves.

Instead of asking, "Why do bad things always happen to me?" or "What did I do to deserve this punishment?" start asking questions like "What can I do today to improve my situation?", "What can I learn from this situation so that it never happens again?", and "What can I learn from this that will help me heal?"

2. Set Positive, Achievable Goals

"Choose always the way that seems the best, however rough it may be. Custom will soon render it easy and agreeable."—Pythagoras

"Sow an act, and you reap a habit. Sow a habit, and you reap a character. Sow a character, and you reap a destiny."—Charles Reade

Achieving goals sets up a "success cycle" similar to the "virtuous cycle" mentioned earlier in this chapter. Success builds upon success until positive achievement is a good habit that is as hard to break as any bad habit.

The key to achieving goals is to set achievable goals and to always state them in positive terms. Never use negative words in your goal statements. For example, it is better to say, "Every Thursday I will try one new recipe using a delicious alternative flour, such as flour made from quinoa, millet, amaranth, teff, milo, barley, rye or yam, until I find several types of baked goods that I enjoy making and eating," than it is to say, "I will not eat bread, pasta, pastries, cookies or any other baked goods because wheat flour makes me ill."

Formulating very specific goals also helps. Vague goals like "I will only eat foods that are healthy for my body" are not as effective as stating, "On Saturday I will purchase and/or prepare enough healthy snack food to last the whole week, including wheat-free baked goods, fresh fruit and fresh vegetables."

Anthony Robbins, in his book *Awaken the Giant Within,* does a great job addressing how to set effective goals. This book is an excellent resource for anyone wishing to make positive life changes.

3. Make Use of Your Resources

"Fortune aids the brave."—Terence

"Do what you can with what you have, where you are."—Theodore Roosevelt

Resources come in all sizes and shapes. Some of your best resources are your friends, neighbors and people you meet through support groups. Other resources are your public library, your own intelligence and your own motivation to get well. If you are so inclined, your resources can also include prayer and/or the support of a religious community.

Use your resources to set yourself up for success. Figure out what you need and then use your resources to get it. Call the Arthritis Foundation for help. Join a support group and find out what has worked best for other people in your situation. Ask friends and your librarian to help you find out everything you can about how other people in your situation were able to get better.

Try asking small groups to help you brainstorm creative solutions to your more difficult problems. Don't censor out the crazy answers. Have someone write down everything, until suddenly something that might have seemed crazy or improbable sparks an answer that just might work. Even if you don't get an immediate answer, this process can be fun.

When you are in too much pain or are too tired to think well, let trusted family and friends help you think about your options.

Learn to ask for help. You don't have to do things that you are physically unable to do. Most people help when given half a chance. Prayer and other contemplative practices help open us to help from within and without.

When you ask for help, be as clear as you can about what you need and, whenever possible, make it easy for others to help you. You might be physically incapacitated. Pain and exhaustion might even make it hard to think clearly. However, if you can accept help from a place of openness and gratitude, you may be surprised at how much others want to be around you. Humans need to be accepted, appreciated and cared about. If you can provide that, no matter how sick you are, others are likely to experience being around you as a blessing.

Learn to use your limited energy for just those things that matter most to you. Let the rest drop away. Say no to "help" that is not helpful. Rest when you need to. If you listen closely to your body it will let you know just how much, or how little, you can do in that moment.

4. Don't Squander Your Most Important Resource

"Your attention—literally whatever you pay attention to—is the tool of creating your world. When it is developed it is one of the most powerful techniques for transformation that you will find. Where ever you focus your attention is where the energy of life takes you."—Brooke Medicine Eagle

Your most important resource is your attention. What you focus your attention on is what shapes your world.

Blame, self-pity, bitterness, refusal to forgive, desire for revenge, and other negative states squander your attention. These unproductive states waste a lot of energy that could be used to have a good life. In fact, you could actually have many of the elements of a good life, but miss out on your blessings because of a negative focus.

Conversely, you can choose to focus on what you love and what makes you feel good. You can choose to focus on the gifts you have to give and that others wish to give to you. These gifts include love, attention, friendliness, help with physical tasks, and most anything else you can think of that makes life easier or better. Paying attention to these blessings amplifies the transformative power of what is good in your life and draws more goodness to you. Even if you have many elements of a bad life in your life, if you can manage to focus on what is good, that which is bad loses its power to make you miserable.

Remember, no matter what happened to you in the past, it is over. You hurt yourself more than anyone else when you fixate your attention on what was negative about the past. Also remember, no matter what is happening to you in the present, if you can find something pleasurable or positive to focus on—no matter how minor—you can use your most important resource—your attention—to leverage yourself into a better life.

Sure, life is ugly, painful and unfair. It is also beautiful, pleasurable and fulfilling. You get what you focus on. You miss what you ignore. The choice is yours.

5. Take an Active Role

"I have heard talk and talk but nothing is done. Good words do not last long unless they amount to something."—Chief Joseph

"Personal power is necessary for health." –Caroline Myss

Take an active role in deciding upon and implementing your treatments. Don't wait around for others to cure you. Take personal responsibility for your choices. Use others as resources and advisors, but always make sure that you are the one making the decisions. When it comes to your body and your health, everyone else is just your support team.

When you take such an active role, you send a strong signal to yourself and others that you are serious about getting well, that you are worth the effort. Often the exact decisions are less important than the fact that you are the one making the decisions.

Healing comes from within, and taking charge of the external process is often just what is needed to tap into those inner healing resources.

Please Write Me

For me, healing from arthritis was a miracle. It was the answer to my prayers. It drastically changed the course of my life.

I wrote this book to share my miracle with others. I hope this book will make it easier for others who are still have arthritis and/or food sensitivities to heal.

If this book helps you conquer arthritis or food sensitivities, please write and share your triumph. I would love to hear what worked for you. If there is anything in the book that is confusing, misleading or unclear to you, also please write and let me know. Your feedback will help me improve future editions.

Please send your comments to Barbara@ConqueringArthritis.com

I will post updates, corrections and clarifications on my Web site, http://www.ConqueringArthritis.com

Resources

Groups and Institutions

Arthritis Foundation
www.arthritis.org
800-283-7800
The Arthritis Foundation provides information and sponsors support groups. Check to see if there is a support group in your area.

Public Libraries, Bookstores and Medical School Libraries
Libraries and bookstores are good sources of books on arthritis. Medical school libraries often have extensive collections of journals that include research articles on arthritis.

Medline
http://www.ncbi.nlm.nih.gov/entrez/query.fcgi?CMD=&DB=PubMed
This free version of Medline allows you to use the internet to search for research articles on arthritis.

The Internet
You can also use search engines to look for arthritis information on the Web.

Prayer Circles and Healing Circles
Inquire at churches, massage schools and New Age bookstores to find prayer circles and healing circles. Ask your friends and acquaintances if they know of any. Look for notices in local publications.

Specific Books

Anthony Robbins, *Awaken the Giant Within* (New York: Fireside, 1992).

Caroline Myss, *Why People Don't Heal and How They Can* (New York: Harmony Books, 1997).

Caroline Myss, *Anatomy of the Spirit: The Seven Stages of Power and Healing* (New York: Harmony Books, 1996).

Appendix A: 4 Factors that Cause Food Sensitivities and Arthritis

The ideas in this appendix bring together many interrelated concepts: circulating immune complexes (CICs), specific antibody types, allergens, autoimmune reactions, different types of immune system cells, including mast cells, T-cells and B-cells.

Unless you are interested in the details it may never be important for you to fully grasp everything in this appendix. What is important is that you and your health care provider realize that there is strong research that supports the relatively inexpensive and relatively low-tech ways to get well that are presented in this book. A large body of work done by careful and well-respected medical researchers solidly supports these ideas.

Four factors that are known to cause food sensitivities and arthritis are:

1. Leaky gut syndrome.
2. Breakdown of oral tolerance.
3. Low levels of certain detoxification enzymes.
4. Dietary lectins.

1. Leaky Gut Syndrome

In leaky gut syndrome, a large number of food particles pass either totally undigested or partially undigested into the bloodstream. This passage of undigested food occurs in the small intestine, where virtually all absorption of fully digested food also occurs. All people, even very healthy people, have some undigested food that leaks into their bloodstream. However, most food-sensitive individuals have much higher levels.[105]

Things that can trigger leaky gut syndrome are use of conventional nonsteroidal anti-inflammatory drugs (NSAIDs), alcohol, anti-ulcer drugs such as Zantac and Tagamet, antacid tablets and/or antibiotics (including antibiotics taken years ago), diets high in simple carbohydrates, gulping

---

[105] Charlotte Cunningham-Rundles, M.D., Ph.D., "Dietary Antigens and Immunologic Disease in Humans," *Rheum Dis Clin North Amer* 17(2) (1991):287-307.

food without chewing thoroughly, presence of parasites in the digestive tract, and a personal or family history of allergies or food sensitivities.

Symptoms can include any of the following: poor digestion, gas and bloating, food sensitivities, yeast infections, fatigue, joint pain, cloudy thinking and difficulty maintaining weight.

A doctor can easily determine if leaky gut syndrome is present using the test described in Chapter 2 in the section called "How to Test for Leaky Gut Syndrome."

The Biology and Biochemistry of Leaky Gut Syndrome

Studies by Dr. Jonathan Brostoff of Middlesex Hospital in London suggest that the **IgE antibody** plays a role in inducing leaky gut syndrome.[106])IgE is pronounced by saying each letter in the name, I-G-E.) Like all antibodies, the IgE antibody class recognizes foreign matter and flags it for removal.

As mentioned in Chapter 2, only low levels of the IgE antibody class circulate in the blood of food-sensitive individuals. However, in food sensitivity reactions the IgE in another location, the small intestine, becomes very important.

Dr. Brostoff's studies indicate that in food-sensitive individuals a three-way interaction between IgE, a type of immune system cell called a **mast cell**, and offending food takes place in the wall of the small intestine. This interaction causes mast cells to release mediators, such as histamine, serotonin and prostaglandins. These mediators cause changes that allow more undigested food to pass through the small intestine.

In Dr. Brostoff's study, the **drug cromolyn sodium** (also called sodium cromoglycase) eliminates food sensitivity symptoms when taken shortly before eating a food that is known to cause symptoms. This drug suppresses the release of mediators from mast cells. It acts without interfering with the binding of the IgE to mast cells and without interfering with the interaction of offending food with IgE bound to mast cells.[107]

---

[106] Linda Gamlin, "Another Man's Poison," *New Scientist* 123 (1989):48-53.

[107] Daniel P. Stites, Abba I. Terr and Tristram G. Parslow, *Basic and Clinical Immunology*, (Norwalk, CT: Appleton & Lange, 1994, 792.)

The mediators released by mast cells have dramatic effects on the body, including intense local inflammation. The resulting local inflammation makes the wall of the small intestine more permeable than is healthy and normal. This increased permeability allows high levels of undigested food molecules to pass into the bloodstream. The release of mediators from mast cells also affects the process of acquiring and maintaining oral tolerance (discussed below).

Once absorbed, food molecules in the bloodstream may cause symptoms by causing high levels of **circulating immune complexes (CICs)** in the bloodstream (discussed below in this section). They may also cause symptoms by provoking T-cell-mediated inflammation throughout the body (discussed below in the section on oral tolerance). **T-cells** are a type of immune system cell.

Leaky gut syndrome also allows parts of the cell walls of bacteria that are living in the small intestine to pass into the bloodstream. In particular, peptidoglycan-polysaccharide fragments from the cell walls of some common, normal intestinal bacteria have been shown to induce severe arthritis. This arthritis can come and go quickly or it can evolve into a chronic condition that destroys the joints.[108]

Although it might seem like a good idea to use cromolyn sodium to treat food sensitivities, in practice it merely masks symptoms without correcting underlying causes. Initially, patients on cromolyn sodium tend to feel better, but their overall condition tends to gradually worsen.

The most effective way to treat leaky gut syndrome is to avoid any foods to which you have an adverse reaction. In addition, steps must be taken to correct underlying problems that contribute to developing food sensitivities. If you don't correct these underlying problems, you run the risk of continuing to develop sensitivities to more foods. Measures for correcting these underlying conditions are described throughout Chapter 2 and in Chapter 13.

How Undigested Food in the Bloodstream Causes Arthritis

When incompletely digested food molecules enter the bloodstream, they usually join with antibodies to form **circulating immune complexes**

---

[108] Stephen A. Stimpson, et al., "Arthropathic Properties of Cell Wall Polymers from Normal Flora Bacteria Infection and Immunity," *Infect.Immun.* 51(1) (1986):240-249.

(CICs). Because everyone absorbs at least a few incompletely digested molecules, even healthy individuals have CICs after a meal. However, food-sensitive individuals tend to absorb much more incompletely digested food and the undigested particles tend to be larger.[109]

Furthermore, the antibodies involved are not exactly the same as in healthy individuals. In healthy individuals, classes of antibodies called **IgA** and **IgG** predominate, whereas in food-sensitive individuals there is less IgA, more IgG and some IgE.[110] The IgG4 subclass of IgG has been implicated in allergic diseases, especially food allergy.[111]

Antibody Classes in Circulating Immune Complexes (CIC's)

Class of Antibody	IgA	IgG	IgE
Action of antibody	Dampens inflammation	The IgG4 subclass can cause food allergy	Can trigger inflammation
Levels in healthy individuals	High	High	Not present
Levels in food-sensitive individuals	Low or moderate	Very High	Some is present

[109] J. Brostoff, C. Carini, D.G. Wraith, et al., "Immune Complexes in Atopy" In *The Mast Cell* edited by J. Pepys and A.M. Edward (London: Pitman, 1979, 380-383.)

[110] Ibid.

[111] E. Savilahi, P. Kuitenen and J.K. Visakorpi, "Cow's Milk Allergy," *In Textbook of Gastroenterology and Nutrition in Infancy*, edited by El Lebenthal, Vol. 2, (New York, Raven Press, 1981, 689-708.)

These differences in the antibody profile are important, because they make the CICs of food-sensitive individuals more likely to promote inflammation. This is so because IgA is low in the CICs of food-sensitive individuals. Therefore, it is not present at normal inflammation-dampening levels. Higher levels of IgG may include higher levels of the IgG4 subclass implicated in food allergy. The IgE present in the CICs of food-sensitive individuals may trigger mast cells and therefore cause inflammation.

Totally apart from causing inflammation, high levels of CICs are a bad thing. CICs are known to do damage in patients with the autoimmune disorder systemic lupus erythematosus (SLE). In the case of lupus, CIC formation is triggered not by food molecules but by an autoimmune reaction against proteins that are a normal part of the body. Patients with SLE have so many CICs in their blood that their body is unable to cope. Anywhere there is turbulent flow through tiny blood vessels, such as in the kidneys, the joints, the skin and around the lungs, painful deposits form.[112] Although it has not been proven, some doctors have suggested that in a much milder form the same phenomenon may be occurring in food-sensitive individuals who suffer from joint pain.[113]

The idea that CICs cause arthritis is also supported by studies showing that arthritis occurs in 28 to 54 percent of recipients of certain types of intestinal bypass operations. Several studies have suggested that CICs are the cause of this arthritis.[114] Surgical reversal of the intestinal bypass is associated with immediate and permanent remission of the arthritis[115] and can produce a prompt decline in CICs.[116]

---

[112] Linda Gamlin, "Another Man's Poison, *New Scientist* 123 (1989):48-53.

[113] Robert D. Inman, M.D., "Antigens, the Gastrointestinal Tract and Arthritis," *Rheum Dis Clin North Am*, 17(2) (1991):309-321.

[114] Ibid.

[115] J. P. Delamere, R. M. Buddeley and K.W. Walton, "Jejunoileal Bypass Arthropathy: Its Clinical Features and Associations," *Ann Rheum Dis* 42 (1983):553-7.

[116] D. O. Clegg, J. J. Zone, C. O. Samuelson, et al., "Circulating Immune Complexes Containing Secretory IgA in Jejunioleal Bypass Disease," *Ann Rheum Dis* 44 (1985):239-244.

The same type of mast cell reaction mentioned above that occurs in the intestines can also occur inside joints. IgE antibody binds to mast cells with extremely high affinity. Upon contact with a specific allergen, it triggers a series of biochemical events. These events culminate in mast cells releasing mediators into the joints and causing inflammation, cartilage degradation, skeletal abnormalities and synovial tissue characteristic of the pathology of RA (rheumatoid arthritis).[117] CICs deposited in joints may well be the source of the allergen that triggers mast cells to release joint-damaging mediators.

In an unfortunate turn of events, the allergens that trigger mast cells to release inflammatory substances in joints may also be the molecules that are a normal part of the body. Sometimes, especially when pathogenic bacteria are involved, an immune system trained to react against bacterial allergens will cross-react to normal body proteins.[118] This type of cross-reaction is believed to be an underlying cause of reactive arthritis (the type of arthritis I had) and at least some cases of RA.[119,120]

Both reactive arthritis and rheumatoid arthritis involve the balance of suppressor and helper T-cells being tipped in favor of too many helper T-cells.[121] This balance is upset, as explained below in the section on oral tolerance, by immature T-cells first encountering an allergen not in the gut but in other parts of the body. CICs traveling through the bloodstream are the cause of this encounter first happening in other parts of the body.

Because CICs carry not only food particles but also bacterial particles, leaky gut syndrome (the reason why so many of these CIC particles are getting into the bloodstream in the first place) causes a wide range of

[117] Barry L. Gerber, M.D., "Immunoglobulin E, Mast Cells, Endogenous Antigens, and Arthritis," *Rheum Dis Clin North Amer* 17(2) (1991):33-341.

[118] Joseph Holoshitz, Irun R. Cohen, et al., "T-Lymphocytes of Rheumatoid Arthritis Patients Show Augmented Reactivity to a Fraction of Mycobacteria Cross-Reactive with Cartilage," *Lancet* (1986):305-309.

[119] P. E. Philips, "How do Bacteria Cause Chronic Arthritis?," *J Rheum* 16: (1989):1017-1019.

[120] J.C. Bennett, "The Infectious Etiology of Rheumatoid Arthritis– New Considerations," *Arthritis Rheum* 21(1989):531-538.

[118] P. C. Res, et al., "Synovial Fluid T-cell Reactivity Against 65 kD Heat Shock Protein of Mycobacteria in Early Chronic Arthritis," *Lancet* 480 (1988):478-480.

problems. It causes food sensitivities, damaging immune system reactions triggered by the bacterial proteins in CICs, and damaging autoimmune reactions originally raised against bacterial proteins but now against the body itself.

See Chapter 2 for ways to prevent and correct leaky gut syndrome.

2. The Breakdown of Oral Tolerance

Another factor that contributes to food intolerance is the breakdown of oral tolerance. Oral tolerance is a term that refers to the training of the immune system **not** to react to molecules of food that leak through the gut into the bloodstream of everyone, even healthy people. In healthy people the training is successful, so food molecules are not attacked. However, for some reason the process of oral tolerance does not work as well in food-sensitive individuals.

The body learns to have oral tolerance in discrete areas of the wall of the small intestine known as Peyer's patches. Cells within each patch actively take up fluid from the gut in a process known as antigen sampling. The term antigen refers to substances that react with antibodies or T-cells. Antibodies and T-cells are both part of the immune system.

When the process of acquiring oral tolerance is successful, sufficient numbers of T-cells are trained in the Peyer's patches **not** to react to a given antigen and then travel all over the body suppressing reactions to that particular antigen. These T-cells are called suppressor T-cells.

Regardless of what happens in the Peyer's patches, other T-cells not trained in the Peyer's patches also travel throughout the body looking for opportunities to instigate reactions. These T-cells are called helper T-cells. In addition to instigating inflammatory reactions, when helper T-cells encounter the antigen to which they react, they proliferate and also cause a proliferation of B-cells that react to this same antigen. B-cells are yet another part of the immune system, a part that makes antibodies.

If suppressor T-cells are more successful in suppressing reactions to a particular food than helper T-cells are in instigating reactions to these particles, then a state of oral tolerance exists. This means the ratio of suppressor T-cells to helper T-cells has to be high enough to suppress reactions.

Important Players in the Process of Maintaining Oral Tolerance

Suppressor T-cells	Helper T-cells	Secretory IgA antibody response
Tilt balance toward oral tolerance	Tilt balance away from oral tolerance	Tilts balance toward oral tolerance
Levels too low (as compared to helper T-cell levels) in food-intolerant individuals	Levels too high in food-intolerant individuals	Levels too low in food-intolerant individuals
Trained in gut but then travel around body suppressing inflammatory reactions to food	Trained in the body at locations outside of the gut to instigate inflammatory reactions to food	Tends to keep food out of bloodstream, thereby lowering levels of inflammatory helper T-cells

Establishing oral tolerance also involves an antibody response. The antibody response is important because it greatly reduces the number of undigested or partially digested food molecules in the bloodstream. This response consists of the production of a type of antibody called secretory IgA (SIgA). This occurs by triggering a proliferation of a type of immune cell called a B-cell that produces SIgA antibody. These B-cells then travel to secretory tissues including those in the small intestine. In this manner, the body's exposed surfaces, including the intestines, receive an ample supply of SIgA.

The binding of SIgA to antigen creates an antigen-antibody complex that tends not to pass through the wall of the small intestine into the bloodstream. This is very good for health. In this manner that SIgA tends to reduce the amount of problem-causing CICs in the bloodstream.

Food-sensitive individuals tend to have less SIgA bound to food molecules that pass into the bloodstream than do healthy individuals. This suggests that part of the mechanism causing food intolerance involves a failure of the immune system to produce adequate amounts of SIgA.

The level of SIgA also affects the suppressor/helper T-cell ratio, a ratio that is out of balance in people with reactive arthritis and rheumatoid arthritis and people with problems with oral tolerance.

This happens because if too little SIgA is bound to food particles, more food particles enter the bloodstream. This results in higher than normal levels of problem-causing CICs in the blood. More T-cells then first encounter antigens in the bloodstream and become reactive, inflammation-causing helper T-cells instead of anti-inflammatory suppressor T-cells. This out-of-kilter T-cell ratio leads to the body waging a war against food particles in the bloodstream and also causes inflammation characteristic of reactive arthritis and rheumatoid arthritis.

Unfortunately, this is not a simple story, and food-intolerant individuals seem to lose out at every turn. To make matters more complicated, some immune system reactions are inflammatory, such as the production of IgG and IgE antibodies (excessive in the CICs of individuals with food intolerances). Other immune system reactions are noninflammatory, such as production of SIgA antibodies (low in the CICs of individuals with food intolerances).

Just the fact that the SIgA level in food-intolerant individuals is low, and does not completely coat the food particles that get into the bloodstream, opens the door to more IgG and IgE antibodies that usual binding to CICs once they reach the bloodstream. That means that not only do food-intolerant individuals have more CICs, but those CICs tend to be more inflammatory.

Delayed Hypersensitivity Reactions

Type IV or delayed hypersensitivity reactions are typically delayed for 48 hours and are known to be caused by lymphocytes (T- and B-cells).[122] Lymphocytes are found in abnormally high numbers in the small intestine in cases of delayed hypersensitivity. Lymphocytes from other parts of the body also proliferate when exposed to the specific foods to which an individual is intolerant. This proliferation indicates that lymphocytes throughout the body are already primed to react against these specific foods. These facts are a very strong indication that the process of oral tolerance is not functioning correctly in cases of delayed hypersensitivity and that the problem beyond a doubt involves the immune system.

---

[122] Sami L. Bahna, MD, Ph.D., and Jayesh Kanuga, M.D., "Food Hypersensitivity," *Rheum Dis Clin North Am*, 17(2) 1991:243-249.

In 1949, Dr. H. S. Lawrence demonstrated that delayed hypersensitivity could be transferred from one person to another by certain low molecular weight fragments from disrupted white blood cells.[123] It was later found that factors that passively transferred antigen-specific reactions from one individual to another come from helper T-cells.[124] Miller and Hanson[125] have further shown transfer of unresponsiveness occurring through transfer of suppressor T-cells. These results further support the central role of helper T-cell/suppressor T-cell ratios in delayed hypersensitivity reactions.

In each of these experiments, transfer occurs through simple injection into the skin of either T-cells, which contain the transfer factor, or the isolated transfer factor itself.

A study reported by Dr. Alan S. Levin[126] is exciting because it offers hope that one day quick and lasting relief from food sensitivities may come through transfer factor therapy. In this study suppressive transfer factors were administered to steroid-dependent asthmatics whose asthma attacks were triggered by food sensitivities. At the time this study was published, these patients had remained symptom-free and off steroids for between five and 18 months.

Interestingly, the initial transfer factor work done by Dr. Lawrence used a tuberculosis protein to induce and to test for delayed hypersensitivity. Coincidentally, later studies have used injections of tuberculosis bacteria to induce a condition known as adjuvant arthritis that is used as an animal model to study rheumatoid arthritis. Adjuvant arthritis studies done by Dr.

---

[123] H. S. Lawrence, "The Cellular Transfer of Cutaneous Hypersensitivity to Tuberculin in Man," *Proc Soc Exp Biol Med* 71 (1949):516-22.

[124] W. Borkowsky and H. S. Lawrence, "Deletion of Antigen-Specific Activity from Leukocyte Dialysates Containing Transfer Factor by Antigen-Coated Polystyrene," *J Immunol* 126 1981): 486-9.

[125] S. D. Miller and D. G. Hanson, "Inhibition of Specific Immune Responses by Feeding Protein Antigens: Evidence for Tolerance and Specific Active Suppression of Cell-Mediated Immune Responses to Ovalbumin," *J Immunol* 123 (1979):2344-2350.

[126] Alan S. Levin, "Transfer Factor and Allergies," *Food Allergy and Intolerance*, edited by Jonathan Brostoff and Stephen J. Challacombe (London: Bailliere Tindall, 1987).

Irun Cohen[127] show that this arthritis is caused by a helper T-cell/ suppressor T-cell ratio that is too high.

Dr. Cohen has also shown that helper T-cells can be taken from the body and engineered to have suppressor activity by certain intentional mechanical disruptions of their cell membranes. Mechanical disruption simply means that mechanical shearing forces like those created by pressure changes were used. These results are very much like the results mentioned above where nonreactiveness to an antigen was transferred from one individual to another. His results are even more promising, however, because a patient's own blood, not someone else's, may eventually become a source of exactly the right transfer factors needed to correct the problem.

Intestinal flora may also be important for establishing oral tolerance. For instance, bacterial lipopolysaccharide taken orally enhances oral tolerance. However, oral tolerance cannot be induced in its absence (in germ-free mice).[128]

More research needs to be done to better understand the process of acquiring oral tolerance and how transfer factors might help in re-establishing this process. Many of the details of acquiring oral tolerance are still poorly understood. It is thought, however, that increased intestinal permeability makes oral tolerance more difficult to achieve and maintain.

The best way to reestablish oral tolerance is likely to be to first correct leaky gut syndrome and then take additional steps, such as transfer factor therapy, if it ever moves from an experimental procedure to an accepted clinical treatment.

How to Reestablish Oral Tolerance

❑ Follow the steps given in Chapter 13 for correcting leaky gut syndrome.

---

[127] Irun R. Cohen, "Regulation of Autoimmune Disease Physiological and Therapeutic," *Immunol Rev.* 94 (1986): 5-21.

[128] S. J. Challacombe and T. B. Tomasi, "Oral Tolerance," *Food Allergy and Intolerance*, edited by Jonathan Brostoff and Stephen J. Challacombe (London: Bailliere Tindall, 1987).

3. Low Levels of Certain Detoxification Enzymes

A series of enzymes has been found to be important in detoxifying certain types of food molecules. These enzymes detoxify by converting a toxic type of chemical group (sulfide groups) into a nontoxic type of chemical group (sulfoxide groups). The name of the reaction that is carried out is sulfoxidation.

According to Dr. Stephen McFadden, among the population as a whole, about 2.5 percent of people cannot carry out this reaction. However, among people with delayed food sensitivity, the percentage of people who cannot carry out this reaction is much higher—about 49 percent. Reduction in the ability to carry out this sulfoxidation reaction is also found much more frequently, as compared to the general population, in cases of systemic lupus erythematosus (SLE), rheumatoid arthritis (RA), Alzheimer's disease, Parkinson's disease, multiple chemical sensitivities, cases of drug intolerance and several other conditions.[129]

Reduced sulfoxidation has been found in 60 percent of people with SLE compared to 4 percent of controls. Reduced sulfoxidation is also found more frequently in people with RA than in controls, although it does not predict disease activity. However, people with both RA and reduced sulfoxidation are 2.5 times more likely to develop joint erosions, 3.9 times more likely to react adversely to the thiol drug D-penicillamine, and 2.5 times more likely to react adversely to the thiol drug sodium aurothiomalate (used in gold treatments) than people with just RA.

Reduced sulfoxidation in individuals with SLE and RA suggests that in subpopulations these conditions may be either produced or exacerbated by metabolic imbalances caused by reduced sulfoxidation.

A related detoxification pathway called sulfation, which detoxifies phenolics, needs sulfate produced by sulfoxidation to work properly. Not surprisingly, impaired sulfation has been found in many of the same conditions associated with poor sulfoxidation. In addition, impaired sulfation may be a factor in the success of the Feingold diet. The Feingold diet is free of salicylates, food colorings and preservatives. It is used to treat behavior disorders such as hyperactivity in children. The first link is that although salicylates themselves are not sulfated, they inhibit sulfate

---

[129] Stephen A. McFadden, "Phenotypic Variation in Xenobiotic Metabolism and Adverse Environmental Response: Focus on Sulfur-Dependent Detoxification Pathways," *Toxicology* 111 (1996):43-65.

transport, thus making it harder for the body to carry out this reaction. The second link is that many food colorings and preservatives are probably ultimately detoxified by sulfation.

The drug acetaminophen is often used to treat rheumatoid arthritis and other arthritic conditions. Acetaminophen is the generic name for a drug sold under 97 brand names, including Tylenol®. It is also sold as a component under in more than 100 brand names in combination with other drugs, including Sinutab®.[130]

For individuals with impaired sulfation this drug is a bad idea. In high doses acetaminophen saturates the sulfation pathway making it impossible for the pathway to handle all the other dietary substances that it should be detoxifying. Saturating the pathway also depletes the amount of sulfate available. Sulfate is required for maintaining the structure of the glycosaminoglycans within joints, and a lack of sulfate may impair joint repair.

Linda Gamlin notes that among people with both food intolerance and intolerance to common synthetic chemicals, such as chlorine, natural gas, exhaust fumes and solvents, about 90 percent have a reduced ability to carry out sulfoxidation reactions.[131] The correlation of difficulty carrying out sulfoxidation reactions with food and chemical sensitivities is interesting because it suggests a possible reason why people with food intolerance are often also chemically sensitive.

Detoxification of synthetic compounds probably relies on both sulfoxidation and sulfation enzymes, whose original function was to break down bacterial products and certain substances in food. Those of us with slightly suboptimal detoxification enzymes do fine as long as our toxic load does not exceed the ability of our enzymes to detoxify it. However, with increased exposure to toxic chemicals in our environment, our enzyme systems become overwhelmed and can no longer detoxify all the chemicals, problematic bacteria and problematic food substances to which we are exposed. Many people find that if they can avoid the chemicals to which they are sensitive, they can better cope with foods that were previously a problem.

---

[130] *1998 Mosby's GenRx: The Complete Reference for Generic and Brand Drugs, 8th Edition* (St. Louis, MO: Mosby, 1998.)

[131] Linda Gamlin, "Another Man's Poison," *New Scientist* 123 (1989):48-53.

Testing for Sulfoxidation and Sulfation

Sulfoxidation capacity is measured with a drug called S-carboxymethyl-L-cysteine (SCMC). The standard protocol is that a dose of SCMC is given at 8 A.M. and urine is collected over the course of the next eight hours, after which the metabolites are evaluated by descending paper chromatography. The "sulfoxidation index" is calculated by dividing the "nonsulfoxide" SCMC metabolites by the "sulfoxide" SCMC metabolites collected in the samples.

Sulfation capacity is measured with acetaminophen. This drug is detoxified by sulfation.

Measurement of sulfoxidation and sulfation are still largely experimental procedures and not yet a part of standard clinical medicine. At present, if you wish to have these levels measured, you will likely have to become part of a clinical research study. Perhaps in the future these tests will become more widely available. Until then, your best bet for testing enzyme levels is to reduce your exposure to substances that require these detoxification systems. To do this, follow the guidelines given in Chapter 13 in the section, "How to Alleviate Symptoms Caused by Overwhelmed Sulfoxidation and Sulfation Detoxification Pathways". If limiting your exposure to the substances listed in Chapter 13 helps your condition, then suboptimal levels of detoxification by these enzyme systems is probably a factor in your condition.

Oral Doses of Sulfoxidation and Sulfation Enzymes

Can the level of detoxifying sulfoxidation and sulfation enzymes in the body be improved by supplementing our diet with these enzymes? This is a logical question, since it is possible to improve other aspects of digestion by taking digestive enzymes.

In the case of sulfoxidation the answer is "no" because this reaction takes place in the liver, not the digestive tract.

In the case of sulfation, all tissues in the body are capable of at least some sulfation, but the most important sulfation occurs in the digestive tract, ensuring that phenolics do not enter systemic circulation. This would imply that taking phenol sulfotransferase enzymes plus sulfate might have a favorable effect on the ability to carry out sulfation. Unfortunately, although sulfate is presumably available through doctors, I am not aware of commercially available phenol sulfotransferase enzyme supplements.

How to Alleviate Symptoms Caused by Overwhelmed Sulfoxidation and Sulfation Detoxification Pathways

See Chapter 13 for steps you can take to reduce toxic loads and increase your body's ability to handle toxic substances.

4. Dietary Lectins and Blood Type Reactions

For a discussion of this factor see Chapter 2.

Appendix B: How Food Sensitivities Cause Pain and Fatigue and How to Stop It

Highlights:

❑ How to stop the pain and fatigue of food sensitivities caused by inappropriate lymphokine release.
❑ 14 things to avoid to heal faster.
❑ 14 proactive steps to take to heal faster.

Effort Involved:

❑ The effort involved is variable.

Payoff:

❑ Less pain and fatigue. More energy.

Inappropriate Lymphokine Release

Lymphokines are a type of molecule which the immune system uses to communicate.

Doctors have noticed that one type of lymphokine called interferon, which is used to treat hepatitis B, has numerous side effects. These include headaches, lethargy, dizziness, abdominal discomfort, bowel disturbance, nausea and joint pain. Many flu symptoms are caused by lymphokine release triggered by the body's response to the influenza virus. The fact that these are some of the same symptoms brought on by food sensitivities suggests that something similar is going on when the body has a food intolerance reaction.

A breakdown in oral tolerance, which is discussed in detail in Chapter 2 and Appendix A, is a likely cause of such lymphokine release.

Steps that heal digestion and bring the immune system back into balance will stop inappropriate lymphokine release caused by food sensitivities. These steps include the strategies given in Chapters 2 and 13 for correcting the four known factors that cause food sensitivities:

1. Leaky gut syndrome.
2. Breakdown of oral tolerance.
3. Low levels of certain detoxification enzymes.
4. Adverse reactions to dietary lectins.

Because these steps promote proper digestion and healthy immune system function, they eliminate the achiness and fatigue caused by food sensitivities.

How to Maximize Healing—14 Things to Avoid

Other strategies that bring the immune system back into balance are mentioned throughout this book. They are powerful healing strategies because they correct underlying problems that cause arthritis and promote overall health.

Fourteen things to avoid (whenever possible) to avoid inappropriate lymphokine release are:

1. Antibiotics
2. Corticosteroid use (including prednisone)
3. Other drugs that suppress the immune system (e.g., chemotherapy drugs, plaquinil and methotrexate)
4. Conventional nonsteroidal anti-inflammatory drugs (NSAIDs)
5. Triggering food sensitivities
6. Stimulants such as caffeine
7. Nutritional deficiencies
8. High-sugar diet
9. High cholesterol levels
10. Being overweight
11. Stress (including overwork, irregular meal times, fretting and social isolation)
12. Not enough sleep and sleep disruptions
13. Smoking
14. Not getting regular exercise

How to Get Well Even Faster—14 Things You Can Do

Avoiding things that are bad for you will help you heal. However, changing your mindset from avoidance to positive action will help you get well even faster. A positive, proactive attitude unleashes additional healing energies.

The 14 things to avoid restated as 14 positive, proactive steps are given below. These steps allow you to take charge. They allow you to stop the inappropriate lymphokine release, improve immune system function and reduce or eliminate food sensitivities that are the underlying causes of many cases of arthritis. The steps are:

1. Whenever practical, treat colds and sniffles with alternative medical treatments that strengthen the immune system, such as those recommended by Dr. Michael Murray, N.D.[132]:
   - *Echinacea* (dried root or as tea: 0.5 to 1 g three times per day or a 1:5 tincture: 2 to 4 ml three times per day) A 1:5 tincture is made with a mixture of 1 part alcohol and 5 parts water.
   - *Astragalus* root (dried root or as decoction: 1 to 2 g three times per day or as a 1:5 tincture: 2 to 4 ml three times per day) A decoction is made by adding cold water to an herb and then heating at a simmer for up to 1 hour.
   - Vitamin C (500 mg every two hours)
   - Zinc lozenges (30 mg per day)
   - Homeopathic remedies
   - Rest
2. Give the remedies in this book a chance before using corticosteroids or other immune-suppressing drugs to treat your arthritis.
3. Test for food sensitivities. If present, identify all foods triggering your sensitivities using the techniques described in Chapters 3 and 4. Use an elimination diet or a rotation diet (see Chapters 5-13) to avoid these foods until your body has healed enough to no longer react adversely.
4. Use the strategies in Chapter 13 to minimize or even eliminate food sensitivities.
5. Give your body what it needs to heal by eating a balanced diet (see Chapter 14) that is rich in whole, natural foods, such as fruit, vegetables, whole grains, beans, seeds and nuts, and low in fats and refined sugars. Eat adequate but not excessive amounts of protein. Substitute water, herbal teas and other caffeine-free beverages for caffeine-containing beverages like coffee, tea and soda.
6. Have set mealtimes and don't skip meals. Chapters 9-12 give many suggestions for eating well despite food sensitivities.
7. Take a multiple vitamin and mineral supplement. Also take an additional supplement high in antioxidant vitamins and minerals. Chapters 14 and 17 explain what to take and why this is important.
8. If overweight, lose weight. The fact that : and fat levels in the blood are usually elevated in obese individuals may explain the impaired

---

[132] Michael Murray and Joseph Pizzorno, *Encyclopedia of Natural Medicine* (Rocklin, CA: Prima Publishing, 1998.)

immune function usually seen in obese people. If you need help losing weight, choose one of the many weight-loss programs that teach you how to lose weight in a slow, healthy manner while eating balanced, nutritious meals. Modify your eating and lifestyle habits so you don't regain the weight after the program is over. You may also want to consider juice fasting as detailed in Chapter 4.

9. Practice daily relaxation exercises (for example, meditation, prayer, tai chi or yoga) to reduce stress. Chapter 15 describes meditation techniques that, among other things, are effective tools for managing pain. Chapter 16 describes meditative forms of exercise that can be used to relax.

10. Have a routine that includes time for meaningful relationships. Make time to give and receive love.

11. Don't fret. Save your energy for those things you can do something about. Take charge of your condition as much as you can. Every time you take a step that improves your ability to cope with your arthritis (or anything else that is stressful to you) you reduce your stress levels, give your immune system a boost, and make it easier to heal.

12. Make it a priority to get as much sleep as you need. Most people need at least seven hours a night. When your arthritis is acting up, you may need 12 or more hours of sleep a night and naps during the day. Avoid working third shift or rotating shifts or being on call at night. Have a regular bedtime and a quiet, dark place to sleep.

13. If you smoke, quit. Studies show that cigarette smoking makes rheumatoid arthritis worse.[133]

14. As your health improves, work up to at least 30 minutes of aerobic exercise four times per week. With arthritis it is important to exercise but not overextend yourself. Chapter 16 explains how to tailor an exercise program to your exact situation, even if you are still very sick.

Long-Term Benefits

Taking the steps suggested in this appendix will likely boost your energy levels and result in lasting improvements in your health.

---

[133] Kenneth G. Saag et al., "Cigarette Smoking and Rheumatoid Arthritis Severity," *Annals of Rheumatic Diseases* 56 (1997):463-469.

Glossary

Agglutination—sticking together

Antibody classes—IgE, IgA, IgG, and SIgA each refer to a specific class of antibodies that the immune system makes. These classes are important because abnormalities in the types or amounts of each one contribute to food sensitivities and abnormal pattern is different from the abnormal pattern found in classical food allergies.

Antibody—is a type of protein made by the immune system. An antibody acts by latching on to a certain, very specific molecular shape that are different for each individual type of antibody. This latching on is how the body identifies things as foreign and it often, but not always, triggers inflammation.

Antigen—the specific molecular section of a substance, usually a stretch of protein, that reacts with antibodies or T-cells. This reaction causes an immune reaction such as either inflammation or tolerazation.

Allergen—a substance, such as cat hair, that carries an antigenic component that gives rise to an immune response.

Allergy—a disease or reaction caused by an immune response to one or more environmental or dietary antigens, resulting in tissue inflammation and organ dysfunction.

Anaphylactic shock—an exaggerated immune response to a foreign protein or other substance to which a person has previously become sensitized. Often the throat constricts, making it difficult or impossible to breathe.

Antioxidants—substances that in small amounts will inhibit the oxidation of other compounds. Oxidation of compounds creates free-radicals, which can damage cells. Antioxidants like vitamin C and E protect the body from damage by free-radicals.

Allopathic—refers to a system of medicinal practice that combats disease by the use of remedies producing effects different from those produced by the disease treated. For example, using anti-inflammatory drugs to treat the inflammation caused by arthritis. So-called Western medicine is generally allopathic.

Amines—a type of organic compound containing nitrogen. Bacterial overgrowth in the intestines can putrefy proteins and form vasoactive amines that in excess can cause leaky gut syndrome.

Aspartate—a chemical used as an artificial sweetener

Autoimmune reaction—a reaction in which the immune system attacks the body.

Autoimmune types of arthritis—types of arthritis such as rheumatoid arthritis, juvenile rheumatoid arthritis, reactive arthritis, Reiter's syndrome, inflammatory bowel disease arthritis, systemic lupus erythematosus, ankylosing spondalytis, psoriatic arthritis, chronic fatigue syndrome and fibromyalgia. In each of these, the body's immune system attacks parts of the body itself, causing arthritis. Over 3.5% of the population of the United States of America or over 9.1 million people suffer from these forms of arthritis. Doctors are just starting to recognize that a sizeable number of these cases are caused by adverse reactions to certain foods.

B-cells—a type of immune system cell that makes antibodies. Some of these antibodies are important in autoimmune reactions and food sensitivities.

Blood type—a characteristic of red blood cells caused by certain molecules on the cell's surface. Human blood types are A, B, O, and AB, each of which can be either Rh+ or Rh-. Blood types can help predict problem foods in the diet that may be perpetuating arthritis.

Circulating immune complexes (CICs)—clumps floating around in the blood steam, formed by antibodies latching on to proteins (often from incompletely digested food).

Classical food allergy—see food allergy

Comprehensive digestive stool analysis (CDSA)—a battery of integrated diagnostic laboratory tests that evaluate digestion, intestinal function, intestinal environment and absorption by carefully examining the stool. It is useful for pinpointing the exact nature of digestive disturbances. In addition to giving a great deal of information on the digestive process itself, CDSA also provides information on the presence of various friendly and/or pathogenic microorganisms in the intestines and on the presence of bacterial overgrowth in the small intestine.

Concomitant reactions—reactions that occur only when another allergen, such as pollen, dust or mold, is present. An example is milk sensitivity or mint sensitivity that occurs only when ragweed pollen is present. Concomitant reactions can occur up to six weeks after pollen season is over. Sometimes prescription drugs can provoke reactions to normally safe foods.

Chondroitin—a substance with a good track record for helping people heal from arthritis. It is usually taken together with glucosamine, because the two work better together than either one alone. Chondroitin stimulates the production of cartilage and stops the action of enzymes that break down cartilage. It also speeds the healing of bones and skin wounds.

Corticosteroids—steroidal compounds with biological properties resembling those of adrenal cortical extract. Used as drugs to combat inflammation. Unfortunately these drugs do not work as well as those substances produced by our own adrenal glands and have many undesirable side effects, including making bones brittle and diminishing adrenal function.

COX-2 inhibitors—a new class of NSAIDs that causes fewer stomach problems than conventional NSAIDs. This is because they inhibit only the inflammation-promoting enzyme COX-2 and not the stomach-acid-regulating enzyme COX-1.

Cross-reactions—reactions that initially develop in response to one substance but are then triggered in response to a different substance. For instance, an immune system trained to react against bacterial allergens will sometimes cross-react to normal body proteins. This type of cross-reaction is believed to be an underlying cause of reactive arthritis and at least some cases of rheumatoid arthritis. Another example: as the use of latex in the health care industry has grown, so have latex allergies and cross-reactions to bananas.

Cyclooxygenase (COX)—two types are found in the body. COX-1 regulates stomach acid. COX-2 promotes inflammation.

Detoxification enzymes—enzymes that convert a toxic type of chemical group into a nontoxic type. For instance, sulfoxidation enzymes convert toxic sulfide groups into nontoxic sulfoxide groups.

Enzymes—proteins that catalyze chemical reactions

Enzyme-potentiated desensitization (EPD)—a treatment based on the ability of enzyme ß-glucuronidase to regulate the immune system cells known as T-cells that would normally facilitate a food sensitivity reaction, in the presence of food allergens. By training T-cells not to react to food

313

allergens, the body learns not to have adverse reactions to these allergens. EPD has been used in England for about 25 years and has recently become available in the United States. It works in about 85 percent of people and treats a wide range of allergens, including food, airborne and chemical allergens.

Fatty acid—a type of molecule that is an important component of oil. Depending on the location of double bonds within a fatty acid, it can be inflammatory (omega-6 fatty acid), anti-inflammatory (omega-3 fatty acids) or neutral with respect to inflammation (omega-9 fatty acids).

Flavinoids—compounds that help give deeply colored fruits and vegetable their color. Generally flavinoids are considered to be quite healthy. However, some flavinoids, especially those in oranges, result in a temporary reduction in sulfation capacity (see sulfation below), which can be a problem for some food sensitive individuals.

Food allergies—generally, an allergic reaction to food. In classical food allergies, a small amount of food, such as peanuts or shrimp, causes a near-immediate response, such as intense local inflammation or anaphylactic shock. These can be fatal. This is what most doctors mean when they say "food allergies." This type of allergic response usually dissipates within a few hours. In classical allergy, laboratory tests also show high levels of the IgE antibody class, both for IgE antibodies that bind specifically to allergy-triggering foods and also for the total amount of IgE antibodies in the bloodstream. This type of allergy is also called a type I or type III immunological reaction to food. For a discussion of another type of food allergy, see the entry under food sensitivities.

Food sensitivities—an adverse reaction to food that is often an underlying cause of autoimmune types of arthritis. Unlike classical food allergies, food sensitivity reactions, 1) usually become noticeable not minutes, but hours to days after ingesting an offending food and may take several days to resolve, 2) patients with food sensitivities do not have high IgE levels in their bloodstream and 3) commonly available allergy skin testing, which is how many people are tested for allergies and which reliably detects classical allergies, is unreliable in cases of food sensitivities.

Food intolerances—a term that broadly means any adverse reaction to food.

Free-radicals—highly reactive chemical groups that react with almost any compound with which they come into contact. These indiscriminate reactions damage the body.

Gastrointestinal—refers to the digestive tract

Glucosamine—a substance with a good track record for helping people heal from arthritis. It is usually taken together with chondroitin. Glucosamine inhibits free-radical production and inflammation. It also speeds wound-healing and reduces scarring. It does this both when placed directly on a wound and when taken orally. It speeds the healing of surgical wounds, traumas such as cuts and bruises, injury to the gastrointestinal tract, and arthritic joints.

Glycemic index—a measure of how much and how quickly a food tends to raise the blood sugar levels after it is eaten.

Gluten—a type of protein that gives texture to kneaded breads. It is allergenic to many people. Gluten is found in wheat, spelt, kamut, rye, oats and barley. Gluten is not found in corn, rice, quinoa and millet.

Insulin resistance—a condition whereby the body is unable to respond properly to normal levels of insulin in the bloodstream.

Intestinal permeability—is a measure of how much stuff intestinal walls allow to pass from the intestines into the bloodstream. Ideally, only fully digested food is allowed to pass. When intestinal permeability is too high, undigested and partially digested food gets into the bloodstream, where it causes problems (see Circulating Immune Complexes).

Ischemic compression—a method for releasing myofascial trigger points (TPs). Ischemia means a lack of blood flow to a body part due to constriction or blocking of a blood vessel. Ischemic compression applies pressure to a TP so it is denied its normal flow of blood. Without the oxygen supplied by the blood, the TP does not have enough energy to maintain its tenseness. It then has no choice but to relax.

Ketosis—an accumulation of ketones in body tissue and fluids, detectable as a slightly sweet odor on the breath. This begins after about three days of fasting. The is metabolism of fat in the absence of carbohydrates produces the ketones, and in the case of a fast, is nothing to worry about.

Leaky gut syndrome—a syndrome in which a large number of food particles pass either totally or partially undigested into the bloodstream. This passage of undigested food occurs in the small intestine, where virtually all absorption of fully digested food also occurs.

Lectins—a type of proteins found in certain foods and viruses that can make cells stick together or agglutinate.

Legumes—the fruit or seed of a pod-bearing plant, such as peas and beans.

Leukotriene B₄—an inflammatory substance made by the enzyme lipoxygenase.

Lipotrophic—refers to certain agents capable of decreasing deposits of fat in the liver.

Lipoxygenase—a type of enzyme in the body that promotes inflammation.

Lymphocytes—a general term that refers to white blood cells and includes T-cells and B-cells.

Lymphokines—a type of molecule which the immune system uses to communicate.

Mannitol/lactulose leaky gut syndrome test—a test which involves administration of two sugars – mannitol and lactulose. Mannitol is a small molecule that is quickly taken up by intestinal cells. Lactulose is a larger molecule that should not be taken up by intestinal cells. However, if leaky gut syndrome is present, lactulose is taken up. Since neither sugar is metabolized, they can be measured by urine analysis of a sample collected six hours later.

Mast cells—immune system cells that trigger inflammation by releasing substances such as histamine.

Meditation—a specific way of focusing attention that, among other things, is very useful in dealing with pain

Monoamine—a compound containing a single amine chemical group. Monoamine-containing foods include cheese, which contains tyramine; chocolate, which contains phenylethamine; and bananas.

Mucins—a type of protein found in cabbage which protects the intestinal tract and promotes healing of digestive problems. Mucins in the body can be increased by glucosamine taken orally.

Myofascial—refers to muscle and fascia, which is a band or sheet of tissue surrounding and connecting muscles

Myofascial trigger point release—releasing pain-causing restrictions in the myofascia known as trigger points.

N.D.—abbreviation for naturopathic doctor

NSAIDs—Non-steroidal anti-inflammatory drugs, including aspirin, ibuprofen, and a host of others. They tend to damage the stomach, because they inhibit not only COX-2, an enzyme that promotes inflammation, but also COX-1, an enzyme that regulates stomach acid.

Omega-3 fatty acids— fatty acid is the chemical name for a type of a molecule that is an important component of oils. Omega-3 fatty acids are anti-inflammatory and found in abundance in cod liver oil and flax seeds. Because food processing tends to destroy these very beneficial components, it is good to supplement your diet with them.

Omega-6 fatty acids— fatty acid is the chemical name for a type of a molecule that is an important component of oils. Omega-6 fatty acids are inflammatory and found in abundance in corn oil, peanut oil and "vegetable oil". It is good to limit your consumption of oils high in omega-6's.

Omega-9 fatty acids— fatty acid is the chemical name for a type of a molecule that is an important component of oils. Omega-9 fatty acids are neutral with respect to inflammation and healthy for the heart. They are found in abundance in extra virgin olive oil.

Oral tolerance— refers to a training of the immune system **not** to react to molecules of food that leak through the gut into the bloodstream. In healthy people the training is successful, so food molecules are not attacked. However, for some reason, the process of oral tolerance does not work as well in food-sensitive individuals.

Osteoarthritis—often known as wear and tear arthritis. Most prevalent in older people and most often found at sites of former injury.

Pathogens—organisms, such as certain bacteria, that cause disease.

Phenolated—refers to substances containing a toxic chemical group called a phenol.

Phenolics—chemical compounds that include a phenol group, which is a group with one or more hydroxyl groups attached to an aromatic or carbon ring. Phenol groups are extremely poisonous. Low doses of phenolics are sometimes added to pharmaceutics to keep bacteria from growing in them.

Prostaglandin E$_2$—an inflammatory substance made by the enzyme COX-2.

Protease inhibitors —substances that inhibit the digestion of proteins. Protease inhibitors are found in the raw and undercooked forms of the following foods: soybeans, peanuts, lentils, rice, corn and potatoes.

Protozoan—a phylum of the animal kingdom made up of microscopic, unicellular organisms. Overgrowths of usually harmless organisms, including protozoans, are often found in the intestines of people with food sensitivities. Proper treatment to correct these overgrowths will often cause food sensitivities to disappear as well.

Provocation-neutralization treatments—a treatment for food sensitivities that involves either subcutaneous (under the skin) injections or sublingual (under the tongue) drops that are carefully measured to contain the exact "neutralizing" dose of food extract needed to "turn off" food intolerance symptoms. Because neutralizing doses change, patients must be retested frequently to keep their neutralizing shots or drops current and working effectively. Although no one knows how these neutralizing doses are able to "turn off" food sensitivity reactions, this phenomenon has been repeatedly observed.

Salicylates—compounds containing a salicylic acid group. These compounds include aspirin and some food additives.

Sprouting—Sprouting is the germination of a seed. Soaking seeds, such as beans or grains, for several hours to overnight induces them to sprout and makes them easier to digest and more nutritious.

Sublingual—under the tongue

Sulfation—a type of reaction that converts a toxic group called a phenolic to a non-toxic type of chemical group. This reaction needs sulfate produced by another type of chemical reaction called sulfoxidation to work properly. Impaired sulfation in the body is one reason why people with food sensitivities often also have problems with chemical sensitivities.

Sulfoxidation—a type of reaction that converts a toxic type of chemical group (sulfide group) into a nontoxic type of chemical group (sulfoxide group). Impaired sulfoxidation in the body is one reason why people with food sensitivities also often have problems with chemical sensitivities.

Synergistic reactions—reactions that occur only when two foods are eaten in the same meal. An example is an allergic reaction to corn and banana when they are eaten together but not when they are eaten separately.

Proven synergistic foods include: corn and banana, beef and yeast, cane sugar and orange, milk and mint, egg and apple, and pork and black pepper.

T-cells—a type of immune system cell produced by an organ called the thymus. These cells come in two types: helper T-cells and suppressor T-cells. Helper T-cells cause inflammation. Suppressor T-cells calm inflammation.

Thymus—an organ of the body found in the chest just above the heart. It is the primary location where T-cells are produced and differentiate. Thymus extracts (thymodulin) have been shown to normalize the ratio of T helper cells to suppressor cells, whether the ratio is low (as in AIDS or cancer) or high (as in allergies or rheumatoid arthritis). A high helper-to-suppressor T-cell ratio is believed to be one of the causes of rheumatoid arthritis (RA) and other types of arthritis such as reactive arthritis. It is not surprising that since thymus extracts improve this ratio, they also improve the clinical symptoms of RA.

Transfer factors—factors found in the blood and associated with T-cells that can transfer delayed hypersensitivity reactions from one person to another. These factors can also transfer non-reactivity to a reactive person. This offers hope that one day transfer factor therapy will be available to treat food sensitivities.

Vasoactive amines—a type of organic compound containing nitrogen that causes changes in the diameter of blood vessels. Bacterial overgrowths in the upper part of the small intestine can lead to the formation of vasoactive amines that can cause leaky gut syndrome.

Vegan—a diet free of all animal products

Index

abdominal discomfort
    interferon side effects, 307
acetaminophen
    alleviating overwhelmed
        detoxification pathways, 207
    detoxified by sulfation, 305
    measuring sulfation capacity, 305
    sulfation, 39, 304
achieving goals, 287
adaptogen, 236
aerobic exercise, 310
agar, 141
agglutination, 40
Airola, Paavo O., 62
alcohol
    corn allergens, 97, 98, 108
    eliminate while fasting, 70
    fermentation products, 57
    food sensitivity reactions, 54
    help quiting, 48
    leaky gut syndrome, 32, 43, 205, 292
    liver function, 209
    need to avoid, 34, 41, 45, 205
    tincture, 309
    triggering sensitivity reactions, 47
    wheat allergens, 102, 115
    yeast allergens, 104
Alexander Technique, 273, 279,
282
alfalfa
    alkalizing, 235
    genetic enginering, 89
    pet food, 84
    sometimes triggers food intolerance
        reaction, 55
    tea, 67, 171
    travel food, 163
allergen
    definition, 311
allergy testing, 31, 314
allopathic medicine, 11, 21, 29,
311
alternative sweeteners
    noncorn sources, 219
Alzheimer's disease
    sulfoxidation, 303
amines

leaky gut syndrome, 36
anaphylactic shock, 30
anemia, 36
    myofascial trigger points, 273
    pork allergens, 112
anger, 244
animal hair
    avoid while testing for food
        sensitivities, 45
    limit exposure while testing for food
        sensitivities, 48
    masking improvement, 49
    minimize exposure while fasting, 70
ankylosing spondalytis
    autoimmune types of arthritis, 18
antacid tablets
    leaky gut syndrome, 32, 205, 292
    need to avoid, 206, 207
antibiotics
    bacterial overgrowths, 36
    increased intestinal permeability, 43
    leaky gut syndrome, 32, 205, 292
    need to avoid, 206, 308
    restoring healthy intestinal flora, 233
    yeast allergens, 54, 116
    yogurt to reseed intestines, 173
antidepressants
    author's experience with, 29
    chronic pain, 274
antigen
    antigen sampling, 298
    binding to antibodies, 299
    blood-type, 40
    definition, 311
    T-cell proliferation, 298
    T-cell training, 298
    transfer factors, 302
antioxidants
    definition, 227
    maximizing thymus function, 211
    onions, 235
    prevent free radical damage, 227
antiperspirants
    hidden allergens, 52
anti-ulcer drugs
    leaky gut syndrome, 32, 205, 292
    need to avoid, 206, 207
    Tagamet, 32, 205, 206, 207, 292
    Zantac, 32, 205, 206, 207, 292

320

McFadden, Stephen A., 207, 209, 219, 303

methionine
  alleviating overwhelmed detoxification pathways, 208
  liver support, 209
  unknown allergens, 123

methotrexate
  need to avoid, 308

milk
  alternatives to cow's milk, 148
  can cause arthritis, 24, 26
  commonly triggers food intolerance reactions, 53
  concomitant reactions with ragweed pollen, 57
  concomitant reactions with viral infections, 57
  corn allergens, 99
  lists of products containing milk allergens, 100, 112
  Norwegian fasting study, 65
  nut and seed milks, 172
  synergistic reaction with mint, 57
  testing for food sensitivity to, 74
  yeast allergens, 104
  yeast overgrowth, 54

milk allergens, 100

milk thistle
  health tonics, 236
  liver support, 209

millet
  alternative flours, 140
  carrot cutlet recipe, 187
  cooking instructions, 144
  corn bread recipe, 151
  flour as thickener or binder, 138
  grain and flour options, 143
  grains in the grass family, 50
  is gluten-free, 137
  pet food, 84

millet bread recipe, 151

miso
  Asian salad dressing recipe, 176
  fermentation products, 57
  good in broth, 170
  healing disgestive tract, 233
  healthy intestinal flora, 168, 206, 233
  Japanese style carrot dressing recipe, 176
  parsley-almond sauce recipe, 159
  rice allergens, 101, 113
  soy allergens, 114

molybdenum
  alleviating overwhelmed detoxification pathways, 208

Mootz, William C., M.D.
  foreword, 11

motor oil, 15

Moyers, Bill, 241, 247

MSG, 80
  allergens introduced into meat by processing, 148
  alleviating overwhelmed detoxification pathways, 208
  alternative names used to hide MSG, 83
  corn allergens, 99
  false advertising on food labels, 121
  foods that include MSG, 121
  names on labels that can indicate MSG, 121
  not regulated as a food additive, 121
  often triggers food intolerance reactions, 54
  overview, 121
  rice allergens, 113
  soy allergens, 102
  wheat allergens, 103, 115
  yeast allergens, 104

mucins
  disrupted in gastrointestinal disturbances, 237
  in cabbage, 233
  in cabbage juice, 67
  increased by glucosamine, 237
  promote healing of stomach, 168

multiple chemical sensitivities
  sulfoxidation, 303

Murray, Michael T., 208, 211, 309

myofascial trigger points
  author's experience with, 270
  body rolling, 278
  chronic infections, 275
  definition, 271
  dull aches eliminated by releasing, 270
  factors that cause, 272
  finding a therapist, 279
  foam roller, 281
  good sports, 275
  hay fever, 275
  how to release, 275
  how to test for, 272
  hypoglycemia, 226

injection and stretch, 276
ischemic compression, 277
mimic arthritis, 230
muscle tension, 274
perpetualted by inadequate levels of
these vitamins, 273
perpetuating factors, 273, 274
posture, 282
recommended dose of vitamin C,
233
referred pain, 271
stretch and spray, 276
thera-cane, 281
vitamins needed for elimination, 230

Nambudripad Allergy
Elimination Technique (NAET)
effort involved, 202
overview, 215

naturopathic doctors, N.D.
how to find, 29

nausea
interferon side effects, 307

Nelson, Miriam, E., 266, 268

nightshade vegetables
often triggers food intolerance
reactions, 55

normal intestinal bacteria, 294

NSAIDs
avoiding to heal digestive tract, 41
biochemical damage, 33
COX-2 inhibitors, 33, 34
definition, 317
glucosamine works better, 237
increase intestinal permeability, 33
leaky gut syndrome, 32, 205, 292
need to avoid, 205, 308

nutritional deficiencies
myofascial trigger points, 273
need to avoid, 308

nuts
commonly trigger food intolerance
reactions, 53
concomitant reactions with viral
infections, 57

oats
contains gluten, 137
grains in the grass family, 50
oat wafers recipe, 192
oatmeal pie crust recipe, 199
oatmeal-flaxseed cookie recipe, 195
pet food, 84
sometimes triggers food intolerance
reaction, 55

omega-3 oils
anti-inflammatory oil and vinegar
dressing recipe, 175
calm inflammation, 225
daily dose, 229
farm-raised fish, 229
flaxseed oil, 169
how to get enough, 225, 229
takes one to two months to work,
230

omega-6 oils
farm-raised fish, 229
how not to get too much, 225
turn on inflammation, 225

omega-9 oils
healthy and non-inflammatory, 225

onions
baked lentils with cheese recipe, 181
carrot cutlet recipe, 188
concomitant reactions with viral
infections, 57
green salad recipe, 175
health tonics, 235
kasha with onions recipe, 161
often triggers food intolerance
reactions, 55

oral tolerance
antibody response, 299
aquiring oral tolerance, 298
CICs, 300
definition of, 38
delayed hypersensitivity reactions,
300
factors known to cause food
sensitivities, 292
how to reestablish, 302
important players, 299
intestinal flora, 302
lectins, 42
lymphokine release, 307
mast cells, 294
overview, 298
Peyer's patches, 298
T-cell ratio, 298, 300
transfer factors, 302

oranges
alleviating overwhelmed
detoxification pathways, 208
cross-reactions, 57
often triggers food intolerance
reactions, 55

organically grown produce, 85

osteoarthritis

benefits from exercise, 252
ginger provides relief, 235
glucosamine, 237
glucosamine and chondroitin, 238
omega-3 oils are effective treatment, 225
vitamin C, 232
vitamins, 230

overweight
impairs immune system, 309

Palmblad, Jan, 62, 63

pancreatin
beef allergens, 107
digestional supplements, 206
pork allergens, 112

papain
allergic reactions to, 120
digestional supplements, 206
range of action, 207

parasites
can increase intestinal permeability, 205
leaky gut syndrome, 32, 36, 205, 293

Parkinson's disease
sulfoxidation, 303

pathogenic bacteria, 34, 297

pathogens
can cause arthritis, 34
can increase intestinal permeability, 34

peanut
list of products containing peanut allergens, 113

peanuts
anaphylactic shock, 30
classical food allergy, 314
commonly trigger food intolerance reactions, 53
cross-reactions, 57
lists of products containing peanut allergens, 101
need to be well cooked, 43
often triggers food intolerance reactions, 55
pet food, 84
protease inhibitors, 41
yeast allergens, 104

pectin
apples high in, 75
citrus allergens, 97, 107
citrus and apple allergens, 120
use as thickener, 142

peppers
can cause arthritis, 26
corn bread recipe, 151
green salad recipe, 175
often triggers food intolerance reactions, 55
pesticides, 85
recipes free of pepper allergens, 105
yeast allergens, 104

peptidoglycan-polysaccharide fragments, 294

pesticides
illegally high levels sometimes go undetected by FDA, 85
more used on genetically altered crops, 89
stress on body to detoxify, 228

pet food
corn allergens, 84
egg allergens, 112
milk allergens, 112
peanut allergens, 113
rice allergens, 113
source of allergens, 84
soy allergens, 114
wheat allergens, 84, 115
yeast allergens, 116

Peyer's patches, 298

phenolics
alleviating overwhelmed detoxification pathways, 208
detoxificed by sulfation enzymes, 303
mostly detoxified in digestive tract, 305

Pioneer HiBred International
transferred a Brazil nut allergen into soybeans using genetic engineering, 88

plaquinil
need to avoid, 308

pollen
allergic cross-reactions, 56
avoid while testing for food senstivitities, 45
concomitant reactions, 57
elimination strategy, 57
limit exposure while testing for food sensitivities, 48
masking improvement, 49
minimize exposure while fasting, 70

poor digestion
bacterial overgrowths, 36

yeast overgrowth, 54

sulfation
  acetaminophen, 39
  alleviating overwhelmed
    detoxification pathways, 207
  definition, 38
  effort involved in alleviating
    symptoms, 201
  link to food sensitivities, 303
  measurement of, 305
  much of it occurs in digestive tract,
    305

sulfation capacity
  testing for, 305

sulfide, 38, 303

sulfoxidation
  alleviating overwhelmed
    detoxification pathways, 207
  definition, 38, 303
  effort involved in alleviating
    symptoms, 201
  in SLE and RA, 303
  involvment in various diseases, 303
  link to chemical sensitivities, 39
  low levels in autoimmune diseases,
    303
  measurement of, 305
  takes place in liver, 305

sulfoxidation capacity
  testing for, 305

sulfoxide, 38, 303

Swami Vishnu-devananda, 261

swimming, 253, 260, 264

synergistic reactions
  definition, 318
  overview, 57

synergy, 22, 283

synovial tissue, 297

systemic lupus erythematosus
  autoimmune types of arthritis, 18
  CICs, 296
  sulfoxidation, 303

Tagamet
  leaky gut syndrome, 292

tai chi, 254
  case history, 263
  helps arthritis, 263

taro, 140

taurine
  alleviating overwhelmed
    detoxification pathways, 208

Taylor, Steve L., 88

T-cell-mediated inflammation, 294

T-cells
  delayed hypersensitivity reactions,
    301
  helper T-cells, 298
  ratio improved by thymus extracts,
    210
  ratio in arthritis, 302
  role in oral tolerance, 299
  SIga affects ratio, 300
  suppressor T-cells, 298
  T-cells ratio, 297

teff
  cooking instructions, 144
  grain and flour options, 143
  grains in the grass family, 50

testing for food sensitivities
  reintroduction phase, 50

thickeners
  alternative flours, 140
  alternatives to white flour, 138
  eggs, 141
  how to modify a recipe, 133
  starch, 139
  wheat allergens, 115

thiol
  low sulfoxidation makes adverse
    reaction to more likely, 303

thymodulin
  thymus extracts, 210

thymus
  function improved by antioxidant
    vitamins and minerals, 210
  pork allergens, 112
  thymus extract, 211

thymus extracts
  improve clinical symptoms of RA,
    210
  improve T-cell ratio, 210
  maximizing thymus function, 211

tomatoes
  baked lentils with cheese recipe, 181
  blood type A reactions, 40
  can cause arthritis, 24, 26
  fresh salsa recipe, 160
  genetic enginering, 89
  green salad recipe, 175
  often triggers food intolerance
    reactions, 55
  pet food, 84

Quick Order Form

📠 **Fax orders**: 1-314-773-1549. Send this form.

📞 **Telephone orders**: Call 1-314-776-4827. Have your credit card ready.

📧 **E-mail orders** orders@ConqueringArthritis.com

📧 **Postal orders**: Conquering Arthritis, PO Box 63353, St. Louis, MO 63163

🖧 **Web Site orders**: Visit our online book store at www.ConqueringArthritis.com

Please send the following books, disks or reports. I understand that I may return any of them for a full refund—for any reason, no questions asked.

_____

_____

_____

Please send more FREE information on:
Other books   Speaking/Seminars   Audio and video tapes

Name:_____

Address:_____

City:_____ State _____ Zip _____-_____

Daytime phone number:_____

Evening phone number:_____

e-mail address:_____

Sales tax: Please add 7.62% for products shipped to Missouri addresses.

Shipping: US $5 for the first book and $2 each additional product. International: $9 for first book, $5 for each additional product (estimate).

Payment: Check or Credit Card: Visa or Mastercard

Card number:_____

Name on card:_____ Exp. Date ____/____

Quick Order Form

✆ **Fax orders**: 1-314-773-1549. Send this form.

📞 **Telephone orders**: Call 1-314-776-4827. Have your credit card ready.

📧 **E-mail orders** orders@ConqueringArthritis.com

📧 **Postal orders**: Conquering Arthritis, PO Box 63353, St. Louis, MO 63163

🖧 **Web Site orders**: Visit our online book store at www.ConqueringArthritis.com

Please send the following books, disks or reports. I understand that I may return any of them for a full refund—for any reason, no questions asked.

_____

_____

_____

Please send more FREE information on:
Other books   Speaking/Seminars   Audio and video tapes

Name:_____

Address:_____

City:_____ State _____ Zip _____-_____

Daytime phone number:_____

Evening phone number:_____

e-mail address:_____

Sales tax: Please add 7.62% for products shipped to Missouri addresses.

Shipping: US $5 for the first book and $2 each additional product. International: $9 for first book, $5 for each additional product (estimate).

Payment: Check or Credit Card: Visa or Mastercard

Card number:_____

Name on card:_____ Exp. Date ____/____

Visit the Conquering Arthritis Web Site

http:\\www.ConqueringArthritis.com

Quick Order Form

 Fax orders: 1-314-773-1549. Send this form.

 Telephone orders: Call 1-314-776-4827. Have your credit card ready.

 E-mail orders orders@ConqueringArthritis.com

 Postal orders: Conquering Arthritis, PO Box 63353, St. Louis, MO 63163

 Web Site orders: Visit our online book store at www.ConqueringArthritis.com

Please send the following books, disks or reports. I understand that I may return any of them for a full refund—for any reason, no questions asked.

_____

_____

_____

Please send more FREE information on:
Other books   Speaking/Seminars   Audio and video tapes

Name:_____

Address:_____

City:_____ State _____ Zip _____-_____

Daytime phone number:_____

Evening phone number:_____

e-mail address:_____

Sales tax: Please add 7.62% for products shipped to Missouri addresses.

Shipping: US $5 for the first book and $2 each additional product. International: $9 for first book, $5 for each additional product (estimate).

Payment: Check or Credit Card: Visa or Mastercard

Card number:_____

Name on card:_____ Exp. Date ____/____